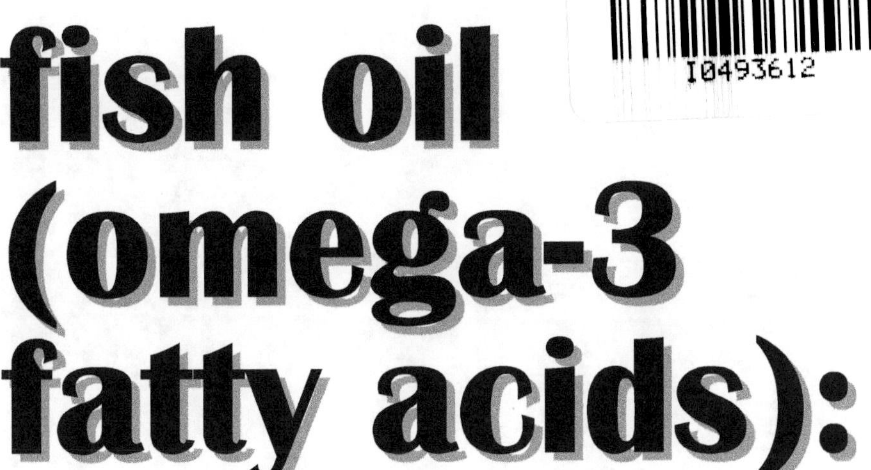

FACTS, FANTASIES & FAILURES

A SELECTIVE REVIEW

Prof Randolph M. Howes MD,PhD
Orthomolecular Scientist, Surgeon, Scholar, Author and Biochemist

Adjunct Assistant Professor of Plastic Surgery, (RET.)
The Johns Hopkins Hospital, Baltimore, MD. USA

Espaldon Professor of Plastic and Reconstructive Surgery,
University of Santo Tomas, Manila, Philippines

Adjunct Professor of Biological Sciences,
Southeastern Louisiana University

Professor of Surgery, Biophysics and Biochemistry,
Louisiana University of Medical Sciences (RET.)

Dean, Louisiana University of Medical Sciences (RET.)

(Also holds an Honorary Doctorate of Humanities)

Free Radical Publishing Co.
ISBN-13: 978-1499567922
ISBN-10: 1499567928

Address for communication: 27439 Highway 441, Kentwood, Louisiana 70444-8152, USA. Email: rhowesmd@hughes.net

DISCLOSURE AND DISCLAIMER

THE CONTENT OF THE MATERIAL PRESENTED HEREIN IS PROVIDED FOR INFORMATIONAL PURPOSES ONLY.

ANY DECISION BY THE READER TO ACT UPON THE MATERIAL PRESENTED HEREIN IS AT THE SOLE DISCRETION OF THE READER. NO ASSURANCE IS GRANTED OR IMPLIED AS TO THE ACCURACY OR COMPLETENESS OF THE MATERIAL HEREIN. ACTUAL PERFORMANCE, OR THE LACK THEREOF, MAY BE DIFFERENT THAN THE ESTIMATED PRESENTATIONS WITHIN THE MATERIAL. IN NO EVENT SHALL THE AUTHOR BE HELD LIABLE FOR DAMAGES, AND/OR ANY ALLEDGED HARM, INCURRED FROM THE USE OF, OR THE RELIANCE ON, THE CONTENT OF THE MATERIAL HEREIN CONTAINED. ALL DECISIONS REGARDING PERSONAL HEALTH AND MEDICAL ISSUES SHOULD BE MADE IN CONSULTATION WITH A LICENSED MEDICAL PRACTIONER.

NOTE: This text is not presented as prescription, diagnosis nor treatment for any disease, illness, infirmity or physical condition. Any form of self-treatment or alternative health program necessarily must involve an individual's acceptance of some risk, and no one should assume otherwise. Persons needing medical care should obtain it from a qualified physician. Always consult your doctor before making any health decision.

It is understood that medicine is an ever-changing science. As new research and clinical experience broaden our knowledge, changes in treatment and drug therapy are required. The author and the publisher of this work have checked with sources believed to be reliable in their efforts to provide information that is complete and generally in accord with the standards accepted at the time of publication. However, in view of the possibility of human error or changes in the medical sciences, neither the authors nor the publisher nor any other party who has been involved in the preparation of publication of this work warrants that the information contained herein is in every respect accurate or complete, and they disclaim all responsibility to any errors or omissions or for the results obtained from use of the information contained in the work. Readers should confirm the information contained herein with other sources. For example and in particular, readers are advised to check the product information sheets (or labels) included in the package of each drug they plan to administer to be certain that the information contained in this work is accurate and that changes have not been made in the recommended dose or in the contraindications for administration. This recommendation is of particular importance in connection with new or infrequently used drugs, additives or supplements.

Disclaimers: Please note: only your personal physician or other health professional you consult can best advise you on matters of your health based on your medical history, your family medical history, your medication history, and how information from any of these databases may apply to you. Neither Dr. Howes nor any party involved in creating, producing or delivering this web site shall be liable for any damages arising out of access to or use of this material or web site, or any errors or omissions in the content thereof.

The information given herein is not intended as medical advice. Always consult with your doctor for underlying illness. Before beginning dietary investigation, consult a dietician or a physician with an interest in nutrition. Information is drawn from the scientific literature, web research, and personal enquiry; while all care is taken, information is not warranted as accurate and the author cannot be held liable for any errors and omissions.

Financial disclosure: Dr. Howes has no financial conflicts of interest and is not involved in the sale of dietary supplements or fitness equipment. The author holds no stocks or interests in companies in the food additive or antioxidant supplement business.

ABOUT THE AUTHOR
Dr. Randolph M. Howes M.D., Ph.D.

Biographical sketch:

As a champion of the people, Dr. Howes anticipates and hopes for the active involvement of all connected parties (patients, caregivers, health-care professionals, etc.) as an integral approach to educating consumers and the public about the potential dangers of excessive antioxidant-containing supplements and "antioxidant stacking."

Some people are born with a silver spoon in their mouth but Dr. Howes had to earn his. Even as a child, Dr. Howes could think with adult clarity. He could envision his future but it would require "decades of dedication" to make it a reality.

From childhood, Dr. Howes was motivated to become a medical doctor and scientist. Assuredly, having been born on a small strawberry farm in rural Louisiana, his journey to the top has proved to be arduous and demanding.

However, he was fortunate to acquire the confidence of Sister Elizabeth at St. Joseph's school and went on to gain the support of his high school speech teacher, Mrs. Iris Brann, who also had strong beliefs in his abilities and potential. Ultimately, with the help of his guitar and his singing ability, he defeated the star quarter back of the high school football team to become the president of the student body.

With the aid of a $25 dollar legislative scholarship, he went on to Southeastern Louisiana College (SLC). At SLC, he was selected for honors chemistry, made the Dean's list, worked at the Psychology Research Lab forty hours a week, maintained a premed study load, and was elected president of the Junior Class and the Interfraternity Council.

To earn badly needed funds, he played music on weekends in a small combo, The Three Blind Mice. Next, he matriculated to Tulane University School of Medicine.

His initial dream was to try to combine both medicine and science. In that regard, he began work as a technician with Dr. Andrew Schally at the Endocrine Polypeptide Lab in the isolation of thyrotropin releasing factor. That work led to a Nobel Prize for Dr. Schally.

Prof Randolph M. Howes MD,PhD

Dr. Howes had been highly impressed with the enthusiasm of biochemist, the late Dr. Richard H. Steele, who accepted him as a doctoral candidate under his tutelage. Dr. Howes graduated in the top 10 of his class, won the Louisiana Pathology Association Award, was elected to the Sigma Xi honor fraternity and was the first in the history of Tulane to become a Doctor of Medicine and a Ph.D. in biochemistry concurrently.

Next, he was selected to pursue a career in surgery at the prestigious Johns Hopkins Hospital.

Unbelievably, at Dr. Howes' urging, he was allowed to operate his own research lab during his surgical internship and residency training while at Johns Hopkins Hospital. He worked hand in hand with the greats in American medicine and surgery.

Independently, he garnered grants, trained lab techs, wrote papers, slept on the cold floor, proudly served as a Captain in the U.S. Army Reserves Medical Corp and finished with board eligibility in both general and plastic surgery in an unheard of six year period.

In another first, he was appointed as an Adjunct Assistant Professor of Plastic Surgery at Johns Hopkins Hospital. He retired from that position in 2013.

For decades, Dr. Howes gave unselfishly to pro bono medical missions in the Philippines and he holds the Ernesto Espaldon Chair as Professor of Plastic Surgery at the University of Santo Tomas.

Upon retirement from a career in cosmetic plastic surgery, he is living his dream of trying to revolutionize the treatment of cancer, heart disease, HIV/AIDS and malaria, with his in depth knowledge of the arcane biochemistry of oxygen metabolism. He is a work in progress! Dedicated and passionate, he is on a mission for mankind.

Dr. Howes invented the triple lumen venous catheter, which has been credited with helping save the lives of over 20 million critically ill patients worldwide. His catheter became the number one venous catheter in the world and his name is well recognized in over 100 countries. He has been recognized as a humanitarian, visionary, entrepreneur, singer, songwriter, inventor and author.

He received the Harper Award for innovative research from the American College for Advancement in Medicine, served as their keynote speaker and his peers refer to him as "a walking encyclopedia on oxygen metabolism."

He is a Dr. Norman Vincent Peale Unsung Hero award winner, which recognized his awesome versatility. Additionally, even though he is humble and does not like talking about it, he is a self made multi-millionaire.

He is currently doing extensive research on cures for cancer and heart disease and development of revolutionary treatment modalities. He has written 20 books over the past 8 years on the subject of antioxidants and oxygen metabolism, as it relates to protection from cancer, heart disease, diabetes, malaria, HIV/AIDS, Alzheimer's disease, aging and arthritis. He has written many scientific and medical papers and has lectured nationally and internationally.

His research has shown that currently common antioxidant vitamins, such as vitamins A & E, (and vitamin C to a lesser extent) can be harmful and that oxygen free radicals protect us from bacterial, fungal and viral infections and they help to control cancer growth and metastasis.

He has developed an effective, inexpensive singlet oxygen generating system, from orthomolecular agents, for the treatment of cancer and heart disease. He is passionate about his research and hopes to have his discoveries at the patient's bedside in his lifetime. Admittedly, this is an extremely ambitious goal.

There are over 8,000 pages in his magnum opus and at the Howes World Selective Library on Oxygen Metabolism. Over 3,000 pages of his opus are available online in a searchable format www.iwillfindthecure.org © by R.M. Howes

NOTE: An avid researcher, Dr. Howes has authored more than 350 original publications, including over 30 medical and scientific books, such as Death In Small Doses (Antioxidant vitamins A, C & E in the 21st Century), Antioxidant Overkill and Dangers of Excessive Antioxidants In Cancer Patients. He has written numerous articles for medical and consumer publications, including The Journal of American Academy of Cosmetic Surgery, Annals of the New York Academy of Science, The Journal of Evidence Based Complementary And Alternative Medicine, The Baton Rouge Advocate, and The Houma Courier. He has a weekly science/medicine column in the Hammond Daily Star, the Independence Times and The Ponchatoula Times. His research interests include truthful reporting of antioxidant dangers, adverse effects of vitamins A, C & E, other antioxidant's deadly unintended consequences, free radicals, oxygen metabolism, and cancer and heart disease treatment and prevention, global health care policy, and oxidative means to revolutionize treating and preventing HIV/AIDS and malaria.

Dr. Howes is also an active and well-known speaker and media personality, having been featured on PBS's The American Health Journal, WWL-TV New Orleans and WDSU-TV New Orleans, Sirius/XM satellite radio, as well as many other national talk and news shows across America.

In 2013, he received from the American College for Advancement In Medicine the first Charles Farr Award for "excellence in oxidative medicine."

After reading Dr. Howes' book, *Dangers of Excessive Antioxidants In Cancer Patients,* Robert C. Allen, M.D., Ph.D., Chairman of the Department of Pathology at Creighton Medical School in Omaha, Nebraska, described Dr. Howes this way, "During my forty-five-year association with Dr. Randolph M. Howes, I've been consistently impressed, and sometimes exhausted, by his brilliance, energy and intensity. Over the past several years his attention has been focused on debunking the meme that oxidants are "bad" and antioxidants are "good". We should all appreciate that oxidation provides the energy that drives all complex life forms. *Dangers of Excessive Antioxidants in Cancer Patients* presents convincing arguments with supporting evidence that simplistically assuming antioxidants are somehow "good" is not valid. Dr. Howes is *The Scientific Voyager* poetically described herein, and this book is the product of his voyage."

Dr. Allen answered the question, "If you or a loved one had cancer, would you now take or recommend antioxidants?" He answered, "If I had cancer and was undergoing chemotherapy, I certainly would not be taking BHT, vitamins A and E, or any "antioxidant" formulation, nor would I recommend antioxidants to my family, loved ones, or anyone else." His support of Dr. Howes' work is clear and undeniable.

Following the same scenario, Dr. Robert Muller, M.D. (Ob-Gyn) answered this way: "Dr Howes book shows the extensive research done on antioxidants, BUT the difficulty lies in overcoming the social norms established by the brainwashing of the public by the pharmaceutical industry. If common sense prevails, the choice becomes very clear—antioxidants are worthless in the prevention and treatment of cancer (and CVD)." Robert Muller, M.D. 5-12-11

These are just two examples of highly qualified, medically-involved, individuals who recognize the innovative brilliance of Dr. Howes' new approach to disease prevention, causation and coexistence.

Dr. Howes' origin from a small Louisiana farming community imbedded in him a unique level of morality, ethical behavior and common sense. He feels that common sense is "commonly missing" in the world of medical science today. True, one must be trained to deal with the arcane biological and physiological sciences but one must also be open-minded and willing to rely on common sense, especially when certain scientific theories go against or fly in the face of inductive/deductive reasoning and clear thinking.

The unanswerable mysteries
of being alive
are surpassed only by
the incomprehensible mysteries
of being dead.
R. M. Howes, M.D., Ph.D.

10/30/11

Dr. Howes spent over a quarter of a century in educational training to prepare himself for the challenging world of medical science. He is fulfilling his dreams of making significant contributions to the prevention and cure of some of mankind's most deadly diseases, such as cancer, heart disease, malaria and HIV/AIDS.

He feels strongly that he must place his innovative ideas onto the public forum, utilizing printed media and the world wide web. Thus, others can evaluate the validity of his contributions and continue in the pursuit of his dreams.

DEDICATION

To the brilliant, but limited, cumulative mind of man.

FISH OIL (OMEGA-3 FATTY ACIDS): FACTS, FANTASIES & FAILURES
TABLE OF CONTENTS:

SECTION ONE

FANTASIES

Introduction

Globally, people spend billions a year on fish oil (omega-3) supplements. According to a 2011 report, Americans alone spent $1.1 billion on fish oil products and their market is estimated to grow 15 percent each year, according to market research studies. In 2012, supplements accounted for 10% of the worldwide retail market for omega-3 products, valued at €26bn.

The global market for omega-3-containing foods is $25 billion, according to Packaged Facts, an industry newsletter.

Advertisers make fish oil sound like food for the gods, but it is not. Yes, it is trendy but consumers have been duped by false advertising campaigns....once again.

The omega-3 fish oil craze has produced a fish oil cult. An increasing amount of products, such as eggs, bread, butters, oils and orange juice, are being "fortified" with omega-3s. This fortified food, coupled with fish oil supplement use, increases the potential for consuming excessively high levels.

Folks are misled to believe the fantasy that fish oil can effectively treat a wide spectrum of diseases, including heart disease, stroke, depression, psychosis, attention deficit-hyperactivity disorder, Alzheimer's disease, dry eyes, glaucoma, age-related macular degeneration, painful periods, breast pain, miscarriage, high blood pressure in pregnancy, diabetes, asthma, developmental coordination disorders, movement disorders, dyslexia, obesity, kidney disease, osteoporosis, certain diseases related to pain and swelling, psoriasis, preventing weight loss, and preventing high blood pressure and kidney damage, childhood behavioral disorders, and yada, yada, yada.

Misinformation and misconceptions dominate the nutritional supplement landscape concerning the scientifically proven benefits omega-3 fish oils. Many books claim fish oil supplements to be "miracles" or "wonder pills."

But, such is far from the scientific reality of failed and disappointing studies conducted on so-called fish oil products, even though many such products actually come from plants.

All studies presented in my book are well referenced and discussion articles are duly credited. This book is the leader in presenting scientifically accurate data and serves to debunk the sea of lies facing the general public regarding an ocean of so-called fish oil products.

Basically, there is "no truth in advertising and "anything goes," because none of these products are government regulated for quality or accuracy of contents and dosage. Sadly, marketers and profiteers will "Tell you anything, to sell you anything." Profit is the muddy waters upon which the fish oil industry bobbles about.

There is a serious down side to these potentially harmful fish oil products, especially if taken in excessive amounts. Our most reliable scientific studies have found that fish oil does not reduce risk or prevent cardiovascular diseases, strokes, dementia, diabetes, macular degeneration or schizophrenia.

Alarmingly, these studies show a significant increased risk of developing prostate cancer.

The truth must be told.

Basically, fish oil have been deemed to be a "miracle." But, just as in the case of many other dietary supplements, fish oil has failed in repeated scientific studies to confer the health benefits so vocally touted by marketers and profiteers.

Sadly, fish oil supplements can contain significant levels of toxins and they can be linked to a spectrum of adverse side effects.

But, a 2012 report in the Journal of the American Medical Association has found that fish oil may not help you live longer. It's a controversial study because so many people take the supplements religiously, but as far as life span is concerned, it does not seem to make that big of a difference.

Fish oil contains high levels of the allegedly magic omega-3 fatty acid ingredients. Omega-3 fatty acids are specific polyunsaturated fatty acids (PUFAs) that cannot be made in the body and consequently they must be consumed via the diet or from a dietary supplement.

I'll try not to overwhelm you with biochemistry at this point but this fatty acid family includes primarily eicosapentaenoic acid (EPA), docosahexaenoic acid (DHA), and alpha-linolenic acid (ALA), but it contains others. EPA and DHA are found predominantly in algae-consuming marine foods (such as fish), which are rendered and extracted into a fish oil product.

The fish oil (omega-3) craze has associated its consumption with a number of health benefits, most notably those involving cardiovascular and heart health, inflammation, and vision and cognitive brain issues. The National Institutes of Health (NIH) notes that omega-3 fatty acids reduce pain and swelling, which may explain why fish oil has been claimed to be effective for psoriasis and dry eyes.

These fatty acids also prevent the blood from clotting quickly, which might make fish oil helpful for some heart conditions. **NIH lists one condition for which fish oil is "effective for" (high triglycerides), and 26 conditions for which omega-3s may be "possibly effective for" (everything from stroke to cancer to psychosis).**

But, as with most dietary supplements, scientific studies of fish oil lacks consistency and leaves the average consumer totally confused by all of the promotional hoopla.

Recent research has raised serious questions, if not totally debunked, previous studies suggesting that the consumption of recommended amounts of DHA and EPA in the form of dietary fish oil supplements lowers triglycerides to safe levels; reduces the risk of death, heart attack, dangerous abnormal heart rhythms, and strokes in people with known cardiovascular disease; slows hardening of the arteries, and lowers blood pressure.

For starters, a Journal of the American Medical Association (JAMA) systematic review of **20 studies found neither eating fish nor taking fish oil supplements reduced the risk of stroke, heart attack or death**.

Also, a British Medical Journal (BMJ) review of 38 studies found that eating two to four servings of fish a week reduced stroke risk by 6 percent compared with eating one serving or less, and having five servings a week reduced the risk by 12 percent. But, the results of the **randomized trials that used fish oil supplements showed no significant effect on risk of stroke.**

And, a review by the respected Cochrane Collaboration group found that **fish oil pills failed to prevent or treat cognitive decline** and a 2011 meta-analysis by Yale University investigators **debunked the claim that omega-3s cured depression**.

Heavy metals such as arsenic, cadmium, lead and mercury end up throughout the environment at low levels, especially in fish and subsequently in fish oil. Heavy metal ingestion can result in cognitive impairments, nervous system dysfunction, blindness, lack of coordination, deafness, development of certain cancers, irreversible liver and kidney damage and death.

Fish oils can also be contaminated with polychlorinated biphenyls (PCBs), which can lead to skin problems, muscle spasms, chronic bronchitis and nervous system disorders; and dioxins and furans have been linked to a number of adverse health effects including skin, liver and immune system problems, endocrine and reproductive disruptions and the development of certain cancers.

So, check with the International Fish Oil Standards Program (IFOS), which is a third party toxin testing and accreditation program for omega-3 fish oil products for more safety information.

The Mayo Clinic website states that fish **oil supplements may cause increased blood sugar levels, nausea, diarrhea, loose stools, decreased appetite, constipation, vomiting and fat in the stool. Restlessness and formication (the sensation of ants crawling on the skin) have also been reported, as has mania in bipolar disorder or severe depression.**

Gastrointestinal side effects may be minimized if fish oils are taken with meals and by using a start low and go slow schedule regarding dosage.

Other downsides include **loss of short-term memory, headache, hemolytic anemia, depression, somatic disorders, increased risk of colon cancer, nasopharyngitis, worsening of asthma**

symptoms, decreased physical activity, increased appetite, increased blood pressure and an uncomfortable feeling.

Additionally, fish oil supplements may increase low-density lipoprotein cholesterol levels, may worsen symptoms for patients with ventricular tachycardia, may increase the risk of bleeding, and may decrease blood pressure.

If taken over a period of months, fish oil may **cause a deficiency of vitamin E and may increase the risk of vitamin A or D toxicity. So, avoid excessively large doses.**

Decreased estrogen receptor production has been associated with fish oil supplementation.

Patients with diabetes, asthma, inflammatory bowel disease or liver disease should use extra caution with fish oil supplementation.

Over fishing of menhaden, a major source of fish oil, has produced endangerment to the species, such that 13 of the 15 Atlantic states have banned Omega Protein of Houston fishing boats from their waters, as they remove half a billion menhaden annually.

As an alternative source of so-called fish oil, flax seed, chia seeds, hemp seeds, and sesame seeds are good vegetarian oil sources of omega-3 fatty acids.

False general overall supplement claims

Profiteers and supplement pushers boast that you can walk into the local nutritional supplements store and achieve and/or secure the following 50 amazing benefits and/or claims by using their array of dietary supplements:

stave off and fight cancer,

bolster your strength and energy,

increase your lifespan,

slow your over all aging process,

minimize infections,

supercharge your sex life, shrink your prostate

block diabetes,

boost heart health, strengthen overall cardiovascular system,

improve digestion,

remove toxins from your body,

improve bowel function,

strengthen your colon,

promote healthy skin,

support your immune system,

power up your reproductive health,

soothe PMS and menstrual imbalances,

enhance memory,

build up brain power and promote an active mind,

help you potentially feel more alert and responsive,

promote heart health, blood circulation and improve heart efficiency,

improve healthy eyesight and eye function,

help maintain cholesterol levels already in normal range,

minimize oxidative stress,

support your brain function,

assist gall bladder function,

help reduce your daily stress,

help support respiratory system health,

provide antioxidant protection against free radicals in your cells, tissues and organs,

help recharge other antioxidant nutrients to their active state,

balance the health of your respiratory system,

help reduce your occasional fatigue,

support your overall heart vitality,

promote improvement in general well-being,

maintain your vitality,

increase antioxidant levels in certain professional athletes,

protect your muscle tissue during and after exercise,

reinforce quicker recovery after workouts,

improve your endurance capacity parameters,

helps build up your overall stamina,

produce more energy for your cells,

acts as an energy production catalyst,

ignite your body's engine.

As long as advertisers of these products do not use the four words, "prevent", "diagnose", "treat" or "cure", made illegal in the 1994 DSHEA law, they can use the following terms to **imply improvement**: bolster, strengthen, reinforce, shore up, support, augment, sustain, increase, build up, upsurge, or multiply.

They can imply that agents can and do supposedly **protect you from diseases or conditions of illness** and they can use: ease, diminish, cut, trim down, lessen, decrease, lower, moderate, condense, suppress, wipe out, erase, deny, repress, blot out, impede, close off, barricade, block out, hide, obscure, or cover….. and **it does not require any scientific proof at all…. and it's all perfectly LEGAL!**

Such is the case with so-called fish oil (omega-3s) supplements.

Krill oil false claims

But, wait, here are more false claims. The list of how krill oil supports you will likely impress you also:

Many Ways Krill Oil Supports You

- A healthy heart
- Support for concentration, memory and learning
- Blood sugar health
- Healthy joints, with an increase in joint comfort
- Fighting your signs of aging
- Healthy brain and nervous system function and development
- Protection for cell membranes
- Cholesterol and other blood lipid health
- Healthy liver function
- Bolstering your immune system
- Healthy mood support
- Optimal skin health

With wild claims of this nature, every person on the planet would want to be taking these potentially dangerous supplements. But many of these claims have sparse scientific support, if any at all.

$25 billion global market for fish oil containing foods

Every year, American consumers spend more than $6 billion on pills and fortified foods containing omega-3 fatty acids. A **new, large study led by researchers at McMaster University** raises questions about whether those dollars are wasted, and whether the fats, usually derived from fish, have any effect on preventing heart attacks.

Investigators found that **the 6,281 patients who got fish oil were no more or less likely to die from cardiovascular causes than the 6,255 who received placebo. Taking fish oil did not lead to fewer heart attacks, fewer strokes, fewer hospitalizations for heart problems, fewer stent procedures, or less chest pain.**

Use in infant formula, is the biggest source of omega-3 sales.

The biggest category of omega-3 products are not drugs or supplements but foods, such as milk, bread, and cereal, to which the oils have been added. **The global market for omega-3-containing foods is $25 billion, according to Packaged Facts**, an industry newsletter.

But 40% of that is for infant formula.

Foods and beverages accounted for about $4 billion in annual sales in the U.S. alone.

Monsanto has been developing a genetically modified soybean that contains the EPA fish oil.

The GISSI-Prevenzione trial, an 11,000-person trial from 1999, found that either eating fish or taking supplements reduced deaths and heart attacks. A 19,000-patient trial of EPA pills from Japan also seemed to show a benefit. In 2008, a 7,000-patient study of people with heart failure seemed to show that 1 gram of fish oil decreased the risk of dying.

But that was then and unsupportive study results are now.

http://www.forbes.com/sites/matthewherper/2012/06/11/fish-oil-or-snake-oil-study-questions-omega-3-benefits/ Accessed 5-8-14.

Today, everything from loaves of bread to frozen fish fingers come with a "RICH IN OMEGA-3" tag. They even have their own international awareness day.

Note: I have included a number of general discussion article in this book. This is to accommodate the lay reader. Out of necessity, I usually have to include a majority of medical science articles, which are predominately biochemical in nature. So, enjoy.

FACTS

Extraordinary theories necessitate extraordinary proof. I have amassed epic support for my innovative prooxidant theories to conquer cancer, heart disease, HIV/AIDS and malaria, the biggest global killers of mankind.

R. M. Howes, M.D., Ph.D.
11/7/10

Here are some of the current misleading or untruthful omega-3 fish oil book titles that perpetuate medical misinformation and misconceptions:

- Omega Rx Zone: The Miracle of the New High-Dose Fish Oil

- The Omega-3 Effect: Everything You Need to Know About the Supernutrient for Living Longer, Happier, and Healthier

- Depression: How to BEAT Depression!: With the power of Omega-3 fish oil tablets

- Fish Oil: The Natural Anti-inflammatory

- The Mystery of Fatty Acids Revealed: Omega-3 Benefits

- The Omega-3 Connection: The Groundbreaking Anti-depression Diet and Brain Program

- Fish Oil Amazing Health Benefits Explained: How Fish Oil Can Help You Fight Diseases, Lose Weight and More

- The Omega-3 Phenomenon

- TheOmega-3 Health Revolution - Why Omega-3 Fatty Acids May be the missing piece of the human health puzzle

- Amazing Fish Benefits Revealed

- Omega-3 - Secrets to a Healthier Life

- Beneficial Effects of Fish Oil on Human Brain

- The Power of Omega-3

- The Ultimate Omega-3 Diet: Maximize the Power of Omega-3s to Supercharge Your Health, Battle Inflammation, and Keep Your Mind Sharp

Here is my first gift to you, the reader. The following statements were taken directly from "disappointing" fish oil scientific studies. Curiously, the average person hears little, if any, truth from the marketers and profiteers selling fish oil supplements or products fortified with omega-3 fatty acids.

****

Go fish

Summary: fish oil (ω-3 FA) study fiascos:
Prof. R.M. Howes, MD, PhD

- ineffective in preventing cancer; increased risk of developing prostate cancer; increased cancer risk among women for ω-3 fatty acid supplementation; fish oil supplements can stop chemotherapy drugs; fish oil did not lead to fewer heart attacks, fewer strokes, fewer hospitalizations for heart problems, fewer stent procedures, or less chest pain; fails heart health benefit; does not reduce risk of heart failure; no statistically significant association was observed with all-cause mortality, cardiac death, sudden death, myocardial infarction, and stroke; no

reduction in heart attack, stroke or heart failure; no significant changes were observed in systolic and diastolic blood pressure; no reduction in cardiovascular events; may cause arrhythmias; did not significantly reduce the rate of major cardiovascular events among patients who had had a myocardial infarction; failing to show additional reductions in adverse cardiovascular events when combined with statins; may also increase LDL-C levels, may have higher risk for hemorrhagic stroke; may increase risk of type 2 diabetes; had no effect on exercise performance; failed to prevent flare-ups of atrial fibrillation; no benefit at all in tests for reaction time, spatial memory, and processing speed measurements; do not slow mental decline in Alzheimer's patients; no better than placebo in improving symptoms of schizophrenia; not found to be significantly more effective in perinatal depression than placebo; ineffective for unipolar depression and obsessive-compulsive disorder patients; non-significant benefit of omega-3 fatty acids (FAs) for major depression; ineffective in treating perinatal depression; performed no better on standard tests of mental abilities, memory or verbal fluency; no difference in cognitive skills between the women with high and low levels of omega-3s in the blood at the time of the first memory tests; no difference between the two groups in how fast their thinking skills declined over time; did not prevent depressive symptoms during pregnancy or postpartum; ADHD have found mixed results; no benefit among individuals who had taken omega-3 or eye vitamins; do not reduce the risk of progression to advanced AMD (macular degeneration); has no effect on serum systemic inflammation markers and oxidative stress in hemodialysis patients; no effect on lupus nephritis; larger study of people with psoriasis found no benefit from fish oil;
feeding mice large amounts of dietary omega-3 fatty acids led to increased risk of colitis and immune alteration and viral or bacterial infection; advice to consume fish and the intake of fish oil capsules was associated with an *increase* in mortality of 20 per cent and 45 per cent respectively!

Yet, use in infant formula, is the biggest source of omega-3 sales.

An increasing amount of products, such as eggs, bread, butters, oils and orange juice, are being "fortified" with omega-3s. This fortified food, coupled with fish oil supplement use, increases the potential for consuming these high levels. Monsanto has been developing a genetically modified soybean that contains

the EPA fish oil. Today, everything from loaves of bread to frozen fish fingers come with a "RICH IN OMEGA-3" tag. Omega-3s even have their own international awareness day.

The global market for omega-3-containing foods is $25 billion, according to Packaged Facts. **A study published in the journal Cancer Research linked fish oil supplements with cancer in mice.** Men with the highest blood levels of omega-3s had a 71% higher risk of aggressive, possibly fatal prostate cancer than those with the lowest levels. Men who had high blood concentrations of omega-3s had **a significant 43% increase in the risk for all grades of prostate cancer. For your safety, eat real fish, don't take a chemically concocted pill or a genetically modified, untested food product.**

The huge profits allow for the continued brain washing of the citizenry and the campaigns of persuasion that "push" these ineffective products on an uninformed public on a daily basis. The truth must be told.

****

Yet, some authors believe that the triglyceride (TG)-lowering benefits of the very-long-chain omega-3 fatty acids eicosapentaenoic acid (EPA) and docosahexaenoic acid (DHA) are well known. Available as prescription formulations and dietary supplements, EPA and DHA are recommended by the American Heart Association for patients with coronary heart disease and hypertriglyceridemia.

Dietary supplements are not subject to the same government regulatory standards for safety, efficacy, and purity as prescription drugs are; moreover, supplements may contain variable concentrations of EPA and DHA and possibly other contaminants. Reducing low-density lipoprotein-cholesterol (LDL-C) levels remains the primary treatment goal in the management of dyslipidemia. **Dietary supplements and prescription formulations that contain both EPA and DHA may lower TG levels, but they may also increase LDL-C (bad cholesterol) levels**. (Bradberry, Hilleman, 2013)

Two prescription formulations of long-chain omega-3 fatty acids are available in the U.S. Although prescription omega-3 acid ethyl esters (OM-3-A EEs, **Lovaza**) contain high-purity EPA and DHA, prescription icosapent ethyl (IPE, **Vascepa**) is a high-purity EPA agent. In clinical trials of statin-treated and non–statin-treated patients with hypertriglyceridemia, **both OM-3-A EE and IPE lowered TG levels and other atherogenic markers;** however, IPE did not increase LDL-C levels. (Bradberry, Hilleman, 2013)

The very-long-chain omega-3 fatty acids EPA and DHA represent viable treatment options for patients with elevated TG levels. The FDA has approved two prescription omega-3 fatty acid agents—OM-3-A EE (Lovaza) and IPE (Vascepa). (Bradberry, Hilleman, 2013)

EPA and DHA are often called very-long-chain omega-3 fatty acids. The typical Western diet is rich in omega-6 fatty acids because of the abundance of linoleic acid present in corn, sunflower, and safflower oils. Conversely, omega-3 fatty acids account for only a small percentage of the daily dietary fat intake and are obtained from two main dietary sources—plants and fish.

Plant oils from walnuts, flaxseed, and canola contain the omega-3 fatty acid ALA, which is a metabolic precursor of the very-long-chain omega-3 fatty acids EPA and DHA; however, the conversion from ALA to EPA and DHA in the body is inefficient. The most concentrated food source of EPA and DHA is fatty fish such as albacore tuna, salmon, mackerel, sardines, and herring.

Following consumption, polyunsaturated fatty acids, such as the omega-3 and omega-6 fatty acids, are incorporated into cell membranes, where they modulate membrane protein function, cellular signaling, and gene expression.

In addition to their anti-inflammatory activity, very-long-chain omega-3 fatty acids have questionable effects on various risk factors for cardiovascular disease. So far, the evidence concerning the role of omega-3 fatty acids in cardiovascular outcomes is conflicting, but recent studies suggest their ineffectiveness.

As regards omega-3 fish oils, I can sum it up this way: **In 20 RCTs data reported on 68,680 patients, no statistically significant association was observed with all-cause mortality, cardiac death, sudden death, myocardial infarction, and stroke when all supplement studies were considered. Overall, omega-3 PUFA supplementation was not associated with a lower risk of all-cause mortality, cardiac death, sudden death, myocardial infarction, or stroke based on relative and absolute measures of association**. (Rizos et al, 2012)

Original Eskimo fish oil consumption study conclusions were wrong

Investigators found something fishy with the classical evidence for dietary fish recommendations

5-5-14

Oily fish are currently recommended as part of a heart healthy diet. This guideline is partially based on the **landmark 1970s study from Bang and Dyerberg that connected the low incidence of coronary artery disease (CAD) among the Eskimos of Greenland to their diet, rich in whale and seal blubber. Now, researchers have found that Eskimos actually suffered from CAD at the same rate as their Caucasian counterparts,** meaning there is insufficient evidence to back Bang and Dyerberg's claims. Their findings are published in the ***Canadian Journal of Cardiology.*** (Fodor et al, 2014)

Using 40 years of new information and research, a team of investigators set out to reexamine Bang and Dyerberg's study of Greenland Eskimos and CAD. This study is still widely cited today when recommending the dietary addition of fish oil supplements (like omega-3 fatty acids) or oily fish to help avoid cardiovascular problems. However, the new review of information has determined that **Bang and Dyerberg failed to actually investigate the cardiovascular health of the Eskimo population**, meaning that the cardioprotective effects of their diet are unsubstantiated.

"Bang and Dyerberg's seminal studies from the 1970s are routinely invoked as 'proof' of low prevalence of CAD in Greenland Eskimos ignoring the fact that **these two Danish investigators did not study the prevalence of CAD**," notes lead investigator George Fodor, MD, PhD, FRCPC, FAHA. "Instead, their research focused on the dietary habits of Eskimos and offered only speculation that the high intake of marine fats exerted a protective effect on coronary arteries."

Bang and Dyerberg relied mainly on annual reports produced by the Chief Medical Officer of Greenland to ascertain CAD deaths in the region. The 2014 study has identified a number of reasons that those records were likely insufficient, mainly that the rural and inaccessible nature of Greenland made it difficult for accurate records to be kept and that many people had inadequate access to medical personnel to report cardiovascular problems or heart attacks. In fact, researchers have now found that **concerns about the validity of Greenland's death certificates have been raised by a number of different reports and that at the time, more than 30% of the population lived in remote outposts where no medical officer was stationed.** This meant that 20% of the death certificates were completed without a doctor having examined the body.

The data collected through this new investigation shows that **Eskimos do have a similar prevalence of CAD to non-Eskimo populations, and in fact, they have very high rates of mortality due to cerebrovascular events (strokes). Overall, their life expectancy is approximately 10 years less than the typical Danish population and their overall mortality is twice as high as that of non-Eskimo populations.**

"Considering the dismal health status of Eskimos, it is remarkable that instead of labeling their diet as dangerous to health, a hypothesis has been construed that dietary intake of marine fats prevents CAD and reduces atherosclerotic burden," remarks Dr. Fodor.

Many recent large and well-designed studies have shown ambiguous or negative results regarding the cardioprotective properties of omega-3 fatty acids and fish oil supplements, and yet partly based on the work of Bang and Dyerberg, they are still widely recommended as part of a heart healthy diet plan.

"Publications still referring to Bang and Dyerberg's nutritional studies as proof that Eskimos have low prevalence of CAD represent either misinterpretation of the original findings or an example of confirmation bias," concludes Dr. Fodor. **"To date, more than 5000 papers have been published studying the alleged beneficial properties of omega-3 fatty acids, not to mention the billion dollar industry producing and selling fish oil capsules based on a hypothesis that was questionable from the beginning."** http://www.eurekalert.org/pub_releases/2014-05/ehs-ifs050114.php

http://www.elsevier.com/about/press-releases/research-and-journals/investigators-find-something-fishy-with-the-classical-evidence-for-dietary-fish-recommendations. Accessed 5-8-14.

This article is incredibly important. It points out the fact that **all of the studies since the 1970s on fish oil and its relation to health**

were erroneously based on a flawed study that produced erroneous conclusions.

Avoid excessive consumption of all supplements

The Food and Drug Administration does not regulate dietary supplements, and they can be sold with little or no research as to their safety, purity, and effectiveness. Dietary supplement manufacturing methods are not always standardized, so how well they work and their side effects can differ between brands or even within a brand. The form of a dietary supplement purchased in a drug store or health food store is likely not the same form used in research. The long-term effects of supplemental antioxidants are not known with certainty.

Despite numerous studies, no substantial health benefits have been demonstrated for supplemental antioxidants, including omega-3 fish oil.

Until there is more conclusive research, the best source of antioxidants is a diet rich in fruits, vegetables, and whole grains. Fish should be eaten twice weekly. Health organizations such as the American Heart Association, the American Cancer Society, and the American Institute for Cancer Research recommend getting antioxidants from food instead of supplements until research determines whether supplements are safe and provide the same benefits as antioxidants found naturally in food. There is plenty of research that suggests that whole grains, fruits, and vegetables, all of which contain extensive networks of antioxidants, are beneficial to health.

Snacking on small amounts of nuts and consuming wine in moderation also contribute to safe antioxidant consumption. Problems develop when excessive supplemental antioxidants are consumed. This directly interferes with at least seven crucial prooxidant protective biochemical pathways.

Some antioxidant supplements may promote disease and increase mortality in humans. Evidence has shown that free radicals induce an endogenous response which protects against exogenous radicals (and possibly other toxic compounds). Recent experimental evidence strongly suggests that such induction of endogenous free radical production extends the life span of *Caenorhabditis elegans*.

Most importantly, this induction of life span is prevented by antioxidants, providing direct evidence that so-called **free radicals (ROS, EMODs) may mitohormetically exert life extending and health promoting effects.** This is just the opposite effect of antioxidant ingestion.

Excessive consumption of supplemental antioxidants, including omega-3 fish oil, has the potential to damage health and do considerable harm.

When it comes to supplement profiteers, here is the way I put it in my 2012 book, *Antioxidants Linked to Deadly Unintended Consequences*, "They'll tell you anything, to sell you anything!"

An increasing number of studies are finding that vitamin supplementation are not only ineffectual but are even dangerous. According to considerable data, **people popping vitamins C and E are predisposing themselves to cancer, according to a study published recently in the journal *Stem Cells*, as high doses of these antioxidants can cause genetic abnormalities. Similarly, a study published in 2010 in the journal *Cancer Research* linked fish oil supplements with cancer in mice. Yet, the supplement craze goes on.**

A little fish oil chronology

Some of the following material was excerpted or modified from: **The Fish Report - Why Public Health Policy Should Promote Plant Omega-3 in Preference to Fish Oils. Dr Justine Butler, 2009**. It is a good overview article. (Butler, 2009)

In the late 1920s the scientists George and Mildred Burr first introduced the idea that specific components of fat could be necessary for normal growth and development (Burr and Burr, 1929).

Since then two specific polyunsaturated fatty acids have been classified as 'essential' as they cannot be manufactured within the body; they must be provided in the diet. Hence, they are called 'essential fatty acids' (EFAs). The two EFAs required for good health are the omega-3 fatty acid alpha linolenic acid (ALA) and the omega-6 fatty acid linoleic acid (LA).

Oily fish first got the nutritional thumbs up when it was erroneously observed that populations such as the Japanese and Inuit (Eskimo) people, with their fish-rich diets, have much lower rates of CVD. However, now we know those studies misled us.

Over the last decade or so, the reputation of fish oils has undergone a meteoric rise from the dreaded cod liver oil of years gone by to the highly esteemed omega-3 fish oil capsules of the new millennia. If you want to keep up with modern nutrition you must be omega-3 savvy! Right?

However, a later review of studies on fish oils and heart health (which included over half a million heart disease patients), showed no clear benefit of omega-3 fats on heart health.

DART – using dietary fish to prevent secondary heart disease

One of the best-known early studies was the Diet and Reinfarcation Trial (DART) (Burr *et al.*, 1989). This study looked at the effects of dietary intervention in the secondary prevention of heart attacks in patients who had previously recovered from one. In this study 2,033 men who had recovered from a heart attack were allocated to receive or not receive advice to eat around 300 grams of oily fish per week, or take fish oil supplements giving an equivalent amount of omega-3 fats.

Results showed that the fish group had a 29 per cent reduction in death during the two year recovery period following a heart attack. So **it was concluded that fish oil may reduce CVD mortality;** the effect being greatest during the period of recovery following a heart attack. It should also be noted that the large amount of omega-3 fats given (1 gram) is the equivalent of consuming a very large amount (around 100 grams) of oily fish per day. This exceeds the 'safe' amount the UK government recommends (FSA, 2009)

No long-term protection against heart disease

A long-term follow-up to the DART study (Ness *et al.*, 2002), showed that **the death rate in the two groups (fish and no fish) after an average follow-up of 15 years was almost identical**. So the dietary advice given to former DART participants, over a decade previously, offered no long-term protective effect. So while fish oil may offer short-term protection to people who have suffered a heart attack, this protection does not appear to stand the test of time.

A further study looked at whether dietary advice (to eat oily fish or fish oil supplements) could reduce the death rate among men with angina (Burr *et al*, 2003). Another surprising result was found: **advice to consume fish and the intake of fish oil capsules was associated with an *increase* in mortality of 20 per cent and 45 per cent respectively**!

This was a truly astounding result.

Furthermore, **this increase was even more prominent for sudden death.** Such results should make health organizations and the Government sit up and rethink their position on fish and fish oil in the primary and secondary prevention of heart disease.

But, more recently, a Finnish study looking at the relationship between omega-3 levels and the five-year risk of heart attack and death in patients with heart disease found that relatively high blood levels of omega-3 fats were associated with a lower risk of death (Erkkilä *et al.*, 2003). However, like the previous trials, **omega-3s did not prevent the recurrence of a heart attack.**

In 2004, the Cochrane Collaboration reviewed the current evidence to see whether dietary or supplemental omega-3 fatty acids alter total mortality (death rate) or cardiovascular events (heart attack and stroke) (Hooper *et al.*, 2004). **They concluded that there was no overall benefit either on heart attacks, deaths from heart disease or overall mortality**.

Another study found fish oil supplements increased life-threatening abnormal heart rhythms in patients with implanted defibrillators (Raitt *et al.*, 2005). This study actually found that **fish oil supplementation did not reduce the risk of abnormal or irregular heart rhythm and may even be pro-arrhythmic in some patients**.

More recently, in 2006, a major review published in the *British Medical Journal* drew the evidence together by reviewing all the relevant studies published over the previous four years (Hooper *et al.*, 2006). It looked at **89 studies** on omega-3 fats and health and concluded that **long chain and shorter chain omega-3 fats do not have a clear effect on total mortality, combined cardiovascular events or cancer**.

Additional treatments

Some arthritis patients have benefited from taking a herbal remedy isolated from *Rosa canina*, a type of rose hip (Winther *et al.*, 2005). In a randomized, double-blind, placebo-controlled trial, published in the

Journal of Rheumatology, 82 per cent of patients reported a reduction in pain after just three weeks of active treatment with this herbal remedy. The authors of the study concluded that it could alleviate symptoms of osteoarthritis. In fact, pain was reduced to such an extent that there was a significant decrease in the consumption of painkillers such as paracetemol, ibuprofen and NSAIDs.

Losing weight, eating a healthy plant-based diet that includes a good supply of omega-3 fatty acids (either though foods or supplements) can help reduce the symptoms of arthritis and may help some people reduce their medication (ARC, 2006). The overall message is that a plant-based diet, low in fat, salt, sugar and processed foods and high in fresh fruit, vegetables, whole grains, nuts and seeds can provide all the nutrients required for good health.

Eczema

The increasing rate of eczema in the West has been linked to a steep rise in the consumption of omega-6 fats and the reduced intake of omega-3s (Koch *et al.*, 2008).

Omega-6 fats favor the formation of specific eicosanoids (hormone-like molecules) that are involved in allergic inflammation. The parent omega-6 fatty acid LA is converted into arachidonic acid, a precursor in the production of eicosanoids (Koch *at al.*, 2008). Consequently, **an increased intake of omega-6 fats can promote allergic reactions**, while increasing omega-3 intake competes with omega-6 metabolism and protects against inflammatory conditions.

Brain food

The human brain grows and develops very rapidly during the first year of life, tripling in size by the age of one. The brain is largely made up of fat (over 60 per cent) and early brain development and function in humans requires a sufficient supply of polyunsaturated EFAs. For humans, the omega-6 fat arachidonic acid and the omega-3 fat DHA are essential for brain development and functioning.

Fish oils for brainy kids?

So, what is the scientific evidence that fish oils can improve cognitive ability and where does the Government stand on this issue? The evidence comes mainly from trials done using children with behavioral problems and is largely anecdotal. Also, what data that does exist is mixed.

The Durham-Oxford Study is the most cited work (Richardson and Montgomery, 2005). In this study, 117 children with developmental co-ordination disorders (DCD) such as attention deficit/hyperactivity disorder (ADHD), dyslexia and dyspraxia were given a daily supplement of fatty acids. The treatment was a supplement containing 80 per cent fish oil and 20 per cent evening primrose oil in gelatine capsules. The daily dose of six capsules provided omega-3 fatty acids (558 mg of EPA and 174 mg of DHA) and the omega-6 fatty acid LA (60 mg), or olive oil (omega-9) as a placebo.

After three months of treatment, results showed **significant improvements in reading, spelling and behavior among those receiving the fish oil supplements.** The researchers concluded that fatty acid supplements may be a safe, tolerable, effective treatment for improving academic progress and behavior among children with DCD. In other words, children who are not fulfilling their potential may benefit from increasing their intake of essential fatty acids.

A follow-up trial was conducted in Durham more recently whereby three million fish oil capsules were given to 2,000 children over eight months to see if their GCSE results improved. Unfortunately **the GCSE results were rather disappointing**, which was not press-released by the County Council. In some very fast back-pedaling they said "...it was never intended, and the County Council never suggested, that it would use this initiative to draw conclusions about the effectiveness or otherwise of using fish oil to boost exam results." So it seems fish oil was not the magic bullet Durham Council was looking for.

Although the Government has refused to shift its position on recommending fish oils for heart health, it is clearly not convinced about cognitive benefits. The FSA (Food Standards Agency) states that: "Evidence on the cognitive benefits of the omega-3 fatty acids, EPA and DHA, which are found in fish oils, is currently uncertain," (FSA, 2008)

Fish oil supplements

Some people prefer to take fish oil supplements rather than eat oily fish. However, fish oil supplements have also been linked to negative health effects in numerous studies. This is particularly worrying as they are increasingly popular as **clever marketing persuades people to buy them.**

Most fish oil supplement manufacturers publicize their meticulous manufacturing techniques reassuring us that all toxins are removed from their products. However, in March 2006, the FSA announced that the fish oil supplement manufacturer Seven Seas Ltd withdrew a number of batches of its own fish oil supplements because the levels of pollutants present (FSA, 2006). Less than a month later Boots withdrew fish oil capsules for the same reason (FSA, 2006a).

In both cases they said although there was no health risk associated with consumption of this product, the level of dioxins found in fish oil used to produce these capsules exceeded statutory limits.

Confused? You will be!

The FSA advises that fish oils protect against CVD and that long chain omega-3s are vital for the development of the central nervous system of the fetus and the breast-feeding infant (SACN, 2004). However, the FSA warns pregnant and breast-feeding women to restrict their intake of oily fish to limit their exposure to harmful toxins. So just when your intake of omega-3 really matters, during pregnancy and when you are breastfeeding, the Government warns you to limit your Intake! Consumers are unsurprisingly confused; the information given is neither comprehensive nor consistent.

In 2002, *Which?* magazine reported the findings of a Consumers' Association survey which asked 972 adults about their awareness of, eating habits and attitudes to oily fish (Consumers' Association, 2002). The survey found that only a sixth of fish-eaters knew that the FSA's advice is to eat oily fish once a week; over half thought the advice was to eat two or more portions. A shocking 61 per cent of people had no idea that oily fish may contain contaminants.

One per cent knew that pregnant women should avoid certain fish but nobody could name them. Most people in the survey were confused by what was meant by oily fish (**14 per cent thought that cod was an oily fish**). It is not just the public who are confused; the Consumers' Association states that the FSA couldn't provide any clear answers about the health implications of eating more than one portion of oily fish per week.

It's no clearer in the US. In 2002 the American Heart Association (AHA) issued a statement supporting the recommendation for at least two servings of fish (particularly oily fish) per week (Kris-Etherton *et al.*, 2002).

However, the AHA warned that the recommendations on fish consumption need to be balanced with concerns over contamination of fish with environmental pollutants (particularly mercury and PCBs). This is an incredibly important proviso which seriously challenges the idea that fish is 'healthy'. It should be noted that the AHA also recommended plant foods that are high in the plant omega-3 ALA such as soy beans, rapeseed, walnuts and flaxseed and oils made from them.

In the joint WHO/FAO 2003 report *Diet, Nutrition and the Prevention of Chronic Diseases*, regular fish consumption of one to two servings per week is recommended to protect against CVD (WHO/FAO, 2003). However, whilst it also states that vegetarians can ensure adequate intakes of the omega-3 fatty acid ALA from plant sources, the report fails to give any warnings about the dangers of environmental contamination.

This conflicting advice has led to much confusion. Who should the public listen to? Who can they believe?

Stop looking for a 'quick miracle fix'

We should **stop looking for a 'quick miracle fix'** and focus on the bigger picture... improving our diets by cutting out the saturated fatty foods laden with animal fats, sugar, salt and cholesterol and eating more fruit, vegetables, pulses, whole grains, nuts and seeds.

Butler says, "Our hearts don't need fish, our brains don't need fish and our health is far better served by plant EFAs as part of a well-balanced plant-based diet. Next time you are told of the magical properties of fish oil, you'll know what to say... fish is not a health food." (Butler, 2009)

Butler gives an interesting spin on the advantages of obtaining omega-3s and PUFA from plant sources, as opposed to using fish as the source.

Fish oil supplements lighten your wallet but do not help your heart
9-11-12

In an analysis of several studies omega-3 fatty acid supplements didn't help prevent heart attack or stroke. Oh, fish oil supplements. We had such high hopes for you and your omega-3 fatty acids—**you were supposed to boost our brain power and make our hearts healthier. Turns out you're pretty much worthless in that regard.**

A study released 9-11-12 in the ***Journal of the American Medical Association*** found that **fish oil supplements weren't linked with a lower risk of death from all causes, cardiac deaths or sudden deaths, nor were they associated with reduced odds of having**

a stroke or heart attack. Researchers scrutinized 20 studies that included 68,680 patients to draw that conclusion. (Rizos et al, 2012)

Omega-3 fatty acids, commonly found in fatty fish such as salmon and some vegetable oils, **may reduce inflammation and lower triglyceride levels, allegedly making them good for cardiovascular health**. Since our bodies can't make them we have to consume them, and there are longstanding debates about whether that's best done through supplements or foods. But in the end, food wins out.

Studies on the benefits of the **Mediterranean diet, which is big on fish and nuts**, have helped push the idea that omega-3 fatty acids are seemingly an essential part of good health.

In the JAMA study all but two of the studies analyzed used supplements, and the average supplement dose was 1.51 grams per day taken for an average of two years. In most studies the supplements were taken by people who already had a heart attack or some form of cardiovascular disease.

"Our findings do not justify the use of omega-3 as a structured intervention in everyday clinical practice or guidelines supporting dietary omega-3 (polyunsaturated fatty acid) administration," the authors of the JAMA article wrote. (Rizos et al, 2012)

So where does that leave us? Back to eating fish, since that may be where the benefits truly are (**By the way, McDonald's Filet-O-Fish doesn't count**.). That's not great news for people who don't love fish—which is a lot of people—and for those who think that taking a pill is the preferred way to solve health problems.

It's also not great news for the supplement industry, if people pay attention to studies like this, which they frequently do not. ***USA Today* reports that sales of fish oil supplements are healthy, with Americans spending $1.1 billion on them in 2011, an increase of 5.4 percent over 2010.**

Dr. Howard Weintraub, clinical director of New York University Center for the Prevention of Cardiovascular Disease, told ABC News, "Patients and doctors like the idea that it is natural and has no real side effects."

On the flip side, **Dr. Steven Nissen, professor of medicine at the Cleveland Clinic Lerner School of Medicine told ABC, "There's never been any compelling evidence of a clinical benefit."**

Of course, there's always the placebo effect, if you don't mind spending $30 a bottle for it.

I like to include multiple discussions on the same research conclusions to present a wide spectrum of opinions. Such will be the case with the work of Rizos. (Rizos et al, 2012)

My Letters to editors over the past 5 years

Letter to the Editor: 4-3-09

"Fish Oils: Is There A Downside?" 4-3-09

Even though there is a current fish oil craze, you can never be too careful about what you put into your body. Fish oil (especially omega-3) proponents have made wild claims for their curative powers for diseases such as cancer, heart disease, dementia, ADD, ADHD, depression, bipolar disorder, dyslexia, dyspraxia, obsessive compulsive disorder, headaches and migraines. They say that they will decrease aggressive behavior, prevent learning disabilities and make kids smarter. One website states that, "Kids will also have better vision, better hearing, better motor skills, more coordination and a friendlier personality, when taking omega-3 fatty acid supplements. It can even help them be leaders in their school and never get picked last in gym class." Such unsupported aggressive advertising has led to "a fish oil gold rush." Unfortunately, most supplements do not hold up under scientific testing and pill-forms of agents such as omega-3, vitamin E, beta carotene and vitamin C do not offer the same benefits as do natural foods containing these same ingredients. A large study at the University of Heidelberg gave fish oil or dummy capsules to more than 3,800 people who had suffered a recent heart attack and found that after a year, there was no difference between fish oil pills or placebo. When it comes to improving brain function, data from a trial of over 800 older people initially showed that those who eat plenty of oily fish seem to have better cognitive function. But factors such as education and mood explained most of the difference and a UK study has cast doubt on claims that eating oily fish can protect against dementia in old age. The American Heart Association (AHA) recommends adults eat fish at least twice a week and for people with heart disease, they advise 1 gram of omega-3 a day. Fish oil capsules are not for children or pregnant women, because the pills pose a bleeding risk and capsules should be stopped a week before any surgery. AHA spokesperson, Dr. Lichtenstein, stated that, "We need to be a little more cautious about the prediction of individual benefit of any nutritional supplements. We see this pattern — people are so willing to embrace the simple answer, as if it's possible to crack a capsule over a hot fudge sundae and undo the harm of harmful diets and lack of exercise."

In the America that I love, we will continue to emphasize the basics of eating a balanced diet, exercising more, avoiding stress, not smoking and not being misled by unscrupulous advertisers. Every time we turn on the TV, we are being oversold on the latest miracle meds or supplements, like they were pitching OxyClean or Sham Wow. So, be on guard and protect your wallet and your health.

Letter to the Editor: The Pundit Speaks 11-2-10

"Fish Oil Does Not Prevent Alzheimer's Disease" 11-2-10

Omega-3 fish oil supplement producers have claimed curative powers for diseases such as cancer, heart disease, dementia, ADD, ADHD, depression, bipolar disorder, dyslexia, dyspraxia, obsessive compulsive disorder, headaches and migraines. Also, it was claimed to decrease aggressive behavior, prevent learning disabilities and make kids smarter. Unsupported aggressive advertising has led to "soaring sales for fish oil." However, disappointing studies are now coming forth and supplements do not have the same benefits as do natural foods containing these same ingredients. Even though claims of being "heart healthy" persist, a large German study gave fish oil or dummy capsules to more than 3,800 people who had suffered a recent heart attack and found that after a year, there was no difference between fish oil pills or placebo. But, there is more bad news for fish oil. Even though data from a trial of over 800 older people initially showed that those who eat plenty of oily fish seem to have better cognitive function, a new study has found that omega-3 pills, promoted as boosting memory, did not slow mental and physical decline in older patients with Alzheimer's disease. This $10 million project studied nearly 300 men and women, aged 76 on average, with mild to moderate Alzheimer's disease. They were randomly assigned to take either the omega-3 fish oil pill (DHA) or dummy pills daily for 18 months. Results were similar in both groups, in that DHA provided no benefits in slowing Alzheimer's symptoms nor did the pills work in a subgroup of participants with the mildest Alzheimer's symptoms. The researchers concluded, "There is no basis for recommending DHA supplementation for patients with Alzheimer disease." Laurie Ryan, program director of Alzheimer's studies at the Institute on Aging, called the results discouraging. Thus, Alzheimer's disease remains basically untreatable and the "fish oil gold rush" may be slowing.

In the America that I love, we realize that generally dietary supplements do not work, except in cases of known deficiencies or malabsorption syndromes. Still, sales of dietary supplements bring in about $23 billion annually. We know that eating more heart-healthy omega-3 fats provided no additional benefit in a study of heart attack survivors who were already getting good care. There is little harm to fish oil when the ratio of omega-6 to omega-3 are properly balanced. Please remember the words of expert, Dr. Lichtenstein, "We need to be a little more cautious about the prediction of individual benefit of any nutritional supplements. People are so willing to embrace the simple answer, as if it's possible to crack a capsule over a hot fudge sundae and undo the harm of harmful diets and lack of exercise." But, give me a chocolate sundae. I'll take my chances.

Letter to the Editor: The Pundit Speaks 5-14-11

"Omega-3 Fish Oil Loses Support" 5-14-11

Things have been getting tough for dietary supplements across the board. The more we submit them to rigorous scientific testing, the more failures we find. Such is becoming the case with omega-3 fish oil. Even recently, we were talking about the "fish oil craze" and the "fish oil gold rush." But, those days are fading fast in light of accumulating studies in which fish oil has failed to live up to its hyped predictions, especially as it relates to cancer, heart disease and Alzheimer's disease. The latest bad news is a Japanese study of over 18,000 men which showed that, "Fish intake was significantly associated with an increased risk of prostate cancer; men who consumed fish more than four times per week had a 54% increased risk of developing prostate cancer compared with men who ate fish less than twice per week." A different study ruled out the presence of mercury, contained in fish as the culprit. Another group of investigators studied 3,461 participants in the Prostate Cancer Prevention Trial and found that "Men with the most DHA (one of the omega-3 fatty acids found in fish oil) in their bloodstreams were two-and-a-half times more likely to have an aggressive form of prostate cancer." These results were supported by the European Prospective Investigation into Cancer and Nutrition study, which showed that men who had the highest omega-3 levels had the highest risk for prostate cancer. Of equal concern, in other studies the fish oil has not lived up to its glowing beneficial claims as it relates to heart patients, stopping Alzheimer's or making babies smarter. Actually, a 2005 study found that fish oil may actually increase the risk of cardiac arrhythmias in some patients. That same year, the Journal of the American Medical Association (JAMA) reported that fish oil does not prevent any type of cancer. A 2006 study in the British Medical Journal reported that omega-3 fatty acids have no heart-health benefit. This is all rather shocking news in light of the widespread exalted claims for fish oil. A 2009 study also found that consuming fish does not reduce the risk of heart failure. And a 2010 article in the New England Journal of Medicine reported that heart patients given omega-3s had no reduction in cardiovascular events and a Harvard study linked intake of omega-3 with an increased risk of developing type 2 diabetes. A study group of 867 elderly adults showed no benefit at all, in tests for reaction time, spatial memory, and mental processing speed measurements and a JAMA report showed that omega-3 supplements do not slow mental decline in Alzheimer's patients.

In the America that I love, we must remain vigilant against deceptive and false advertising of dietary supplements. Enough already!

Letter to the editor: 9-13-11

"Fish Oil Heart Claims Debunked" 9-13-11

In recent times, nothing has been more aggressively marketed than fish oil (omega-3 polyunsaturated fats), with glowing claims which sound nearly miraculous. Advertisements and endless promotions by Dr. Oz and Dr. Andrew Weil have convinced many people that fish oil will protect them for nearly all forms of cancer, heart disease, Alzheimer's disease, all forms of dementia, ADD, ADHD, depression, bipolar disorder, dyslexia, dyspraxia, obsessive compulsive disorder, headaches and migraines. Yet, study after study have failed to support these unsubstantiated claims. Still, sales of fish oils go through the economic roof. The *Nutrition Business Journal* showed Americans spent $1.1 billion on fish oil supplements in 2011. A 2012 report in the *Journal of the American Medical Association* presented data showing fish oil supplements weren't linked with a lower risk of death from all causes, cardiac deaths or sudden deaths, nor were they associated with reduced odds of having a stroke or heart attack. Many recent studies have failed to find much benefit from dietary supplements, whether taken as a single vitamin or multivitamin. High doses of vitamin E, vitamin C, beta carotene, selenium and B vitamins all failed to prevent cancer, according to recent carefully done studies. According to industry figures, more than half of adults take at least one dietary supplement and 10% take more than five. It seems that folks only listen to advertisements and not to the result of well conducted scientific studies. Admittedly, the commercials pushing supplements are very powerful and carefully crafted influences. Figures show that dietary supplements have grown from $4 billion a year in 1994 to nearly $24 billion in 2008. Yet, no credible government agency recommends routine supplement use for preventing chronic diseases. Two studies found fish oil failed to prevent an irregular heartbeat condition called atrial fibrillation, which is found in one third of heart surgery patients. Additionally, a new meta-analysis looking at the effects of omega-3 fatty acids in patients at high risk for cardiovascular events has shown that the supplements have no effect on hard clinical outcomes, including all-cause mortality, cardiac death, sudden death, myocardial infarction (MI), or stroke.

In the America that I love, we realize that life style management and diet are very important for our overall well being and the Lyon Heart Study, published in 1999, found that heart attack survivors who ate a Mediterranean diet reduced their risk of another heart attack or death by 70% in just two years. Good health comes from keeping weight down, no smoking, daily exercise and a well balanced diet including fresh fruits and vegetables. At this point, most supplements, which have been scientifically tested, do not come anywhere close to the benefits of nutrients obtained from one's diet.

Letter to the editor: 9-16-12

"Fish Oil Supplements Appear Worthless" 9-16-12

American pill poppers will be disbelieving of the recent studies coming out against the claimed benefits of omega-3 fish oil supplements. Tell people anything but do not tell them fish oil supplements are worthless, because they will refuse to believe it. Fish oil has been promoted as if it was some kind of wonder drug or magic potion. False claims have been made that it can prevent cancer, heart disease, Alzheiner's disease, all forms of dementia, ADD, ADHD, depression, bipolar disorder, dyslexia, dyspraxia, obsessive compulsive disorder, headaches and migraines. Also, it was claimed to decrease aggressive behavior, prevent learning disabilities and make kids smarter. Consequently, sales of fish oil soared. In 2011, the *Nutrition Business Journal* showed Americans spent $1.1 billion on fish oil supplements. The *Journal of the American Medical Association* just published data showing fish oil supplements weren't linked with a lower risk of death from all causes, cardiac deaths or sudden deaths, nor were they associated with reduced odds of having a stroke or heart attack. Researchers scrutinized 20 studies that included 68,680 patients to draw that conclusion. Experts concluded, "Our findings do not justify the use of omega-3 as a structured intervention in everyday clinical practice or guidelines supporting dietary omega-3 (polyunsaturated fatty acid) administration." Citizens will scream out that they have been assured by highly promoted advertisements that fish oil supplements are basically a cure-all with no harmful downside. I have been telling you about the ineffectiveness of fish oil supplements for the past four years. The supplements do not work and you are wasting your money. To do the right thing, simply include fish in your balanced diet and that is as good as it is going to get. And for God's sake, do not listen to or be misled by the likes of Dr. Oz or by his hour long supplement infomercials. Additionally, fish oils do have a downside. A Japanese study of over 18,000 men showed that, "Fish intake was significantly associated with an increased risk of prostate cancer; men who consumed fish more than four times per week had a 54% increased risk of developing prostate cancer." Other experts found, "Men with the most DHA (one of the omega-3 fatty acids found in fish oil) in their bloodstreams were two-and-a-half times more likely to have an aggressive form of prostate cancer." Others found fish oils can block chemotherapy used to treat and kill cancer. The best scientific studies show fish oil supplements do not prevent cancer, heart disease, strokes or dementia.

In the America that I love, there is convincing evidence that supplements are basically ineffective in health maintenance or disease prevention. So, eat fish and throw away the pills.

Letter to the Editor: 10-9-12

"Fish Consumption Can Be Good and Bad" 10-9-12

According to the scientific literature, consumption of fish continues to have up sides and down sides. It is no wonder that consumers are so confused. An October 2012 study found, "Elevated mercury levels, which can come from eating more fish - depending on the fish species - were tied to a higher risk of developing symptoms, such as hyperactivity, impulsiveness or inattentiveness (ADHD, attention deficit/hyperactivity disorder)." Investigators found that I microgram of mercury per gram of a mother's hair - about eight times the average levels found in similar women's hair in another analysis - was tied to about a 60 percent increase in the risk of their child exhibiting ADHD-like behaviors. Please remember that mercury has been implicated in autism as a result of the use of mercury containing vaccines. Any level of mercury is considered to be toxic to human brain cells. Experts recommend, "Staying away from 'big fishes,' such as tuna and swordfish, which typically contain the most mercury. Instead, stick to fishes such as haddock and salmon." But, there is also a good side to eating fish. An article in the Archives of Pediatrics & Adolescent Medicine found that eating at least two servings of fish per week was linked to about a 60 percent lower risk of kids developing certain ADHD-like symptoms. However, please remember that most of these studies do not prove cause and effect and are not designed to do so. So, please do not jump to conclusions upon reading about these potentially alarming studies. Conflicting research conclusions are as common as conflicting and unreliable political speeches. Unfortunately, interpretations of data is erroneously assumed to be fact, but that is rarely the case. Also, please remember that about half (50%) of so called scientific studies will be shown to be flawed or incorrect. Even past studies looking at the link between mercury and ADHD have produced conflicting results. Inconsistencies are everywhere, as I have found in the glowing claims made for dietary supplements and antioxidants.

Case in point is the one involving the benefits versus the harmful potential of omega-3 fish oil supplements. American television is saturated with convincing complimentary ads for fish oil supplementation, but studies show a downside relating to increased risk for prostate cancer and blockage of chemotherapy drugs.

In the America that I love, we must view new scientific data with a skeptical eye. We must apply good ole' common sense to the many alarming headlines regarding the benefits or harmful effects of common foods, vitamins and supplements. Avoid knee-jerk reactions to bold headlines and enjoy eating some fish, including some fried catfish. Additionally, watch marketers and always follow the money. And, please use your judgment wisely.

Letter to the editor: The Pundit Speaks 4-16-13

"Fish Oil Failures" 4-16-13

Attention, pill poppers of America! Television, radio and printed advertising is saturated with convincing complimentary ads for fish oil supplementation, but scientific studies are showing either no beneficial effects or they show a downside. When scientifically tested, fish oil supplements (omega-3, PUFA) does not live up to the exalted claims of advertisers. In 2005, the Journal of the American Medical Association (JAMA) reported that fish oil does not prevent cancer. In 2006, the British Medical Journal (BMJ) reported that omega-3 fatty acids have no heart-health benefit. Among nearly 4,000 heart attack patients, no difference was seen between those who consumed omega-3 supplements and those who took dummy pills. In 2009, other investigators agreed, when they found that consuming fish does not reduce the risk of heart failure. In 2010, the New England Journal of Medicine (NEJM) reported similarly dismal results with heart patients given omega-3 fatty acids in addition to standard drug therapy, in that there was no reduction in cardiovascular events. In 2010, a study on elderly adults showed no benefit at all in tests for reaction time, spatial memory, and processing speed measurements (brain function). And, later in 2010, a JAMA report showed that omega-3 supplements do not slow mental decline in Alzheimer's patients. Also, a 2010 JAMA report showed that consumption of fish oil during pregnancy does not benefit babies' cognitive development. In short, fish oil is no help for heart patients, does not forestall Alzheimer's disease, does not prevent depression, and does not make babies smarter. Here is the kicker! In 20 randomized controlled trials (RCTs) data was reported on 68,680 patients in a JAMA review study in 2012. Overall, omega-3 PUFA (fish oil) supplementation was not associated with a lower risk of all-cause mortality, cardiac death, sudden death, myocardial infarction, or stroke based on relative and absolute measures of association. Experts stated, "Our findings do not justify the use of omega-3 fish oil as a structured intervention in everyday clinical practice or guidelines supporting dietary omega-3 (polyunsaturated fatty acid) administration." But, that is not the end of the story. There is a downside, in spite of the heavy marketing. Fish oil increased the risk for an aggressive form of prostate cancer and fish oil has been shown to block some forms of chemotherapy from killing cancer cells. A 2005 JAMA report showed that fish oil may actually increase the risk of cardiac arrhythmias in some patients.

In the America that I love, the more we submit dietary supplements to rigorous scientific testing, the more failures we find. In 2011, "campaigns of persuasion" had people dole out $1.1 billion on fish oil supplements. Please, turn off Dr. Oz, toss the pills and eat real fish instead.

Letter to the Editor: The Pundit Speaks

"Fish Oils are Sounding Fishy" 4-27-14

For decades, we have been scolded and warned to avoid eating saturated fats because of their presumed link to heart disease. But, not so fast. Until now, doctors have said that saturated fats increase "bad" LDL cholesterol, which can cause plaques to form in your arteries and raise your risk of a heart attack or stroke. At the same time, omega-3 fish oils were said to improve heart health because they allegedly increase "good" HDL cholesterol. Good cholesterol is believed to help the body rid itself of bad cholesterol. Saturated fats are solid at room temperature. They can be found in butter, lard, cheese and cream, as well as the fatty white areas on cuts of meat. By contrast, unsaturated fats are liquid at room temperature, such as those seen in vegetable cooking oil or olive oil. Amazingly, Dr. Rajiv Chowdhury, a cardiovascular epidemiologist at the University of Cambridge and lead author of a comprehensive review of nutrition research related to fats, and his team found that neither effect seemed to make much difference for overall cardiac risk. In short, fish oil supplements do not protect your heart. Their meta-analysis study involved data from 72 studies with more than 600,000 participants from 18 nations. The team combined study findings to assess the heart health benefits of all types of dietary fat, including saturated fat, unsaturated fat, and the omega-3 (fish oils) and omega-6 fatty acids. Saturated fats, long considered a dietary no-no, appeared to pose no additional risk for heart disease according to recent research. Shockingly, saturated fats carried about the same cardiac risk as unsaturated fats, omega-3 and omega-6 fatty acids. Thus, people who take fish oil capsules may not be getting the heart-health benefits they desired, according to a pair of new research reports. Sadly, both studies found the omega-3 fatty acids in fish oil supplements do not provide any significant protection against heart disease, when compared to other types of dietary fats. Researchers looked at the 17 randomized clinical trials and found they showed consistently little or no significant effect on reducing coronary heart disease events." A second study also came to the same disappointing conclusion regarding omega-3 fatty acid fish oils. This study had been reviewing the use of omega-3s for eye health, but researchers used their data to look at whether the supplements also helped prevent heart disease. Bad trans fats can still be found in processed foods, which are "hydrogenated" or "partially hydrogenated" in the ingredient list.

In the America that I love, people should get their omega-3 fatty acids and fish oil from food rather than through supplements. All supplements should be used with caution. Please eat a balanced diet and exercise regularly.

RMH Note: A study found that "reducing the intake of CHO with high glycemic index is more effective in the prevention of CVD than reducing SAFA intake per se."

From a 2010 study out of Japan, saturated fat intake "was inversely associated with mortality from total stroke."

A 2010 meta-analysis found "that there is no significant evidence for concluding that dietary saturated fat is associated with an increased risk of CHD or CVD."

Polar bears have levels of Low Density Lipoprotein (LDL) and have a diet consisting of mainly blubber that would cause cardiovascular disease in humans, but their genetic changes seem to have taken care of the problem with atherosclerosis.

Saturated fat is not the villain that the AMA and the FDA have made it out to be. In fact, a low carbohydrate and high fat diet (LCHF) seems to work well to keep weight down and increase longevity.

If you live a LCHF lifestyle, you lose weight or maintain a healthy weight, your cholesterol, LDL, and triglycerides go down, and your HDL goes up. Your body adjusts from using glucose for energy to using ketones for energy. Ketones are the byproduct from burning fat.

It's the high carb lifestyle pushed by the FDA that is partially responsible for the obesity epidemic in this country. Walk down almost any isle in the grocery store and you will find almost nothing except highly processed carbs. Carbs are SUGAR, whether in bread, pasta, or rice, and all are detrimental to your metabolism.

SUMMARY: Omega-3 fish oil facts and failures

Based on earlier studies, many claimed that a diet that's rich in omega-3s can protect you against certain cancers, heart disease and strokes. But, many well designed current scientific studies show no benefit. In fact, supplements don't seem to protect against cancer, strokes, dementia or heart disease. Some antioxidants, including fish oil, may even increase the risk of certain cancers. Experts also worry that high doses of antioxidants, including fish oil, reduce the effectiveness of chemotherapy.

Therefore, fish oil does not live up to its claims and the facts are as follows:

- These data do reinforce the results of other studies of omega-3 fatty acids (fish oil) in unipolar depression patients (Marangell et al, 2003) and in obsessive-compulsive disorder patients (Fux et al, 2004) where placebo-controlled crossover trials found **that EPA is virtually ineffective**.

- in 2005, JAMA reported that **fish oil does not prevent cancer**. (MacLean et al, 2005)

- in 2005, a JAMA report showed that **fish oil may actually increase the risk of cardiac arrhythmias** in some patients. (Raitt, 2005) a randomized, double-blind, controlled trial

- The following year in 2006, the "British Medical Journal reported that **omega-3 fatty acids have no heart-health benefit.** Among nearly 4,000 heart attack patients, no difference was seen between those who consumed omega-3 supplements and those who took placebo pills. (Hooper et al, 2006)

- Trial evidence that examines the effects of n–3 PUFAs on depressed mood is limited and is difficult to summarize and evaluate because of considerable heterogeneity. **The evidence available provides little**

support for the use of n–3 PUFAs (fish oil) to improve depressed mood. (Appleton et al, 2006)

- In 2009, other investigators agreed when they found that **consuming fish does not reduce the risk of heart failure.** (Dijkstra et al, 2009, the Rotterdam Study) a randomized, double-blind, controlled trial.

- Then in 2010, the New England Journal of Medicine reported **similarly dismal results with heart patients given omega-3 fatty acids in addition to standard drug therapy.** They had **no reduction in cardiovascular events.** (Krombout et al, 2010)

- In the **Alpha Omega Trial**, as reported by Kromhout et al supplementation with a combination of n–3 eicosapentaenoic acid (EPA) and n–3 docosahexaenoic acid (DHA), n–3 alpha-linolenic acid (ALA), or both EPA–DHA and ALA **did not significantly reduce the rate of major cardiovascular events among patients who had had a myocardial infarction** and who were receiving conventional state-of-the-art therapy. (Krombout et al, 2010)

- in 2010, researchers dashed those hopes also. A group of **867 elderly people** were randomly assigned to either **a fish-oil supplement** or placebo. After two years of supplementation, **elderly adults showed no benefit at all in tests for reaction time, spatial memory, and processing speed measurements.** (Dangour et al, 2010) a randomized, double-blind, controlled trial.

- A later 2010 JAMA report showed that **omega-3 supplements do not slow mental decline in Alzheimer's patients.** (Quinn et al, 2010)

- babies get no benefit either from omega-3s. A JAMA report showed that **consumption of fish oil during pregnancy does not benefit babies' cognitive development.** (Makrides et al, 2010)

- **Fish oil supplementation was not found to be significantly more effective in perinatal depression than placebo at post-treatment with a pooled effect size using a fixed-effects model.** (Jans et al, 2010)

- **In 13 randomized, placebo-controlled trials examining the efficacy of omega-3 FAs involving 731 participants, meta-analysis demonstrated no significant benefit of omega-3 FA treatment for major depression compared with placebo. Meta-analysis**

demonstrated significant heterogeneity and publication bias. Current published trials suggest a small, non-significant benefit of omega-3 FAs for major depression. Nearly all of the treatment efficacy observed in the published literature may be attributable to publication bias. (Bloch, Hannestad, 2012)

- **No evidence was found for those exploring their efficacy** (of omega-3 Fatty acids) **on depressive symptoms in young populations, perinatal depression, primary disease other than depression and healthy subjects.** (Grosso et al, 2014)

- In these reports, **fish oil is sounding more like snake oil.** The new findings linking higher DHA levels to cancer add yet another reason to use caution with fish oil supplements.

- **Fish oil has failed its marketing claims.** Specifically, **it is no help for heart patients, does not forestall Alzheimer's disease, does not prevent depression, and does not make babies smarter.**

Thus, here is a chronological account showing fish oil (omega-3s) has harmful potential as follows:

- In earlier studies, **animals fed high-erucic-acid rape seed oil showed growth retardation and undesirable changes in various organs, especially the heart, a discovery that touched off the so-called "erucic acid crisis"** and spurred plant geneticists to develop new versions of the seed. (Vles et al, 1978) **Rats genetically selected to be prone to heart lesions developed more lesions on the LEAR oil and the flax oil, than those on olive oil or sunflower oil, leading researchers to speculate that the omega-3 fatty acids (not erucic acid) in LEAR and flax oil might be the culprit.**

- **saturated fats (palmitic and stearic acids) were protective against heart lesions but that high levels of omega-3 fatty acids correlated with high levels of lesions.** They found a lesser correlation with heart lesions and erucic acid. (Trenholm et al, 1979)

- Studies carried out at the Health Research and Toxicology Research Divisions in Ottawa, Canada discovered that **rats bred to have high blood pressure and proneness to stroke had shortened life-spans when fed canola oil as the sole source of fat.** The results of a later study suggested that **the culprit was the sterol compounds** in the oil, which "make the cell membrane more rigid" and contribute to the shortened life-span of the animals. (Wallsundera et al, 2000)

- studies carried out at the Health Research and Toxicology Research Divisions in Ottawa, Canada discovered that **rats bred to have high blood pressure and proneness to stroke had shortened life-spans when fed canola oil as the sole source of fat.** (Ratnayake et al, 2000)

- **there is evidence that over consumption of omega-3 fatty acids in a diet lacking in saturated fats may actually be bad for the heart.** In test animals, diets high in canola oil, which is **relatively high in omega-3 fatty acids but low in saturated fats, caused fibrotic heart lesions, vitamin E deficiencies and abnormal changes to the blood platelets.** (Sauer et al, 1997) (Kramer et al, 1982) (Trenholm et al, 1979)

-These studies all point in the same direction -- that **canola oil is definitely not healthy for the cardiovascular system.** Like rapeseed oil, its predecessor, **canola oil is associated with fibrotic lesions of the heart.** It also causes vitamin E deficiency, undesirable changes in the blood platelets and shortened life-span in stroke-prone rats when it was the only oil in the animals' diet. Furthermore, it seems to retard growth, which is why **the FDA does not allow the use of canola oil in infant formula**. (Federal Register, 1985)

- **many studies show that the problems with canola oil are not related to the content of erucic acid, but more with the high levels of omega-3 fatty acids and low levels of saturated fats**. (http://www.dcnutrition.com/news/Detail.CFM?RecordNumber=639. Accessed 6-4-11) We have been repeatedly advised to avoid saturated fats because they were allegedly bad for us.

- Surprisingly, in 2009, **Harvard linked fish and omega-3 fats to type 2 diabetes**. Following **195,204 adults** for 14 to 18 years, researchers reported in 2009 that they had found that **the more fish or long-chain omega-3 fatty acids participants consumed, the higher their risk of developing diabetes**. (Kaushik et al, 2009)

- **Supplementation with n-3 PUFA resulted in a significant increase in plasma EPA and DHA but had no effect on 10-km time-trial performance; preexercise outcome measures; exercise-induced increases in plasma cytokines, myeloperoxidase, blood total leukocytes, serum C-reactive protein, and creatine kinase; or the decrease in the salivary**

IgA:protein ratio. In conclusion, **6 wk supplementation with a large daily dose of n-3 PUFAs increased plasma EPA and DHA but had no effect on exercise performance** or in countering measures of inflammation and immunity before or after a 3-d period of 9 hr of heavy exertion. (Nieman et al, 2009)

- A group of 867 elderly people were randomly assigned to either a fish-oil supplement or placebo. After two years of supplementation, elderly adults showed **no benefit at all in tests for reaction time, spatial memory, and processing speed measurements**. (Dangour et al, 2010)

- A *JAMA* report showed that consumption of **fish oil during pregnancy does not benefit babies' cognitive development.** (Makrides et al, 2010)

- **Fish oil capsules failed to prevent flare-ups of atrial fibrillation, a common heart rhythm problem, in a large study in 2010.**

- In the journal *Cancer Cell*, September 2011, investigators in the Netherlands reported **fish oil supplements can stop chemotherapy drugs from working. They advise cancer patients undergoing chemotherapy not to take fish oil supplements. The two fatty acids involved, KHT and 16:4(n-3), which are also produced by stem cells in the blood, lead to tumors becoming immune to treatment. Using drugs to block the production of the fatty acids prevented this form of resistance which "significantly enhances the chemotherapy,"** the study says. **They showed that off-the-shelf fish oil supplements, given to mice, could stop chemotherapy working against some tumors.**

- the *American Journal of Epidemiology* reports that **men with higher levels of DHA, one of the omega-3 fatty acids found in fish oil, were at increased risk of developing** prostate cancer. Men with the most DHA in their bloodstreams were two-and-a-half times more likely to have an aggressive form of prostate cancer. (Brasky et al, 2011) Prostate Cancer Prevention Trial.

Similar results were found in the European Prospective Investigation into Cancer and Nutrition study, where **men who had the highest omega-3 levels had the highest risk for prostate cancer.**

- **In hemodialysis patients, 2,080 mg marine omega-3 fatty acids has no effect on serum systemic inflammation markers and oxidative stress in hemodialysis patients.** (Kooshki et al, 2011)

- **In a 2012 review by the Cochrane Library, researchers found participants taking omega-3 scored no better in standard tests of memory and mental performance than a placebo.** They called the studies "disappointing."

- **In two studies, Cochrane researchers compared the effects of omega-3 (fish oil) capsules versus placebo capsules containing olive or sunflower oil. In the third study, participants used either omega-3-fortified margarine or a regular margarine spread. In the end (**a total of **3,536 people** over the age of 60 were studied, which lasted between six and 40 months**), the 2012 data showed that participants who got extra omega-3s performed no better on standard tests of mental abilities, memory or verbal fluency than those who took placebos.** http://summaries.cochrane.org/CD005379/fish-oils-for-the-prevention-of-dementia-in-older-people. Accessed 5-8-14.

- **In 20 RCTs data reported in 2012, on 68,680 patients, no statistically significant association was observed with all-cause mortality, cardiac death, sudden death, myocardial infarction, and stroke when all supplement studies were considered. Overall, omega-3 PUFA supplementation was not associated with a lower risk of all-cause mortality, cardiac death, sudden death, myocardial infarction, or stroke based on relative and absolute measures of association.** (Rizos et al, 2012)

- **three recent randomized trials in high-risk populations (those with either multiple risk factors or a history of cardiovascular disease) have suggested very little benefit from omega-3 fatty acids.** (Roncaglioni, Tombesi et al, 2013) (Kotwal et al, 2012) (Rizos et al, 2012)

- **In type II diabetes, no significant changes were observed in systolic and diastolic blood pressure before and after daily consumption of omega-3 capsules.** (Hosseinzadeh et al, 2012)

- A new study looked at the effects of giving **321 schoolchildren** in South Africa either supplements containing iron, omega-3s or both and **there was no overall benefit linked to omega-3 supplements. And when the researchers zeroed in on kids with anemia,**

those who used omega-3s did worse than before on one test of memory. (Baumgartner et al, 2012) a randomized, double-blind, placebo-controlled intervention.

- **The researchers found no difference in cognitive skills between the women with high and low levels of omega-3s in the blood at the time of the first memory tests. There was also no difference between the two groups in how fast their thinking skills declined over time.** (Ammann et al, 2013)

- **In a clinical study of 30 people with bipolar disorder, those who took fish oil in addition to standard prescription treatments for bipolar disorder for 4 months experienced fewer mood swings and relapse than those who received placebo. But another 4 month long clinical study treating people with bipolar depression and rapid cycling bipolar disorder did not find that EPA helped reduce symptoms.**

Source: Omega-3 fatty acids | University of Maryland Medical Center http://umm.edu/health/medical/altmed/supplement/omega3-fatty-acids#ixzz2h9cLWE78. University of Maryland Medical Center

- **EPA-rich fish oil and DHA-rich fish oil supplementation did not prevent depressive symptoms during pregnancy or postpartum.** (Mozurkewich et al, 2013) a double-blind, randomized controlled trial.

- **Results of recent outcomes trials of long-chain omega-3 fatty acids, fibrates, and niacin have been disappointing, failing to show additional reductions in adverse cardiovascular events when combined with statins.** (Bradberry, Hilleman, 2013)

- "**Looking at the 17 randomized clinical trials that we combined, the majority of the trials -- especially the more recent and large-scale ones -- showed consistently little or no significant effect on reducing coronary heart disease events**," said Dr. Rajiv Chowdhury, 2014.

- **That study found no reduction in heart attack, stroke or heart failure among almost 1,100 people taking omega-3 supplements, compared to similar numbers of people taking other supplements for eye health or just an inactive placebo. It appeared online March 17, 2014 in *JAMA Internal Medicine*. The**

meta-analysis performed by Chowdhury's team involved data from 72 studies with more than 600,000 participants from 18 nations. (Chowdhury,Van Horn,AHA, 2014)

- Researchers found no benefit among individuals who had taken omega-3 or eye vitamins; they were as likely to have experienced a heart problem during the study period as people who took a placebo, according to the study published in (March 17, 2014) in the journal JAMA Internal Medicine. "Also, **omega-3 or omega-6 fatty acids have no or little impact on reducing cardiovascular disease outcomes.**"

(Chowdhury,Van Horn,AHA, 2014)

Omega-3s do not prevent progression of AMD

5-5-13 ***Journal of the American Medical Association*** **online. Simply adding omega-3s or lutein and zeaxanthin to the standard AREDS formula did not help or hurt the progression of age-related macular degeneration (AMD).** These **popular supplements are commonly sold as the "AREDS" formula — short for the Age-Related Eye Disease Study. In short, the antioxidants omega-3, lutein and zeaxanthin were ineffective in delaying the progression of AMD.** (AREDS, JAMA, 2013)

Omega-3 fatty acids and beta-carotene clearly do not reduce the risk of progression to advanced AMD; however, adding lutein and zeaxanthin in place of beta-carotene may further improve the formulation. (Chew et al, 2013)

While a healthy diet promotes good eye health and general well-being, based on overall AREDS2 data, **regular high doses of antioxidant supplements do not prevent cataract**. (Chew et al, 2013)

Many high quality clinical trials on antioxidant supplements have shown no effect or adverse outcomes ranging from morbidity to all cause mortality. Theoretically, such antioxidants may do more harm than good. Ironically, the health and therapeutic power of antioxidants were overly magnified by the pharmaceutical industry for self-gain profit rather than concern for human health.

For example: The Selenium and Vitamin E Cancer Prevention Trial (SELECT), using oral selenium and vitamin E antioxidant supplementation in disease-free volunteers, was designed to test a prostate cancer chemoprevention hypothesis. SELECT was terminated early because of both harm being done to those receiving antioxidants and negative data for the formulations and doses given.

The view of Singh et al on harmful antioxidants (similar to omega-3s)

Singh et al wrote a 2010 paper entitled, Reconvene and reconnect the antioxidant hypothesis in human health and disease. It has been included to give another view on antioxidants, which includes omega-3s.

Also, for my additional views, please refer to **my companion books** as follows:

- Death In Small Doses? Trafford Publishing, © 2010

- Antioxidant Overkill, CreateSpace and Free Radical Publishing, © 2011

- Dangers of Excessive Antioxidants in Cancer Patients, CreateSpace and Free Radical Publishing, © 2011

- Heart Disease and Antioxidant Failures, CreateSpace and Free Radical Publishing, © 2011

- Antioxidant Failures and Dangers, CreateSpace and Free Radical Publishing, © 2011

- Anti-Aging Anti-oxidant Scams, CreateSpace and Free Radical Publishing, © 2011

- Sports, Athletes, Exercise Facts and Antioxidant Myths, CreateSpace and Free Radical Publishing, © 2011

- Alzheimer's Disease: Forget Antioxidants and Supplements, CreateSpace and Free Radical Publishing, © 2012

- Sex, Performance, Reproduction, Naked Radicals And Antioxidants, CreateSpace and Free Radical Publishing, © 2012

- Antioxidants Linked To Deadly Unintended Consequences, CreateSpace and Free Radical Publishing, © 2013

- Diabetes and Oxygen Free Radical Sophistry, CreateSpace and Free Radical Publishing, © 2014, revised

- Hydrogen Peroxide: A Health, Homeostatic and Protective Essentiality, CreateSpace and Free Radical Publishing, © 2014

- Reactive Oxygen Species vs. Antioxidants: The Oxypocalypse or The War That Never Was, CreateSpace and Free Radical Publishing, © 2014

Several **Cochrane Meta-analysis and Markov Model techniques, which are presently best available statistical models to derive conclusive answers for comparing large number of trials**, offers some support for beneficial claims. (Singh et al, 2010)

However, **the reputation of antioxidants began to slump with adverse outcomes in clinical trials** (Pazdro, Burges, 2010) (Murray et al, 2006) (Nathan, 2003) (Gulshan et al, 2005) (Bjalakovic et al, JAMA, 2007) (Pocobelli et al, 2009) (Miller et al, 2005)

(Blomhoff, 2005) (Lichtenstein, 2005) (Johansen et al, 2005) (Williams, Fisher, 2005) (Singh et al, J Physiol. 2009) (Sokol, 1984)

In due course of time, their role as "Elixirs of Life" was summarily rejected. In midst of massive literature piling up with **superlative praises of AO**, it is indeed commendable that **Halliwell and his group kept on issuing warning against exaggerated praises, which is now quite justified.**

Ironically, the initial juggernaut image of antioxidants, as impeccable devotee of health and longevity, without considering their merit, started crumbling.

Suddenly, antioxidant supplements are reported as wearing black hats.

The toxicity of high doses of some vitamins has been well known for a long time. The human body has good tolerance of vitamin-C and E but prolonged intake of **high doses of these vitamins has now been demonstrated to have many ill effects including increased mortality.** (Nathan, 2003) (Gulshan et al, 2005)

(Bjalakovic et al, JAMA, 2007)

Feinendegen has claimed that **low ROS (EMOD) concentration during antioxidant supplementation may prevent apoptosis in favor of cell survival and proliferation also in neoplastic cells and thus rather promote cancer than protect against it.** (Finendegen, 2002)

For an in depth discussion, please refer to my books entitled, *Dangers Of Excessive Antioxidants In Cancer Patients* and *Anti-oxidant, Anti-aging Scams.*

Contrary to earlier prevailing concept that supplementation with alpha-tocopherol confers protection against a large spectrum of diseases such as CVD, cancer, diabetes mellitus, Parkinsonism, Alzheimer disease pre-eclampsia and aging, the recent observations from large prospective, randomized placebo controlled trials have largely been negative.

William and Fisher critically analyzed the benefits and harms of various dietary antioxidants in relation to CVD. **They concluded: "Guidelines for diet should adhere closely to what has been clinically proved and by this standard there is no basis to recommended antioxidant use, beyond what is inherent to the "heart healthy" diet in order to benefit cardiovascular health".** (Williams, Fisher, 2005)

In an article by Verrax and Calderon, **they said, "Thus, for many people, vitamin C is believed to prevent or cure viral respiratory infections and to be beneficial in both cardiovascular diseases and cancer. Although there is no clinical evidence, as yet, that vitamin C can be beneficial in any one of these indications, it is still perceived by the public as a miracle-pill."** They are frank enough to confess that the popularity of vitamin C has been exaggerated and over embroidered by expensive advertising campaigns.

In summary, the current opinion is that **as long as body has adequate levels of antioxidants and that the dietary intake is normal, additional supplement are not needed.** On the contrary, **such supplements may do more harm than good.**

Background on fish oil - Wikipedia

Fish Oil Background: Wikipedia http://en.wikipedia.org/wiki/Fish_oil accessed 2013

Fish oil is oil derived from the tissues of oily fish. Fish oils contain the omega-3 fatty acids eicosapentaenoic acid (EPA), and docosahexaenoic acid (DHA), precursors of certain eicosanoids that are believed to reduce inflammation throughout the body. (Moghadasian, 2008) (Cleland, James, Proudman, 2006)

Fish do not actually produce omega-3 fatty acids, but instead accumulate them by consuming either microalgae or prey fish that have accumulated omega-3 fatty acids, together with a high quantity of antioxidants such as iodide and selenium, from microalgae, where these antioxidants are able to protect the fragile polyunsaturated lipids from peroxidation. (Venturi, Donati, et al. 2000) (Venturi, Venturi, 2007)

Fatty predatory fish likc sharks, swordish, tilefish, and albacore tuma may be high in omega-3 fatty acids, but due to their position at the top of the food chain, these species can also accumulate toxic substances through biomagnification. For this reason, **the U.S. Food and Drug Administration recommends limiting consumption of certain (predatory) fish species (e.g. albacore tuna, shark, king mackerel, tilefish and swordfish) due to high levels of toxic contaminants such as mercury, dioxin, PCB's and chlordane.** (EPA, 2007)

Marine and freshwater fish oil vary in contents of arachidonic acid, EPA and DHA. (Innis, rioux, et al. 1995)

The various species range from lean to fatty and their oil content in the tissues has been shown to vary from 0.7–15.5%. (Gruger, Nelson, et al, 1964)

They also differ in their effects on organ lipids. (Innis, Rioux, et al. 1995)

Studies have revealed that there is no relation between total fish intake or estimated omega–3 fatty acid intake from all fish and serum omega–3 fatty acid concentrations. (Philibert, Vanier, et al, 2006)

Only fatty fish intake, particularly salmonid, and estimated EPA + DHA intake from fatty fish has been observed to be significantly associated with increase in serum EPA + DHA. (Philibert, Vanier, et al. 2006)

The omega-3 fatty acids in fish oil are thought to be beneficial in treating hypertriglyceridemia, and possibly beneficial in preventing heart disease. (NIH, 2006)

Fish oil and omega-3 fatty acids have been studied in a wide variety of other conditions, such as clinical depression, (Su, Huang, et al. 2003) (Naliwaiko, Araujo, et al. 2004) **anxiety**, (Green, Hermesh, et al, 2006) (Yehuda, Rabinovitz, 2005) (Nemets, Stahl, et al. 2002) **cancer, and macular degeneration, although benefit in these conditions remains to be proven**. (NIH, 2006) Actually, they have been debunked.

Omega-3 fatty acids overview (Univ Maryland Med Ctr. 2011)

The following section was excerpted or modified from the article by the **Univ Maryland Med Ctr. accessed 11-9-11 http://www.umm.edu/altmed/articles/omega-3-000316.htm.** It is included for those new to the field of omega-3s.

Overview:

Omega-3 fatty acids are considered essential fatty acids: They are necessary for human health but **the body can't make them** -- you have to get them through food. Omega-3 fatty acids can be found in fish, such as salmon, tuna, and halibut, other seafood including algae and krill, some plants, and nut oils. **Also known as polyunsaturated fatty acids (PUFAs), omega-3 fatty acids** play a crucial role in brain function, as well as normal growth and development. They have also become popular because they may reduce the risk of heart disease. The American Heart Association recommends eating fish (particularly fatty fish such as mackerel, lake trout, herring, sardines, albacore tuna, and salmon) at least 2 times a week.

PUFAs serve as antioxidants, including omega-3 fish oils. The unsaturated double bonds trap EMODs (electronically modified oxygen derivatives; formerly known as reactive oxygen species, ROS).

Omega-3 fatty acids are highly concentrated in the brain and appear to be important for cognitive (brain memory and performance) and behavioral function. In fact, **infants who do not get enough omega-3 fatty acids from their mothers during pregnancy are at risk for developing vision and nerve problems. Symptoms of omega-3 fatty acid deficiency include fatigue, poor memory, dry skin, heart problems, mood swings or depression, and poor circulation.**

It is important to have the proper ratio of omega-3 and omega-6 (another essential fatty acid) in the diet. **Omega-3 fatty acids may help reduce inflammation, and most omega-6 fatty acids tend to promote inflammation. The typical American diet tends to contain 14 - 25 times more omega-6 fatty acids than omega-3 fatty acids,** which many nutritionally oriented physicians consider to be way too high on the omega-6 side.

The Mediterranean diet, on the other hand, has a healthier balance between omega-3 and omega-6 fatty acids. Many studies have suggested that people who follow this diet are less likely to develop heart disease. The Mediterranean diet emphasizes foods rich in omega-3 fatty acids, including whole grains, fresh fruits and vegetables, fish, olive oil, garlic, as well as moderate wine consumption.

Uses:

Clinical evidence was previously suggested for heart disease and problems that contribute to heart disease, but omega-3 fatty acids may also possibly be used for:

High cholesterol

People who follow a Mediterranean style diet **tend to have** higher HDL or "good" cholesterol levels, which help promote heart health. Inuit Eskimos, who get high amounts of omega-3 fatty acids from eating fatty fish, also tend to have increased HDL cholesterol and decreased triglycerides (fats in the blood). Several studies have shown that fish oil supplements reduce triglyceride levels. Finally, walnuts (which are rich in alpha linolenic acid or ALA, which converts to omega-3s in the body) have been reported to lower total cholesterol and triglycerides in people with high cholesterol levels.

High blood pressure

Several clinical studies suggest that diets rich in omega-3 fatty acids lower blood pressure in people with hypertension. An analysis of 17 clinical studies using fish oil supplements found that taking 3 or more grams of fish oil daily **may** reduce blood pressure in people with untreated hypertension. Doses this high, however, should only be taken under the direction of a physician.

Heart disease

The role of omega-3 fatty acids in cardiovascular disease is *well established (?)*. One of the best ways to help prevent heart disease is to eat a diet low in saturated fat and to eat foods that are rich in monounsaturated and polyunsaturated fats (including omega-3 fatty acids). Clinical evidence **suggests** that EPA and DHA (eicosapentaenoic acid and docosahexaenoic acid, the 2 omega-3 fatty acids found in fish oil) help reduce risk factors for heart disease, including high cholesterol and high blood pressure. Fish oil has been shown (in the estimation of some) to lower levels of triglycerides (fats in the blood), and to lower the risk of death, heart attack, stroke, and abnormal heart rhythms in people who have already had a heart attack. Fish oil also **appears** to help prevent and treat atherosclerosis (hardening of the arteries) by slowing the development of plaque and blood clots, which can clog arteries. **DEBUNKED.**

Large population studies **suggest** that getting omega-3 fatty acids in the diet, primarily from fish, helps protect against stroke caused by plaque buildup and blood clots in the arteries that lead to the brain. Eating at least 2 servings of fish per week can reduce the risk of stroke by as much as 50% (in select studies). **DEBUNKED.**

However, high doses of fish oil and omega-3 fatty acids may increase the risk of bleeding. People who eat more than 3 grams of omega-3 fatty acids per day (equivalent to 3 servings of fish per day) may have higher risk for hemorrhagic stroke, a potentially fatal type of stroke in which an artery in the brain leaks or ruptures.

Diabetes

People with diabetes often have high triglyceride and low HDL levels. Omega-3 fatty acids from fish oil can help lower triglycerides and apoproteins (markers of diabetes), and raise HDL, so eating foods or taking fish oil supplements **may** help people with diabetes. Another type of omega-3 fatty acid, ALA (from flaxseed, for example) may not have the same benefit as fish oil. Some people with diabetes can' t efficiently convert ALA to a form of omega-3 fatty acids that the body can use. Also, **some people with type 2 diabetes may have slight increases in**

fasting blood sugar when taking fish oil, so talk to your doctor to see if fish oil is right for you.

Rheumatoid arthritis

Most clinical studies examining omega-3 fatty acid supplements for arthritis have focused on rheumatoid arthritis (RA), an autoimmune disease that causes inflammation in the joints. A number of small studies have found that fish oil helps reduce symptoms of RA, including joint pain and morning stiffness. One study suggests that people with RA who take fish oil may be able to lower their dose of non-steroidal anti-inflammatory drugs (NSAIDs). **However, unlike prescription medications, fish oil does not appear to slow progression of RA, only to treat the symptoms. Joint damage still occurs.**

Laboratory studies suggest that diets rich in omega-3 fatty acids (and low in the inflammatory omega-6 fatty acids) may help people with osteoarthritis, although more study is needed. New Zealand green lipped mussel (Perna canaliculus), another potential source of omega-3 fatty acids, has been reported to reduce joint stiffness and pain, increase grip strength, and improve walking pace in a small group of people with osteoarthritis. For some people, symptoms got worse before they improved.

An analysis of 17 randomized, controlled clinical trials looked at the pain relieving effects of omega-3 fatty acid supplements in people with RA or joint pain caused by inflammatory bowel disease (IBS) and painful menstruation (dysmenorrhea). The results suggest that omega-3 fatty acids, along with conventional therapies such as NSAIDs, may help relieve joint pain associated with these conditions.

Systemic lupus erythematosus (SLE)

Several small studies suggest that EPA and fish oil may help reduce symptoms of lupus, an autoimmune condition characterized by fatigue and joint pain. **However, 2 small studies found fish oil had no effect on lupus nephritis (kidney disease caused by lupus, a frequent complication of the disease).**

Osteoporosis

Some studies suggest that omega-3 fatty acids **may** help increase levels of calcium in the body and improve bone strength, although not all results were positive. Some studies also suggest that people who don' t get enough of some essential fatty acids (particularly EPA and gamma-linolenic acid [GLA], an omega-6 fatty acid) are more likely to have bone loss than those with normal levels of these fatty acids. In a study of women over 65 with osteoporosis, those who took EPA and GLA supplements had less bone loss over 3 years than those who took placebo. Many of these women also experienced an increase in bone density.

Depression

Studies have found mixed results as to whether taking omega-3 fatty acids can help depression symptoms. Several studies have found that people who took omega-3 fatty acids in addition to prescription antidepressants had a greater improvement in symptoms than those who took antidepressants alone. Other studies show that omega-3 fatty acid intake helps protect against postpartum depression, among other benefits. However, **other studies have found no benefit**.

Studies are also mixed on whether omega-3 fatty acids alone have any effect on depression.

Bipolar disorder

In a clinical study of 30 people with bipolar disorder, those who took fish oil in addition to standard prescription treatments for bipolar disorder for 4 months experienced fewer mood swings and relapse than those who received placebo. **But another 4 month long clinical study treating people with bipolar depression and rapid cycling bipolar disorder did not find that EPA helped reduce symptoms.**

Schizophrenia

Preliminary clinical evidence suggests that people with schizophrenia may have an improvement in symptoms when given omega-3 fatty acids. **However, a recent well designed study concluded that EPA supplements are no better than placebo in improving symptoms of schizophrenia.**

Attention deficit/hyperactivity disorder (ADHD)

Children with attention deficit/hyperactivity disorder (ADHD) may have low levels of certain essential fatty acids (including EPA and DHA). In a clinical study of nearly 100 boys, those with lower levels of omega-3 fatty acids had more learning and behavioral problems (such as temper tantrums and sleep disturbances) than boys with normal omega-3 fatty acid levels.

However, studies examining whether omega-3 fatty acids help improve symptoms of ADHD have found mixed results. A few studies have found that omega-3 fatty acids helped improve behavioral symptoms, but most were not well designed. One study that looked at DHA in addition to stimulant therapy (standard therapy for ADHD) found no effect. More research is needed, but eating foods that are high in omega-3 fatty acids is a reasonable approach for someone with ADHD.

Cognitive decline

A number of studies show that reduced intake of omega-3 fatty acids is associated with increased risk of age related cognitive decline or dementia, including Alzheimer's disease. Scientists believe the omega-3 fatty acid DHA is protective against Alzheimer's disease and dementia. **But studies have not proved that fish oil will treat Alzheimer's disease.**

Skin disorders

In one clinical study, 13 people with sun sensitivity known as photo dermatitis showed less sensitivity to UV rays after taking fish oil supplements. However, topical sunscreens are much better at protecting the skin from damaging effects of the sun than omega-3 fatty acids. In another study of 40 people with psoriasis, those who took EPA with their prescription medications did better than those treated with the medications alone. **However, a larger study of people with psoriasis found no benefit from fish oil.**

Inflammatory bowel disease (IBD)

Results are mixed as to whether omega-3 fatty acids can help reduce symptoms of Crohn' s disease and ulcerative colitis, the 2 types of IBD. Some studies suggest that omega-3 fatty acids may help when added to medication, such as sulfasalazine (a standard medication for IBD). **Others find no effect.** More studies are needed. **Fish oil supplements can cause side effects that are similar to symptoms of IBD (such as flatulence, belching, bloating, and diarrhea).**

Asthma

Studies examining omega-3 fatty acids for **asthma** are mixed. In one small, well designed clinical study of 29 children with asthma, those who took fish oil supplements rich in EPA and DHA for 10 months reduced their symptoms compared to children who took placebo. **However, most studies have shown no effect.**

Macular Degeneration

A questionnaire given to more than 3,000 people over the age of 49 found that those who ate more fish were less likely to have macular degeneration (a serious age related eye condition that can progress to blindness) than those who ate less fish. Similarly, a clinical study comparing 350 people with macular degeneration to 500 without the eye disease found that those with a healthy dietary balance of omega-3 and omega-6 fatty acids and more fish in their diets were less likely to have macular degeneration. **AREDS2 debunked this notion.**

Menstrual pain

In one study of 42 women, they had less menstrual pain when they took fish oil supplements than when they took placebo.

Colon cancer

Eating foods rich in omega-3 fatty acids seems to reduce the risk of colorectal cancer. For example, Eskimos, who tend to have a high fat diet, but eat significant amounts of fish rich in omega-3 fatty acids, have a low rate of colorectal cancer. Animal studies and laboratory studies have found that omega-3 fatty acids prevent worsening of colon cancer. Preliminary studies **suggest** that taking fish oil daily may help slow the progression of colon cancer in people with early stages of the disease.

Breast cancer

Although not all experts agree, women who eat foods rich in omega-3 fatty acids over many years **may be** less likely to develop breast cancer. More research is needed to understand the effect that omega-3 fatty acids may have on the prevention of breast cancer.

Prostate cancer

Population based studies of groups of men suggest that **a low fat diet including omega-3 fatty acids from fish or fish oil help prevent the development of prostate cancer**.Actually, recent studies **show increased risk of aggressive prostatic cancer linked to fish oil consumption**.

Dietary Sources:

Fish, plant, and nut oils are the primary dietary source of omega-3 fatty acids. Eicosapentaenoic acid (EPA) and docosahexaenoic acid (DHA) are found in cold water fish such as salmon, mackerel, halibut, sardines, tuna, and herring. ALA is found in flaxseeds, flaxseed oil, canola (rapeseed) oil, soybeans, soybean oil, pumpkin seeds, pumpkin seed oil, purslane, perilla seed oil, walnuts, and walnut oil. **The health effects of omega-3 fatty acids come mostly from EPA and DHA.** ALA from flax and other vegetarian sources needs to be converted in the body to EPA and DHA. Many people do not make these conversions very effectively, however. This remains an ongoing debate in the nutrition community; fish and sea vegetable sources of EPA and DHA versus vegetarian sources of ALA. Other sources of omega-3 fatty acids include sea life such as krill and algae.

Available Forms:

Both EPA and DHA can be taken in the form of fish oil capsules. Flaxseed, flaxseed oil, fish, and krill oils should be kept refrigerated. Whole flaxseeds must be ground within 24 hours of use, so the ingredients stay active. Flaxseeds are also available in ground form in a special mylar package so the components in the flaxseeds stay active.

Be sure to buy omega-3 fatty acid supplements made by established companies who certify that their products are free of heavy metals such as mercury, lead, and cadmium.

How to Take It:

Dosing for fish oil supplements should be based on the amount of EPA and DHA, not on the total amount of fish oil. Supplements vary in the amounts and ratios of EPA and DHA. A common amount of omega-3 fatty acids in fish oil capsules is 0.18 grams (180 mg) of EPA and 0.12 grams (120 mg) of DHA. Different types of fish contain variable amounts of omega-3 fatty acids, and different types of nuts or oil contain variable amounts of ALA. Fish oils contain approximately 9 calories per gram of oil.

Children (18 years and younger)

There is no established dose for children. Omega-3 fatty acids are used in some infant formulas. Fish oil capsules should not be used in children except under the direction of a health care provider. **Children should avoid eating fish that may be high in mercury, such as shark, swordfish, king mackerel, and tilefish**.

Adults

Do not take more than 3 grams daily of omega-3 fatty acids from capsules without the supervision of a health care provider, due to an increased risk of bleeding.

- For healthy adults with no history of heart disease: The American Heart Association (AHA) recommends eating fish at least 2 times per week.
- For adults with coronary heart disease: The AHA recommends an omega-3 fatty acid supplement (as fish oils), 1 gram daily of EPA and DHA. It may take 2 - 3 weeks for benefits of fish oil supplements to be seen. Supplements should be taken under the direction of a physician.
- For adults with high cholesterol levels: The AHA recommends an omega-3 fatty acid supplement (as fish oils), 2 - 4 grams daily of EPA and DHA. It may take 2 - 3 weeks for benefits of fish oil supplements to be seen. Supplements should be taken under the direction of a physician.
- For adults with high blood pressure, scientists generally recommend 3 - 4 grams per day, but you should only take under the supervision of a health care provider.

Precautions:

Because of the potential for side effects and interactions with medications, you should only take dietary supplements only under the supervision of a knowledgeable health care provider.

Omega-3 fatty acids should be used cautiously by people who bruise easily, have a bleeding disorder, or take blood thinning medications including warfarin (Coumadin), clopidogrel (Plavix), or aspirin. High doses of omega-3 fatty acids may increase the risk of bleeding, even in people without a history of bleeding disorders -- and even in those who are not taking other medications.

Fish oil can cause gas, bloating, belching, and diarrhea. Time release preparations may reduce these side effects, however.

People with either diabetes or schizophrenia may lack the ability to convert alpha-linolenic acid (ALA) to eicosapentaenoic acid (EPA) and docosahexaenoic acid (DHA), the forms more readily used in the body. People with these conditions should be sure to get enough EPA and DHA from their diets.Also, people with type 2 diabetes may experience increases in fasting blood sugar levels while taking fish oil supplements. If you have type 2 diabetes, use fish oil supplements only under the supervision of a health care provider.

Although studies suggest that eating fish (which includes the omega-3 fatty acids EPA and DHA) may reduce the risk of macular degeneration, a recent study including 2 large groups of men and women found that diets rich in ALA may increase the risk of this disease. Until more information becomes available, people with macular degeneration should get omega-3 fatty acids from sources of EPA and DHA, rather than ALA.

Fish and fish oil may protect against prostate cancer, but some suggest that ALA may be associated with increased risk of prostate cancer in men. More research in this area is needed.

Some fish may contain potentially harmful contaminants, such as heavy metals (including mercury), dioxins, and polychlorinated biphenyls (PCBs). For sport caught fish, the U.S. Environmental Protection Agency (EPA) recommends that pregnant or nursing women eat no more than a single 6 ounce meal per week, and young children less than 2 ounces per week. For farm raised, imported, or marine fish, the U.S. Food and Drug Administration recommends that pregnant or nursing women and young children avoid eating types with higher levels of mercury (such as mackerel, shark, swordfish, or tilefish), and eat up to 12 ounces per week of other fish types.

Buy fish oil from a reputable source that tests to make sure there is no mercury or pesticide residues in its products.

Possible Interactions:

If you are currently being treated with any of the following medications, you should not use omega-3 fatty acid supplements, including eicosapentaenoic acid (EPA), docosahexaenoic acid (DHA), and alpha-linolenic acid (ALA), without first talking to your health care provider.

Blood thinning medications -- Omega-3 fatty acids may increase the effects of blood thinning medications, including aspirin, warfarin (Coumadin), and clopedigrel (Plavix). Taking aspirin and omega-3 fatty acids may be helpful in some circumstances (such as in heart disease), but they should only be taken together under the supervision of a health care provider.

Diabetes medications -- Taking omega-3 fatty acid supplements may increase fasting blood sugar levels. Use with caution if taking medications to lower blood sugar, such as glipizide (Glucotrol and Glucotrol XL), glyburide (Micronase or Diabeta), glucophage (Metformin), or insulin. Your doctor may need to increase your medication dose. These drugs include:

- Glipizide (Glucotrol and Glucotrol XL)
- Glyburide (Micronase or Diabeta)
- Metformin (Glucophage)
- Insulin

Cyclosporine -- Cyclosporine is a medication given to people with organ transplants. Taking omega-3 fatty acids during cyclosporine (Sandimmune) therapy may reduce toxic side effects, such as high blood pressure and kidney damage, associated with this medication.

Etretinate and topical steroids -- Adding omega-3 fatty acids (specifically EPA) to the drug therapy etretinate (Tegison) and topical corticosteroids may improve symptoms of psoriasis.

Cholesterol-lowering medications -- Following dietary guidelines, including increasing the amount of omega-3 fatty acids in your diet and reducing the omega-6 to omega-3 ratio, may help a group of cholesterol lowering medications known as statins to work more effectively. These medications include:

- Atorvastatin (Liptor)
- Lovastatin (Mevacor)
- Simvastatin (Zocor)

Nonsteroidal anti-inflammatory drugs (NSAIDs) -- In an animal study, treatment with omega-3 fatty acids reduced the risk of ulcers from nonsteroidal anti-inflammatory drugs (NSAIDs). NSAIDs include ibuprofen (Motrin or Advil) and naproxen (Aleve or Naprosyn). More research is needed to see whether omega-3 fatty acids would have the same effects in people.

Reviewed last on: 5/10/2011. Accessed 5-5-14.

Supporting Research (references)

(Aben, Danckaerts, 2010) (Angerer, von Schacky, 2000) (Aronson et al, 2001) (Bahadori, et al, 2010) (Balk et al, 2006) (Bays, 2007) (Belluzzi et al, 2000) (Berbert et al, 2005) (Berson et al, 2004) (Boelsma et al, 2001) (Boskou, 2000) (Bradbury et al, 2004) (Buckley et al, 2004) (Burgess et al, 2000) (Burr et al, 2006) (Calo et al, 2005) (Caron, White, et al, 2001) (Chan, Cho, 2009) (Chattipakorn et al, 2009) (Cho et al, 2001) (Christensen et al, 2001) (Cole, 2009) (Compl., 2010) (Daniel et al, 2009) (Dewailly et al, 2001) (Dichi et al, 2000) (Dopheide, Pliszka, 2009) (AHA 41st conf, 2001) (Fenton et al, 2001) (Firestein, 2008) (Fotuhi et al, 2009) (Frangou et al, 2006) (Freeman et al, 2000) (Freund-Levi, Meydani et al, 2006) (Freund-Leve, Hjorth et al, 2009) (Galli, Rise, 2009) (Geelen et al, 2005) (Geerling et al, 2000) (Goldberg, Katz et al, 2007) (Hagen et al, 2009) (Hall et al, 2007) (Hartweg et al, 2009) (Hooper et al, 2004) (Iso et al, 2001) (Itomura et al, 2005) (Jeschke et al, 2001) (Joy et al, 2006) (Kelley et al, 2009) (Krauss et al, 2000) (Kremer, 2000) (Kris-Etherton et al, 2001) (Lee et al, 2009) (Mattar, Obeid, 2009) (Mitchell et al, 1987) (Montori et al, 2000) (Mori, 2010) (Moxaffarian et al, 2005) (Nagakura et al, 2000) (Newcomer et al, 2001) (Okamoto et al, 2000) (Olsen, Secher, 2002) (Rakel, 2007) (Riediger et al, 2009) (Richardson, Puri, 2000) (Rocha et al, 2010) (Romano et al, 2006) (Sarris et al, 2009) (Seddon et al, 2001) (Silvers et al, 2005) (Smith et al, 2000) (Stark et al, 2000) (Sundstrom et al, 2006) (Terry et al, 2001) (Weinstock-Guttman, 2005) (Yashodhara, 2009) (Yuen et al, 2005)

Nutritional Recommendations for Cardiovascular Disease Prevention

This recent article offers a well-rounded picture and background of the current status of omega-3 fish oil studies. This excerpted and modified review article best describes the conflicted and confusing data on the effects of fish oils and omega-3 fatty acids. **The lack of consistently reproducible data considerably weakens the evidence which attributes some cardiovascular benefits to these agents**.

(Sigal Eilat-Adar, et al, 2013)

Omega-3 and Fish Oil

Polyunsaturated fatty acids are characterized according to the position of the first double bond. **In omega-3 (also called ω-3 or *n*-3) fatty acids the first double bond is situated after the third carbon atom from the methyl end of the carbon chain.**

Humans cannot synthesize short-chain fatty acids and therefore need to consume them in their diet.

They include the plant-derived **alpha-linolenic acid (ALA**, 18:3*n*-3), and the fish-oil-derived **eicosapentaenoic acid (EPA**, 20:5*n*-3) and **docosahexaenoic acid (DHA**, 22:6*n*-3).

Dietary Sources

ALA is found in seeds, vegetable oils (especially canola and flaxseed), green leafy vegetables, walnuts, and beans. Although some ALA can be transformed in the human body to EPA and DHA, such conversion appears to be inefficient, and **the majority of these fatty acids are consumed from cold water oily fish, such as salmon, herring, mackerel, anchovies, tuna, and sardines.**

Omega-3 Supplements

Various sources of omega-3 fatty acids are used as supplements for commercial use, including fish oil, flaxseed oil, and walnut oil. Although the FDA has concluded that omega-3 dietary supplements from fish are "generally recognized as safe", **some have questioned the safety of fish oil supplements because some species of fish can contain high levels of mercury, pesticides, or polychlorinated biphenyls (PCBs).**

Most fish oil supplements undergo purification processes and do not appear to contain these substances in appreciable quantities. **Many clinical trials have used an ethyl-ester form of omega-3 fatty acids, which may affect the product's bioavailability and metabolism.** (Neubronner et al, 2011)

Commonly used doses of omega-3 supplements (up to 1 g daily) do not appear to have significant side effects. However, **larger doses may cause minor gastrointestinal upsets, worsening of glycemia control, and a rise in LDL-C levels.** (Kris-Etherton *et al.*, 2002)

Observational Studies

Most observational studies show an inverse correlation between fish consumption and cardiovascular CVD. **A review of 11 cohort studies involving 116,764 individuals suggested that fish consumption at 40–60 g daily is associated with markedly reduced CHD mortality in high-risk**, but not in low-risk populations. (Gronbaek, 1999)

Intervention Studies (EPA, DHA)

A meta-analysis of intervention trials including 7951 individuals treated with omega-3 compared to 7855 controls found **a significant decrease in mortality from MI but not in non-lethal MI.** (Bucher et al, 2002)

In another meta-analysis of 97 studies using different types of lipid management strategies, **the most effective combination was that of statins with omega-3, which resulted in a relative-risk reduction of 23% in total mortality** and 32% in cardiac mortality. (Studer et al, 2005)

However, more recent studies looking at the benefit of omega-3 treatment in high-risk patients (CHD and/or diabetes mellitus) receiving optimal medical therapy, including statins, have shown **mixed results with some showing significant benefit.** (Rauch et al, 2010)

Yet, **others show little additional benefit.** (Bosch et al, 2012) (Kromhout et al, 2010) (Galan et al, 2010)

Recent meta-analyses of randomized controlled trials found little evidence of a protective effect of omega-3 supplementation on the incidence of CVD (Kwak et al, 2012), **cerebrovascular disease** (Chowdhury et al, 2012), **or atrial fibrillation** (Liu et al, 2011).

In a meta-analysis of 20 studies of 68,680 patients (13 on secondary prevention), omega-3 PUFA supplementation was not associated with a lower risk of all-cause mortality, cardiac death, sudden death, myocardial infarction, or stroke based on relative and absolute measures of association. (Rizos et al, 2012)

Possible Mechanisms (EPA, DHA)

The long-chain omega-3 fatty acids EPA and DHA compete with arachidonic acid (a long chain omega-6 fatty acid) in the synthesis of prostaglandins and leukotrienes involved in inflammation and thrombogenesis.

Omega-3 fatty acids have been shown to increase arrhythmic thresholds, reduce blood pressure, improve endothelial function, reduce inflammation and platelet aggregation, enhance plaque stabilization, and favorably affect autonomic tone. (Kromhout et al, 2012)

At high doses (2–6 g daily) they can significantly reduce the serum triglyceride levels, but the long-term clinical outcome of such treatment in hypertriglyceridemic individuals has not been evaluated. (Lau, 2006)

Phytosterols

Sterols constitute an important constituent of plant cellular membranes, in a manner similar to the role of cholesterol in human cells. (Moreau et al, 2002)

RMH Note: Both cholesterol and the omega-3 fatty acids function as antioxidants. Please read my companion books regarding the potential dangers of excessive antioxidant ingestion. Please see the list of my companion books at the end of this text.

They are found at low concentrations in most plant-derived nutrients but at somewhat higher concentrations in some grains. **Despite their structural similarities to cholesterol, plant sterols are not synthesized in the human body and are only minimally absorbed**

from the human intestinal tract. The average western diet contains approximately 200–500 mg of cholesterol, approximately 200–400 mg of plant sterols, and 20–50 mg of plant stanols. Amongst the best known plant sterols are sitosterol, campesterol, and stigmasterol. Those that are incorporated in food are usually esterified. Hydrogenation converts sterols into stanols (e.g., sitostanol and campestanol), which can also be esterified.

Intervention Studies (sterol esters)

Evaluation of intervention studies with sterol esters and stanol esters suggest a reduction in LDL-C level of approximately 10%, without specific differences between the type of sterol or stanol or the method by which it was administered (immersed in a food product or as a separate supplement).

Similar results were obtained in the different populations studied (children, healthy adults, or patients with diabetes and/or CHD). **The optimal dose appears to be 1.5–2.5 g/day, with no additional benefit at higher doses.**

Addition to statins resulted in a further 10% reduction in LDL-C beyond that achieved with the statins alone. To date, no long-term intervention studies of sterol/stanol treatment evaluating clinical endpoints have been published.

Possible Mechanisms (sterol esters)

Due to their biochemical similarity, plant sterols and stanols can displace cholesterol from mixed micelles in the intestine, thus reducing the absorption of dietary cholesterol. Although they have significant atherogenic potential, **the intestinal absorption of sterols and stanols is poor, resulting in very low serum concentrations.**

An exception to this rule is patients with sitosterolemia, a rare genetic disorder in which the absorption of sterols is enhanced, resulting in significant damage to various organs. RMH Note: again, this indicates that excessive levels of antioxidants (sterols) are harmful.

Safety

Sterol supplementation at the recommended doses is generally considered safe. (Hendriks et al, 2003)

However, several potential **risks** need to be considered. **In addition to inhibiting cholesterol absorption, some (though not all) studies suggest that sterols and stanols can reduce the blood levels of antioxidants such as lycopene and beta-carotene.**

This can be counteracted, at least partly, by the ingestion of a diet reach in vegetables and fruits. Despite the low serum concentration of sterols and stanols, **some concern has been raised that even the slight increase associated with dietary supplementation of sterols might increase the risk for atherosclerosis.** (Weingartner et al, 2009)

RMH Note:This is in direct contradistinction to the many claims of omega-3 fatty acids reducing the risk of atherosclerosis.

Eating fish is good, pills are bad

5-8-13 Eating fish is good for your heart but taking fish oil capsules does not help people at high risk of heart problems who are already taking medicines to prevent them, a large study in Italy found. **Fish oil supplements in high risk patients does not prevent heart attacks.**

The work makes clearer who does and does not benefit from taking supplements of omega-3 fatty acids, the good oils found in fish such as salmon, tuna and sardines.

Previous studies have suggested that fish oil capsules could lower heart risks in people with heart failure or who have already suffered a heart attack. **The American Heart Association recommends them only for people who have high levels of fats called triglycerides in their blood,** says the group's president, Dr. Donna Arnett of the University of Alabama at Birmingham.

Fish oil capsules failed to prevent flare-ups of atrial fibrillation, a common heart rhythm problem, in a large study in 2010.

The new study was led by the Mario Negri Institute for Pharmacological Research in Milan. It tested 1 **gram a day of fish oil versus dummy capsules in 12,513 people throughout Italy. They had not suffered a heart attack but were at high risk of having one because of diabetes, high blood pressure, high cholesterol, smoking, obesity or other conditions.** Most already were taking cholesterol-lowering statins, aspirin and other medicines to lower their chances of heart problems.

Researchers at first planned to compare the rate of death, heart attacks and strokes in the two groups, but these were less frequent than anticipated. So they started measuring how long it was before people in either group suffered one of these fates or was hospitalized for heart-related reasons. After five years, the rate was the same — about 12 percent of each group had one of these problems.

"They're very high-risk people and so the level of other treatments was very high," Arnett said. "When you're being aggressively treated for all of your other risk factors, **adding fish oil yielded no additional benefits."**

Results are published in **5-9-13 New England Journal of Medicine**. Makers of fish oil supplements helped pay for the study.

Eating fish is thought to help protect against heart disease, and the Heart Association recommends it at least twice a week.

"People who choose to eat more fish are more likely to eat heart healthier diets and engage in more physical activity," and studies testing the benefit of supplements may not be able to completely adjust for differences like these, said **Alice Lichtenstein**, director of the cardiovascular nutrition lab at Tufts University in Boston.

The results do show that **people can't rely on a pill to make up for a bad diet**, she said.

"It is sort of like breaking a fish oil capsule over a hot fudge sundae and expecting the effect of the calories and saturated fat to go away," she said.

Eating fish is good for your heart but taking fish oil capsules does not help people at high risk of heart problems who are already taking medicines to prevent them, a large study in

Italy found. The work, published on May 9, 2013 in the New England Journal of Medicine, makes clearer who does and does not benefit from taking supplements of omega-3 fatty acids.

Conclusions

A healthy diet should include diversity of foods and to maintain a healthy weight. It is preferable to eat fresh or frozen food without additional sugar, salt or high-calorie gravies, using cooking methods that retain the original nutrients undestroyed. It should contain a variety of vegetables and fruits, legumes, whole grains, whole wheat bread and high-fiber low-salt food items. Vegetable oils, (especially olive and canola oils, excluding palm and coconut oils), should be preferred over animal fat. **RMH Note: Studies in 2014 indicate that animal fats may not be as problematic as they were once thought to be. In fact, they indicate that they may not increase the risk of vessel blockage to any degree.**

Additional elements that may confer health benefits include avocado, nuts, almonds and tahini, low-fat dairy products, green tea and 2 to 3 servings of fatty fish per week.

It is recommended to minimize consumption of high-fat meat (especially processed meats that are high in fat and sodium), hard margarines and pastries with hydrogenated fat, and foods that are high in sodium and sugar. It is recommended to drink a lot of water, and reduce consumption of sweetened beverages as well as fresh juices. The Mediterranean diet has been shown to reduce cardiovascular morbidity and mortality in both primary and secondary prevention. Other dietary patterns that have been shown to confer advantage in specific medical situations include low-fat diet for individuals at high cardiovascular risk, DASH diet for people with hypertension, and low-carbohydrate diets for overweight people and for the metabolic syndrome.

Please remember that studies of this nature are all over the map and consistent results are not available in the literature.

National Institutes of Health: Omega-3 supplements - an introduction

Key facts

- There has been a substantial amount of research on supplements of omega-3s, particularly those found in seafood and fish oil, and heart disease. The findings of individual studies have been inconsistent. In 2012, two combined analyses of the results of these studies did not find convincing evidence these omega-3s protect against heart disease.
- There is some evidence that omega-3s found in seafood and fish oil may be modestly helpful in relieving symptoms in rheumatoid arthritis. For most other conditions for which omega-3s have been studied, definitive conclusions cannot yet be reached, or studies have not shown omega-3s to be beneficial.
- Omega-3 supplements may interact with drugs that affect blood clotting.
- It is uncertain whether people with fish or shellfish allergies can safely consume fish oil supplements.
- Fish liver oils (which are not the same as fish oils) contain vitamins A and D as well as omega-3 fatty acids; these vitamins can be toxic in high doses.
- Tell all your health care providers about any complementary health approaches you use. Give them a full picture of what you do to manage your health. This will help ensure coordinated and safe care.

Commonly used dietary supplements that contain omega-3s include fish oil (which provides EPA and DHA) and flaxseed oil (which provides ALA). **Algae oils are a vegetarian source of DHA.**

Omega-3 fatty acids are important for a number of bodily functions, including muscle activity, blood clotting, digestion, fertility, and cell division and growth. DHA is important for brain development and function. ALA is an "essential" fatty acid, meaning that people must obtain it from food or supplements because the human body cannot manufacture it.

Safety

- Omega-3 fatty acid supplements usually do not have negative side effects. When side effects do occur, they typically consist of minor gastrointestinal symptoms, such as belching, indigestion, or diarrhea.
- Omega-3 supplements may extend bleeding time (the time it takes for a cut to stop bleeding). People who take drugs that affect bleeding time, such as anticoagulants ("blood thinners") or nonsteroidal anti-inflammatory drugs (NSAIDs), should discuss the use of omega-3 fatty acid supplements with a health care provider.
- Fish liver oils, such as cod liver oil, are not the same as fish oil. Fish liver oils contain vitamins A and D as well as omega-3 fatty acids. Both of these vitamins can be toxic in large doses. The amounts of vitamins in fish liver oil supplements vary from one product to another.
- There is conflicting evidence about whether omega-3 fatty acids found in seafood and fish oil might increase the risk of prostate cancer. Additional research on the association of omega-3 consumption and prostate cancer risk is under way.

Use of Omega-3 supplements in the United States

According to the 2007 National Health Interview Survey, which included a comprehensive survey on the use of complementary health approaches by Americans, fish oil/omega-3/DHA supplements are the nonvitamin/nonmineral natural product most commonly taken by adults, and the second most commonly taken by children. Among survey participants who had used selected natural products in the last 30 days, about 37 percent of adults (10.9 million) and 31 percent of children (441,000) had taken an omega-3 supplement for health reasons.

What the science says

Moderate evidence has emerged about the health benefits of eating seafood. **The health benefits of omega-3 dietary supplements are unclear.**

Cardiovascular disease

Evidence suggests that seafood rich in omega-3 fatty acids should be included in a heart-healthy diet. However, **omega-3s in supplement form have not been shown to protect against heart disease.**

- Epidemiological studies done more than 30 years ago noted relatively low death rates due to cardiovascular disease in Eskimo populations with high seafood consumption. Since then, much research has been done on seafood and heart disease. The results provide moderate evidence that people who eat seafood at least once a week are less likely to die of heart disease than those who rarely or never eat seafood.
- The Federal Government's Dietary Guidelines for Americans, 2010 includes a new recommendation that adults eat 8 or more ounces of a variety of seafood (fish or shellfish) per week because it provides a range of nutrients, including omega-3 fatty acids. (Smaller amounts are recommended for young children.)
- Many studies have evaluated the effects of supplements rich in EPA and DHA, such as fish oil, on heart disease risk. In these studies, researchers compared the number of cardiovascular events (such as heart attacks or strokes) or the number of deaths in people who were given the supplements with those in people who were given inactive substances (placebos) or standard care. Most of these studies involved people who already had evidence of heart disease. A smaller number of studies included people with no history of heart disease. The results of individual studies were inconsistent; some indicated that the supplements were protective, but others did not. In 2012, two groups of scientists conducted meta-analyses of these studies; one group analyzed only studies in people with a history of heart disease, and the other group analyzed studies in people both with and without a

history of heart disease. Neither meta-analysis found convincing evidence of a protective effect.

- There are several reasons why supplements that contain EPA and DHA may not help to prevent heart disease even though a diet rich in seafood may. Eating seafood a few times a week might provide enough of these omega-3s to protect the heart; more may not be better. Some of the benefits of seafood may result from people eating it in place of less healthful foods. There is also evidence that people who eat seafood have generally healthier lifestyles, and these other lifestyle characteristics may be responsible for the lower incidence of cardiovascular disease.

Rheumatoid arthritis

A 2012 systematic review concluded that the types of omega-3s found in seafood and fish oil **may be modestly helpful in relieving symptoms of rheumatoid arthritis.** In the studies included in the review, many of the participants reported that when they were taking fish oil they had briefer morning stiffness, less joint swelling and pain, and less need for anti-inflammatory drugs to control their symptoms.

Infant development

The nutritional value of seafood is particularly important during early development. The Dietary Guidelines recommend that women who are pregnant or breastfeeding consume at least 8 ounces but no more than 12 ounces of seafood each week and not eat certain types of seafood that are high in mercury—a toxin that can harm the nervous system of a fetus or young child.

Diseases of the brain and the eye

DHA plays important roles in the functioning of the brain and the eye. Research is being conducted on DHA and other omega-3 fatty acids and diseases of the brain and eye, but there is not enough evidence to draw conclusions about the effectiveness of omega-3s for these conditions.

Research is looking at:

- Diseases of the brain or nervous system, such as cognitive decline and multiple sclerosis.
- Mental and behavioral health problems, such as depression, attention-deficit hyperactivity disorder, autism, bipolar disorder, borderline personality disorder, and schizophrenia.
- Diseases of the eye, such as age-related macular degeneration (AMD; an eye disease that can cause vision loss in older people) and dry eye syndrome. Studies have shown that people who eat diets rich in seafood are less likely to develop the advanced stage of AMD. However, a large National Institutes of Health (NIH)–sponsored study, called Age-Related Eye Disease Study 2 **(AREDS2), indicated that supplements containing EPA and DHA did not slow the progression of AMD** in people who were at high risk of developing the advanced stage of this disease.

Other conditions

Omega-3 supplements (primarily fish oil supplements) also have been studied for preventing or treating a variety of other conditions such as allergies, asthma, cachexia (severe weight loss) associated with advanced cancer, Crohn's disease, cystic fibrosis, diabetes, kidney disease, lupus, menstrual cramps, obesity, osteoporosis, and ulcerative colitis, as well as organ transplantation outcomes (e.g., decreasing the likelihood of rejection). No conclusions can be drawn about whether omega-3s are helpful for these conditions based on currently available evidence.

Fish oil: http://nccam.nih.gov/health/omega3/introduction.htm. NCCAM Pub No.:

D482 Date Created: July 2009 Last Updated: June 2013.

References to the above NIH article

(AREDS2, 2013) (Anandan et al, 2009) (Appleton et al, 2010) (Bent et al, 2009) (Brasky et al, 2011) (Buckley, Howe, 2009) (Calder, Yaqoob, 2009) (Chong et al, 2008) (Covington, 2004) (De Ley et al, 2007) (Farinotte et al, 2007) (Fassett et a, 2010) (Filion et al, 2010) (Hooper *et al.*, 2004) (Hu, Manson, 2012) (Huang, 2010) (Irving et al, 2012) (Kris-Etherton *et al.*, 2002) (Kwak et al, 2012) (Lee et al, 2009) (Miles, Calder, 2012) (Oh, 2005) (Oliver et al, 2007) (Raz, Gabis, 2009) (Riediger et al, 2009) (Rizos et al, 2012) (Salari et al, 2008) (Saravanan et al, 2010) (Szymanski et al, Am J Clin Nut. 2010) (Turner et al, 2009) (Weitz et al, 2010)

Potential risk in consuming excess omega-3 fatty acids

October 30, 2013

A new review suggests that omega-3 fatty acids taken in excess could have unintended health consequences in certain situations, and that dietary standards based on the best available evidence need to be established.

"What looked like a slam dunk a few years ago may not be as clear cut as we thought," said Norman Hord, associate professor in OSU's College of Public Health and Human Sciences and a coauthor on the paper.

"We are seeing the potential for negative effects at really high levels of omega-3 fatty acid consumption. Because we lack valid biomarkers for exposure and knowledge of who might be at risk if consuming excessive amounts, it isn't possible to determine an upper limit at this time."

Previous research led by Michigan State University's Jenifer Fenton and her collaborators found that **feeding mice large amounts of dietary omega-3 fatty acids led to <u>increased risk of colitis and immune alteration</u>. Those results were published in *Cancer Research* in 2010.**

As a follow-up, published online in the **journal *Prostaglandins, Leukotrienes & Essential Fatty Acids,*** Fenton and her co-authors, including Hord, reviewed the literature and discuss the potential adverse health outcomes that could result from excess consumption of omega-3 fatty acids.

Studies have shown that omega-3s, also known as long chain polyunsaturated fatty acids (LCPUFAs), were allegedly associated with lower risk of sudden cardiac death and other cardiovascular disease outcomes.

"We were inspired to review the literature based on our findings **after recent publications showed increased risk of advanced prostate cancer and atrial fibrillation in those with high blood levels of LCPUFAs,**" Fenton said.

Omega-3 fatty acids have anti-inflammatory properties, which is one of the reasons they can be beneficial to heart health and inflammatory issues. However, the researchers said **excess amounts of omega-3 fatty acids can alter immune function sometimes in ways that may lead to a dysfunctional immune response to a viral or bacterial infection.**

"**The dysfunctional immune response to excessive omega-3 fatty acid consumption can affect the body's ability to fight microbial pathogens, like bacteria**," Hord said.

Generally, the researchers point out that the amounts of fish oil used in most studies are typically above what one could consume from foods or usual dosage of a dietary supplement. However, **an increasing amount of products, such as eggs, bread, butters, oils and orange juice, are being "fortified" with omega-3s**. Hord said **this fortified food, coupled with fish oil supplement use, increases the potential for consuming these high levels**.

"Overall, we support the dietary recommendations from the American Heart Association to eat fish, particularly fatty fish like salmon, mackerel, lake trout or sardines, at least two times a week, and for those at risk of coronary artery disease to talk to their doctor about supplements," he said.

"Our main concern here is the hyper-supplemented individual, who may be taking high-dose omega-3 supplements and eating four to five omega-3-enriched foods per day," Hord added. "This could potentially get someone to an excessive amount. As our paper indicates, there may be subgroups of those who may be at risk from consuming excess amounts of these fatty acids."

Hord said there are no evidence-based standards for omega-3 intake and no way to tell who might be at health risk if they consume too high a level of these fatty acids.

"We're not against using fish oil supplements appropriately, but **there is a potential for risk,**" Hord said. "**As is all true with any nutrient, taking too much can have negative effects.** We need to establish clear biomarkers through clinical trials. This is necessary in order for us to know who is eating adequate amounts of these nutrients and who may be deficient or eating too much.

"Until we establish valid biomarkers of omega-3 exposure, making good evidence-based dietary recommendations across potential dietary exposure ranges will not be possible." (Medical News Today, 2013)

New warning about omega-3 supplements

"Still Taking Fish Oil? Check Out This NEW Warning..."

Omega-3s are crucial for supporting heart health, your immune function, and a positive mood, but you may want to think twice about the source you're getting them from... especially when you read about this new warning.*

Now in a perfect world, you would be able to get all the omega-3s you need by eating fish. Unfortunately, **studies show that eating fish can potentially expose you to a high degree of contamination with industrial pollutants and toxins like mercury, PCBs, heavy metals and radioactive poisons.**

In fact, the FDA and EPA have put out health advisories warning against certain fish and shellfish consumption for young children, women who are pregnant or may become pregnant, and nursing mothers.

New lab testing from **Consumer Lab** reveals some disturbing lapses in quality among popular fish oil and krill oil supplements.

These **problems ranged from inaccurate labels, spoilage (including one in a children's product), and enteric-coated products that released too early. And sky-high PCBs in one designed for pets.**

Why EFA balance is critical to your health

Essential fatty acids (EFAs) include both omega-3 fats (high in the vital compounds EPA and DHA) and omega-6 fats. **EFAs cannot be manufactured in your body** but are beneficial to normal health and metabolism.* Therefore, **EFAs must be obtained through your diet.**

Although some omega-6 fats are good for your health, **the balance of omega-6s to omega-3s is crucial.** Unfortunately, **most people consume an overabundance of omega-6 fats.**

Your ancestors embraced a diet with a healthy balance of approximately equal omega-6 and omega-3 fats. But the **current Western diet is far too high in omega-6 fats. The average omega-6 to omega-3 ratio is now closer to 20:1**, and in some cases even 50:1. According to some, this can keep you from optimal health.

Myth: Supplements always make you healthier

An increasing number of studies are finding that vitamin supplementation may not only be ineffectual but may even be dangerous. For example, **people downing vitamins C and E may be predisposing themselves to cancer, according to a study published earlier this year in the journal Stem Cells**, as high doses of these antioxidants can cause genetic abnormalities. Similarly, **a study published this year in the journal Cancer Research linked fish oil supplements with cancer in mice.** "The FDA does not require supplements to be regulated in the same way that drugs are, which can be a real problem," Vreeman said. As a result, the safety of many supplements has not been rigorously studied. Furthermore, the **bottles can sport unsubstantiated claims and even make errors in dosage recommendations**, she said. There is no need to worry about overdosing, however, if the good-for-you compound is coming from real food, rather than a pill. "**A vitamin pill is not the answer,**" Vreeman said. "Eating more healthily in general is the answer." http://www.livescience.com/36100-10-medical-myths.html

The SELECT Trial

As reported, **the study found that men who had high concentrations of omega-3s in their blood had a risk of developing prostate cancer that was 43 percent higher than men who had the lowest blood levels of these fatty acids. Even more alarming was the finding that men with the highest blood levels of omega-3s had a 71 percent higher risk of aggressive, possibly fatal prostate cancer than those with the lowest levels. The study was published online on July 10, 2013, in the *Journal of the National Cancer Institute*.**

The team looked at blood levels of omega-3s among men who were enrolled in the **Selenium and Vitamin E Cancer Prevention Trial (SELECT), a large National Cancer Institute trial** aimed at determining whether either of those supplements alone or in combination lowered the risk of prostate cancer. More than **35,000 men** enrolled in SELECT starting in 2001. The authors of this recent study based their conclusions on the analysis of a single blood sample from each of 834 men in the study diagnosed with prostate cancer through 2007 and from a corresponding group of 1,393 healthy men who participated in the SELECT study and were matched by age and race to the men who developed the disease. The blood samples were taken when the men entered SELECT. Later, the researchers added in 75 men who were diagnosed with high-grade prostate cancer in the 8th and 9th year of SELECT.

The investigators found that men eating the most fatty fish and taking the most fish oil supplements had an overall 43 percent increase in risk for all prostate cancer, compared with men eating the least fish or taking the fewest supplements. The risk for aggressive prostate cancer was 71 percent higher; for non-aggressive prostate cancer, the risk was 44 percent greater. (Brasky, 2013)

Andrew Weil Responds

The fats the research team focused on were plasma phospholipid fatty acids, which tell you that an individual recently consumed fish or fish oil but don't really give you an accurate indication of the long term use of fish oil supplements or a diet that includes regular servings of fish. **Blood levels of these fatty acids will rise and stay high for four to 12 hours after a single dose of fish oil or a meal containing**

fish. Unless you eat more fish or take another supplement, blood levels of omega-3s will wash out in about 48 hours.

The study found that the mean blood level of plasma phospholipid fatty acids were 4.66 percent in the men with prostate cancer and 4.48 percent in the healthy controls, a difference of not quite 0.2 percent. That's a very small difference on which to base the suggestion, as these researchers did, that omega-3s "are involved in prostate tumorigenesis" and that those who recommend that men increase consumption of omega-3s "should consider its potential risks."

Bottom line: this appears to be an unfortunate combination of questionable science, unwarranted conclusions, and dreadful media coverage. The well documented evidence for myriad benefits of high dietary intake of omega-3 fatty acids on both physical and mental health is very strong.

Please remember, Dr. Weil sells these fish oil products.

Andrew Weil, M.D. Published 7/26/2013

Paul Offit Chimes In

Dr. Paul Offit interview on Oct 2, 2013 by Dr. Topol

Medscape One-on-One

http://www.medscape.com/viewarticle/811569_6

A look at fish oil

Dr. Topol: You gave a pass to certain things in your book, which I was a little surprised about. For example, you were kind to fish oil. And you probably saw the big paper in the New England Journal of Medicine? **It was a big Italian study that showed that fish oil didn't do anything for preventing heart disease**. Would you revise? Would you be a little tougher on fish oils if you were to get the most updated information, or do you still think there is a place for fish oil?

Dr. Offit: Absolutely. Harper Collins is the publisher; it is a big publisher. This book was written a year and a half ago, so it takes a while to get those books out. I absolutely would revise it, and there were some recent studies that showed that at least the antioxidant part of omega-3 fatty acids actually could increase your risk for such things as cancer, so I absolutely would revise it. That is the problem with books -- they are written at a specific point in time.

Dr. Topol: You know, out here in California, my patients come in and they typically have a list of 20 or 30 supplements and vitamins that they're taking.

SECTION TWO

CANCER

A study published this year in the journal *Cancer Research* linked fish oil supplements with cancer in mice.

Hold the salmon: omega-3 fatty acids linked to higher risk of cancer

By **Claire Groden**, TIME.com July 12, 2013

What's good for the heart may not be so healthy for other organs, says **the latest study that links omega-3 fatty acids to an elevated risk of prostate cancer.**

It's not just an apple a day that keeps the doctor away anymore — recently, fish oils found in species like salmon, trout and tuna have been associated with a lower risk of heart disease and even Alzheimer's. In fact, **the most recent revisions to the Dietary Guidelines for Americans in 2010 recommended consumers substitute high-fat protein sources with more seafood, including fatty fish**.

Not surprisingly, fish oil has since skyrocketed to be the most popular supplement in the United States.

A new study in the Journal of the National Cancer Institute, however, shows that these fish fats may not be improving everyone's health — in the trial, those with high concentrations of marine-derived omega-3s in their blood showed a 43% higher risk of developing prostate cancer than those with the

lowest levels. This is discussed in more detail elsewhere in this text (Brasky, 2013).

Fish oil may favorably alter biology of prostate cancer

Excerpted from Roxanne Nelson - November 20, 2013

A low-fat diet and supplementation with fish oil appears to reduce proinflammatory substances in the blood of prostate cancer patients, according to a new study. It also decreased the cell cycle progression (CCP) score, which is a measure used to predict cancer recurrence.

The study was published online October 29, 2013 in *Cancer Prevention Research*.

It is a follow-up to an earlier clinical trial conducted by the same team, which found that **men who ate a low-fat diet with fish oil supplements, consumed for 4 to 6 weeks prior to prostate removal, slowed the growth of cancer cells, compared with men in the control group who ate a traditional high-fat Western diet (*Cancer Prev Res (Phila)*. 2011;4:2062-2071).**

"**We found that CCP scores were significantly lower in men who consumed the low-fat fish oil diet**," said lead author William Aronson, MD, clinical professor of urology at the University of California, Los Angeles, and chief of urologic oncology at the West Los Angeles Veterans Affairs Medical Center. "We also found that **men on the low-fat fish oil diet had reduced blood levels of proinflammatory substances that have been associated with cancer.**"

A number studies have investigated the relation between prostate cancer and omega-3 fatty acids. "**To my knowledge, all preclinical studies suggest a potential benefit of fish oil and omega-3 fatty acids for the prevention and treatment of prostate cancer**," Dr. Aronson told *Medscape Medical News*.

In preclinical studies, reducing dietary fat from corn oil (omega-6 fatty acids) and increasing fish oil intake (omega-3 fatty acids) has been shown to delay the development and progression of prostate cancer, the authors note.

But epidemiologic studies are mixed with regard to the benefit of fish oil for prevention and treatment, Dr. Aronson explained.

Mixed results

A 2007 study found that for men with a genetic predisposition to prostate cancer, the consumption of a diet rich in omega-3 fatty acids might lower the risk for disease.

A more recent study found that men who had high blood concentrations of long-chain omega-3 polyunsaturated fatty acids had a significant 43% increase in the risk for all grades of prostate cancer, compared with men who had the lowest concentrations, although that study was criticized as being flawed.

The study suggesting an increased risk with fish oil "received an enormous amount of press, but that is just one piece of the puzzle," Dr. Aronson noted. "Other studies show the opposite or a beneficial effect."

"There are contradictions and, clearly, further prospective randomized trials are indicated, given the numerous articles suggesting potential benefits of fish oil," he continued. "In our study, we combined fish oil with a low-fat diet. This allows for a reduction in intake of **omega-6 fatty acids, which stimulate cancer development and growth in preclinical studies,** and an increase in omega-3 fatty acids."

He added that they believe this is a novel and rational approach. **"Just taking a nutritional supplement or vitamin pill alone, without also changing the diet, may not effectively prevent or treat prostate cancer."**

The previous phase 2 randomized trial by Dr. Aronson's team involved **55 patients undergoing radical prostatectomy**. One group ate a low-fat diet with 5 g of fish oil daily (2:1 ratio of dietary omega-6/omega-3) or a control Western diet (15:1 ratio of omega-6/omega-3) for 4 to 6 weeks prior to surgery. The primary end point was change in serum insulin-like growth factor 1 (IGF-1) between the study groups. Secondary end points were changes in serum IGFBP-1, prostate prostaglandin E2 levels, omega-6/omega-3 fatty acid ratios, COX-2, and markers of proliferation and apoptosis.

The primary outcome (serum IFG-1 levels) was negative, but positive secondary outcomes with the low-fat fish oil diet included reduced benign and malignant prostate tissue omega-6/omega-3 ratios, reduced proliferation (Ki-67 index), and reduced proliferation in an ex vivo bioassay when patient serum was applied to prostate cancer cells in vitro.

Intervention lowered markers

In the current study, Dr.Aronson's team evaluated the effect of the low-fat fish oil diet on 2 serum proinflammatory eicosanoids — 15(S)-HETE and leukotriene B4 (LTB4) — and the CCP score. They measured serum fatty acids and eicosanoids with gas chromatography and ELISA, and measured the CCP score with reverse transcriptase-polymerase chain reaction.

In addition, the associations between serum eicosanoids, Ki67, and CCP score were evaluated using partial correlation analyses, and BLT1 (LTB4 receptor) expression was determined in prostate cancer cell lines and prostatectomy specimens.

This post hoc analysis used serum and prostate tissue obtained in the original study.

The majority of men in the 2 groups were either overweight or obese, and the average diet duration was 28 to 30 days. Patients in both groups were compliant with the diet, and those in the low-fat group were compliant with fish oil capsule consumption.

CCP score was significantly lower with the low-fat fish oil diet than with the control diet (*P* = .03).

In men who ate the low-fat fish oil diet, there was a significant decrease in the mean level of total omega-6 fatty acids, an increase in the level of total omega-3 fatty acids, and a decrease in the omega-6/omega-3 fatty acid ratio.

There was also a significant decrease in circulating levels of the proinflammatory eicosanoid 15(S)-HETE with the low-fat fish oil diet. In addition, postintervention 15(S)-HETE circulating levels were significantly lower than preintervention levels.

Even though there was no difference in LTB4 levels between the low-fat fish oil group and the control group, postintervention LTB4 levels in the low-fat fish oil group were significantly lower than preintervention levels.

The LTB4 receptor BLT1 was detected in prostate cancer cell lines and human prostate cancer specimens. In a statement, Dr.Aronson said that the team plans to conduct further studies to determine the importance of this novel receptor in prostate cancer progression.

No clinical recommendations yet

"We are extremely encouraged by our findings, but at this time, would not make clinical recommendations with regard to a low-fat diet or fish oil capsules for the prevention or treatment of prostate cancer," Dr. Aronson said. "Based on our positive findings, the National Institutes of Health has provided funding for a 1-year trial, which we will begin in early 2014."

Cancer Prev Res. Published online October 29, 2013. Abstract

High levels of fish oil may boost risk for prostate cancer

Roxanne Nelson Jul 19, 2013 http://www.medscape.com/viewarticle/808139

August 1, 2013 — **A high intake of omega-3 fatty acid, which is found in fish oil, might significantly boost the risk of developing prostate cancer**, according to **a prospective study**.

Overall, **men who had high blood concentrations of long-chain omega-3 polyunsaturated fatty acids (PUFA) had a significant 43% increase in the risk for all grades of prostate cancer, compared with men who had the lowest concentrations. The risk for high-grade disease was increased by 71%.**

The results of the study, led by Theodore M. Brasky, PhD, from the Ohio State University Comprehensive Cancer Center in Columbus, were published online **July 11 in the *Journal of the National Cancer Institute*.** (Brasky, 2013)

However, **the study design has serious flaws, and the conclusions about prostate cancer are not valid,** according to urology expert Gerald Chodak, MD, director of the Midwest Prostate and Urology Health Center in Michiana Shores, Indiana. In a recent expert video commentary on Medscape's Chodak on Urology, he discusses the design of the study in some detail, and raises questions about the control group and the way in which prostate cancer was diagnosed.

Previous findings

According to Dr. Brasky and colleagues, **their study confirms previous reports of increased prostate cancer risk in men with high blood concentrations of omega-3 fatty acids.**

A previous study by the same team in a different cohort of men found a similar link between high serum concentrations of omega-3 fatty acids and a large increase in the risk for high-grade prostate cancer. (Szymanski et al, 2011)

The men in the current study were participants in SELECT (**Selenium and Vitamin E Cancer Prevention Trial), which is a large randomized trial.**

We recommended moderating fish intake and avoiding supplements.

"The 2 sources of these fatty acids in blood are food and supplements, so the blood samples represent total exposure," Dr. Brasky told *Medscape Medical News*. "The results shouldn't change with the source of the fats," he said.

However, "given that **supplements represent mega doses of omega-3s**, we recommended moderating fish intake and avoiding supplements," he added.

Conflicting data

Previous studies have reported conflicting results on the benefits and risks of fish oils, either consumed as fish or in supplements, in cancer patients.

Fish oil supplements were associated with a lower risk for breast cancer in postmenopausal women in the Vitamins and Lifestyle (VITAL) cohort study (Brasky et al, 2010), as previously reported by *Medscape Medical News*. Although that study, which was also led by Dr. Brasky, found that "fish oil is a potential candidate for chemoprevention studies," it is currently "not recommended for individual use for breast cancer prevention."

Another study found that in men with a genetic predisposition to prostate cancer, the consumption of a diet rich in omega-3 fatty acids can lower the risk for disease (Berquin et al, 2007). **In**

that study, a diet high in omega-3 fatty acid reduced prostate tumor growth and increased survival, but omega-6 fatty acids had the opposite effects.

Omega-3 vs omega-6

Chronic inflammation has been associated with cancer risk, and omega-3 fatty acids, which are found primarily in fatty fish and fish oil supplements, have anti-inflammatory effects. In contrast, other fats, such as the omega-6 fats in vegetable oil and the *trans*-fats commonly found in fast food, can promote inflammation.

Eicosapentaenoic acid (EPA), docosapentaenoic acid, and docosahexaenoic acid (DHA) are anti-inflammatory and metabolically related fatty acids derived from fatty fish and fish oil supplements. **However, in the current study, they were associated with statistically significant increases in prostate cancer risk.**

In contrast, linoleic and arachidonic acids, which are the primary omega-6 fatty acids associated with increased inflammation, were inconsistent, Dr. Brasky and his team note.

In fact, in the current study, concentrations of linoleic acid above the lowest quartile were associated with a lower cancer risk, without any evidence of a linear trend, whereas concentrations of arachidonic acid were not associated with cancer risk. Findings for *trans*-fatty acids, which are also associated with increased inflammation, were also inconsistent.

More definitive research needed

Eliot Brinton, MD, director of atherometabolic research at the Utah Foundation for Biomedical Research in Salt Lake City, who was asked by *Medscape Medical News* to comment on the findings, said the data suggest that there might be an effect.

However, "this is an **observational study**, and these studies usually generate rather than confirm hypotheses," he explained. "For observational data, they came to a fairly strong conclusion. It is a little puzzling, interesting, and provocative. It raises questions but is a long way from being definitive."

"It highlights the potential differences between DHA and EPA," Dr. Brinton added. "More definitive studies are needed that address that."

Dr. Brinton pointed out that recent observational data have shown a benefit in breast cancer, so the effect doesn't appear to be uniform across cancer types. There is also limited information about how the blood levels were reached. "We don't know if it was from supplementation, a prescription for fish oil, or diet," he said, "or possibly the manner in which the omega-3 fatty acids were metabolized."

He noted that many population studies have shown the benefits of fish intake. "There remains a consensus among nutrition scientists that eating fish remains healthy, with caveats," he said. "However, the results of this study might 'temper the enthusiasm' for dietary supplements."

"Many have been guilty of pushing fish oil supplements, and physicians often misunderstand them," he said. "They may be good for some people, but it doesn't mean we should be putting everyone on fish oil. It should give us some hesitation about rubber stamping low-dose fish oil."

"Of course, it's not always harmful, but we probably shouldn't be assuming that it is healthy for everyone," Dr. Brinton added. "But we don't know at this point who it is healthy for, and that is what we need to find out."

Study details

In the current study, Dr. Brasky and colleagues examined the association between plasma phospholipid fatty acids and prostate cancer risk in men who participated in **SELECT**. The **randomized placebo-controlled trial** was designed to evaluate whether selenium and vitamin E, alone or in combination, could reduce the risk for prostate cancer. The study population of **35,533 involved black men 50 years or older or men of another race 55 years or older who had no history of prostate cancer and a serum prostate-specific antigen (PSA) level of 4 ng/mL**.

The case–cohort study was nested within SELECT. Cases were men with baseline blood samples available for analysis who were diagnosed with incident primary prostate cancer before July 31, 2009. This analysis was one of the secondary aims of the original trial, explained Dr. Brasky.

In continuous models, the researchers found that **with each 50% increase in total long-chain omega-3 PUFA, there was an**

associated 22% to 25% increased cancer risk. Results for the individual long-chain omega-3 PUFA were similar, but the effect sizes tended to be smaller, and not all reached statistical significance.

Of the major omega-6 PUFA, higher levels of linoleic acid were associated with a 25% reduced risk for low-grade cancer and a 23% reduced risk for total cancer, but there was no dose response.

The researchers explored the possibly that the higher risk for prostate cancer might be explained by increased screening among those who consume high amounts of omega-3 PUFA. In a separate sensitivity analysis, they censored noncase individuals at the date of their last screening test, but found the results largely unchanged. Hazard ratios for associations between total long-chain omega-3 PUFA and total, low-grade, and high-grade prostate cancer were 1.44, 1.44, and 1.67, respectively. (Brasky, 2013)

The controversy over the Brasky data is somewhat typical of responses seen in other studies demeaning the alleged benefits of fish oil.

Plasma phospholipid fatty acids and prostate cancer risk

SELECT Trial

Background Studies of dietary ω-3 fatty acid intake and prostate cancer risk are inconsistent; however, recent large prospective studies have found increased risk of prostate cancer among men with high blood concentrations of long-chain ω-3 polyunsaturated fatty acids ([LCω-3PUFA] 20:5ω3; 22:5ω3; 22:6ω3]. This case–cohort study examines associations between plasma phospholipid fatty acids and prostate cancer risk among participants in the Selenium and Vitamin E Cancer Prevention Trial.

Methods Case subjects were 834 men diagnosed with prostate cancer, of which 156 had high-grade cancer. The subcohort consisted of 1,393 men selected randomly at baseline and from within strata frequency matched to case subjects on age and race. Proportional hazards models estimated hazard ratios (HR) and 95% confidence intervals (CI) for associations between fatty acids and prostate cancer risk overall and by grade. All statistical tests were two-sided.

Results Compared with men in the lowest quartiles of LCω-3PUFA, men in the highest quartile had increased risks for low-grade, high-grade, and total prostate cancer. Associations were similar for individual long-chain ω-3 fatty acids. Higher linoleic acid (ω-6) was associated with reduced risks of low-grade and total prostate cancer; however, there was no dose response.

Conclusions: **This study by Brasky et al. confirms previous reports of increased prostate cancer risk among men with high blood concentrations of LCω-3PUFA.** The consistency of these findings suggests that these fatty acids are involved in prostate tumorigenesis. Recommendations to increase LCω-3PUFA intake should consider its potential risks. (Brasky et al, 2013) (Nordqvist, 2013)

Omega-3 Fatty Acids May Lower Genetic Risk for Prostate Cancer

Roxanne Nelson Jun 21, 2007 http://www.medscape.com/viewarticle/558671

June 21, 2007 — **In men with a genetic predisposition to prostate cancer, the consumption of a diet rich in omega-3 fatty acids may lower the risk for disease.** Results of an experimental study, published online June 21, 2007 in the *Journal of Clinical Investigation*, show that **a diet high in omega-3 fatty acid reduced prostate tumor growth and increased survival, while omega-6 fatty acids had the opposite effects.**

Increasing evidence suggests that omega-3 fatty acids, which are commonly found in fatty fish and fish oils, inhibit carcinogenesis. Specifically, write the authors, data from epidemiological studies suggest that the consumption of fish or fish oil may reduce the incidence of prostate cancer. As an example, a large prospective study of **6272 men** who were followed for 30 years found that **the consumption of fatty fish was associated with a lower risk for prostate cancer.** (Terry et al, 2001)

Other studies have reported significantly lower levels of omega-3 polyunsaturated fatty acids in men with benign prostate hyperplasia and prostate cancer, as compared with a control population. **Conversely, levels of omega-6 fatty acids were higher in patients with prostate cancer.**

The researchers point out that while the causal role of genetic alterations in human cancer has been established, the influence of environmental factors on cancer risk is still not well understood. Yong Q. Chen, PhD, a professor of cancer biology at Wake Forest University, in Winston-Salem, North Carolina, and colleagues examined the influence of both omega-3 and -6 essential fatty acids on a **mouse model of prostate cancer** to evaluate whether a diet rich in omega-3 polyunsaturated fatty acids can lower the incidence of cancer. The study was carried out in *PTEN*-knockout mice, which are bred to be predisposed to developing prostate tumors.

Overall, diets rich in omega-3 fatty acids reduced prostate tumor growth, slowed histopathological progression, and increased survival, the researchers write. The 12-month survival rate was 60% for mice fed a diet high in omega-3, 10% on the low–omega-3 diet, and 0% on the high–omega-6 diet. **The ideal ratio of omega-6 to omega-3 fatty acids is 1:1,** and mice fed diets with this ratio of fatty acids were able to delay both the formation and progression of prostate tumors and prolong their survival, they comment.

The researchers also noted that animals fed a diet low in omega-3 fatty acids and with an omega-6/omega-3 ratio of 20 (rather than a ratio of 1 in the recommended diet) had intermediary tumor growth, progression, and survival. "Therefore, **the omega-6/omega-3 ratio appears to be a critical factor in the effectiveness of prostate cancer suppression**, with a higher proportion of omega-3 being more effective," they write.

The introduction of the enzyme omega-3 desaturase, which is able to convert omega-6 to omega-3, reduced the growth of tumors in a fashion similar to a diet rich in omega-3 fatty acids. The investigators also found that the effect of polyunsaturated fatty acids on the development of prostate cancer is partially mediated by the protein BAD. **The omega-3 fatty acids, but not omega-6, appear to induce apoptosis of prostate cancer cells through regulation of BAD**.

Dr. Chen and his team also note that the absolute amount of polyunsaturated fatty acids may also play a role, **as high fat intake has been associated with the risk for cancer. All of the diets initiated in this study contained 13% fat with 30% energy from fat, which is similar to the average Western diet**. In control mice, normal prostate development was unaffected by the fatty-acid ratio, which suggests the importance of interactions between genes and diet and that a genetic cancer risk can be favorably modified by dietary intervention.

"Clinically, **prostate cancer is usually diagnosed in men age 60 or older**, and cancer cells proliferate slowly," they write. "Therefore, dietary and/or chemoprevention are of particular importance for the management of prostate cancer."

However, it has not yet been determined, they add, whether beneficial effects can also be achieved by supplementing the diet with omega-3 fatty acids in patients who have already developed the disease.

Dr. Oz says fish oil gives you "burp back" and krill oil does not, for whatever that is worth.

Omega-3 role in preventing oral and skin cancers

http://www.fish-oil-advice.com/benefits-of-fish-oil/

8-2-13 **Foods containing omega-3 fatty acids may help in the prevention of early- and late-stage oral and skin cancers, according to a study published in the journal *Carcinogenesis*.**

UK researchers from Queen Mary, University of London grew cell cultures in the laboratory from several different cell lines. These included both malignant oral and skin cancers, alongside pre-malignant cells and normal skin and oral cells.

The focus was mainly on a type of cancer called squamous-cell carcinoma. This is one of the major forms of skin cancer affecting the outer layers of the skin (mainly made up of squamous cells). The researchers point out that squamous-cell carcinoma can also occur in the lining of the digestive tract, lungs and other areas of the body.

Oral squamous cell carcinomas are the sixth most common skin cancer worldwide, the researchers say, and are difficult and expensive to treat.

Omega-3 induced cancer cell death

When the researchers carried out *in vitro* tests by adding fatty acids into the cell cultures, results showed that omega-3 fatty acids induced cell death in malignant and pre-malignant cells in doses that did not affect normal cells.

Professor Kenneth Parkinson, head of the oral cancer research group at Queen Mary's Institute of Dentistry, says:

"We found that the omega-3 fatty acid selectively inhibited the growth of the malignant and pre-malignant cells at doses which did not affect the normal cells."

"Surprisingly, we discovered this was partly due to an over-stimulation of a key growth factor (epidermal growth factor) which triggered cell death. This is a novel mechanism of action of these fatty acids," Prof. Parkinson adds.

Potential cure for oral and skin cancers?

The scientists say that because the doses needed to kill the cancer cells did not affect normal cells, this means **Omega-3 fatty acids could be used for the prevention and treatment of oral and skin cancers.**

Omega-3 polyunsaturated fatty acids are found mainly in oily, fatty fish. Previous research has found that omega-3 may have numerous health benefits, including helping to prevent cardiovascular disease.

Research from the University of Pittsburgh has also suggested that high consumption of the fatty acids can improve memory in young adults.

Increasing omega-3 levels 'may reduce cancer risk'

Because omega-3 cannot be made in large quantities by the human body, the main way to increase levels is to consume foods that are rich in it. Advice on fish and omega-3 fatty acids from the American Heart Association recommends at least two servings (3.5 ounces for each) of oily fish every week.

Many other foods also contain high levels of omega-3, including:

- Salmon
- Walnuts
- Ground flax seeds
- Sardines

- Beef (from grass-fed cows)
- Soybeans
- Halibut
- Scallops
- Shrimp
- Tofu.

One of the authors of the study into skin and oral cancers, Dr. Zacharoula Nikolakopoulou from the London School of Medicine and Dentistry, says higher omega-3 intake may be particularly worthwhile for some people:

"It **may be** that those at an increased risk of such cancers - or their reccurrence - could benefit from increased omega-3 fatty acids. Moreover, as the skin and oral cancers are often easily accessible, there is the potential to deliver targeted doses locally via aerosols or gels. However, further research is needed to define the appropriate therapeutic doses.

Medical News Today spoke exclusively to Dr. Zacharoula Nikolakopoulou about this study and what it means for potential cancer sufferers.

Interview with Dr. Zacharoula Nikolakopoulou

How was the study conducted?

In this study we used several cancer (squamous cell carcinoma) and pre-malignant oral and skin cell lines in culture, which we treated with omega-3 fatty acids.

The effect of the fatty acids on the cell growth and death was assessed, and also the mechanism of action was investigated. We also used normal oral and skin cells to compare the effect.

What did your findings show?

We showed that low doses of Eicosapentanoic acid (EPA), in particular, selectively inhibited the growth of pre-malignant and malignant skin and oral cells more than the normal cells in culture, by a combination of growth arrest and apoptosis.

This was partly accomplished by the overstimulation of a cellular pathway triggered by the over-activation of the epidermal growth factor in the malignant and pre-malignant cells.

How could this research be used in the prevention and treatment of oral and skin cancers?

This study suggests that there is a great potential in the use of these fatty acids in the prevention and treatment of these cancers. Together with many other studies done in different types of cancer, our study suggests that the omega-3 fatty acids in diet might protect from oral and skin cancer.

As regards the therapeutic potential, they could also be delivered locally on the tumors in the form of sprays or gels, as these cancers are usually easily accessible.

What are the next steps for this research?

After the initial step, which was to study the effects in vitro, the research should continue by assessing the effects in model organisms in vivo and then in humans in clinical trials, in order to examine the exact effect of these fatty acids and define the appropriate therapeutic doses.

Written by Honor Whiteman

B vitamin and/or ω-3 fatty acid supplementation and cancer

Abstract

BACKGROUND:

To advance knowledge about the cancer-chemopreventive potential of individual nutrients, we investigated the effects of B vitamin and/or ω-3 fatty acid supplements on cancer outcomes among survivors of cardiovascular disease.

METHODS:

This was an ancillary study of the Supplementation With Folate, Vitamins B(6) and B(12) and/or Omega-3 Fatty Acids (SU.FOL.OM3) secondary prevention trial (2003-2009). In all, 2501 individuals aged 45 to 80 years were randomized in a 2 × 2 factorial design to one of the following 4 daily supplementation groups: (1) 5-methyltetrahydrofolate (0.56 mg), pyridoxine hydrochloride (vitamin B(6); 3 mg) and cyanocobalamin (vitamin B(12); 0.02 mg); (2) eicosapentaenoic and docosahexaenoic acid (600 mg) in a 2:1 ratio; (3) B vitamins and ω-3 fatty acids; or (4) placebo. Overall and sex-specific hazard ratios (HRs) and 95% CIs regarding the cancer outcomes were estimated with Cox proportional hazards models.

RESULTS:

After 5 years of supplementation, incident cancer was validated in 7.0% of the sample (145 events in men and 29 in women), and death from cancer occurred in 2.3% of the sample. **There was no association between cancer outcomes and supplementation with B vitamins and/or ω-3 fatty acids.**

There was a statistically significant interaction of treatment by sex, with no effect of treatment on cancer risk among men and increased cancer risk among women for ω-3 fatty acid supplementation.

CONCLUSION:

Andreeva VA, et al found no beneficial effects of supplementation with relatively low doses of B vitamins and/or ω-3 fatty acids on cancer outcomes in individuals with prior cardiovascular disease. There was a statistically significant interaction of treatment by sex, with no effect of treatment on cancer risk among men and increased cancer risk among women for ω-3 fatty acid supplementation. (Andreeva et al, 2012)

Fish oils can block chemotherapy drugs

9-12-11 Fats found in fish oil supplements can stop chemotherapy drugs working, according to researchers. Writing in the journal **Cancer Cell, they advise cancer patients not to take the supplements.**

The two fatty acids involved, which are also produced by stem cells in the blood, lead to tumors becoming immune to treatment.

Cancer Research UK advised patients to ask their doctor whether they would be affected.

Scientists in the Netherlands were investigating how tumors develop resistance to treatments.

Fat shield

Experiments on mice showed that stem cells in the blood responded to the widely-used cancer drug cisplatin. The cells started producing two fatty acids, known as **KHT and 16:4(n-3).**

These fatty acids begin a series of chemical reactions, which mean cancerous cells become resistant to chemotherapy.

"We currently recommend that these products should not be used whilst people are undergoing chemotherapy"

End Quote Prof Emile Voest University Medical Centre Utrecht

Using drugs to block the production of the fatty acids prevented this form of resistance which "significantly enhances the chemotherapy," the study says.

However, researchers warned that these fatty acids were "abundantly present in commercially available fish oil products". **They showed that off-the-shelf fish oil supplements, given to mice, could stop chemotherapy working against some tumors**.

Prof Emile Voest, lead researcher at University Medical Centre Utrecht, said: "We show that the body itself secretes protective substances into the blood that are powerful enough to block the effect of chemotherapy.

"These substances can be found in some types of fish oil.

"Whilst waiting for the results of further research, we currently recommend that these products should not be used while people are undergoing chemotherapy."

Jessica Harris, health information manager for Cancer Research UK, said: "This interesting study suggests one possible option for stopping cancers becoming resistant to treatment, but it is at an early stage and much more research would be needed to develop ways to halt resistance.

"The results also suggest that fish oil preparations may reduce the effectiveness of chemotherapy drugs.

"Cancer patients who are taking or thinking of taking these supplements should talk to their doctors to find out whether they could affect their treatments."

This next paper next article presents the other side of the argument.

Fish oil's link to prostate cancer unproven

July 26, 2013

This is included to present an opposing view.

Dr. Gerald Chodak for Medscape presents his side of the story in which a controversial study that suggested that the intake of omega-3 fatty acids increased a man's risk of developing prostate cancer. Brasky and coworkers published a study in the *Journal of the National Cancer Institute* in which they measured levels of omega-3 and omega-6 fatty acids in a group of men who had participated in the SELECT trial. SELECT was a study testing whether vitamin E alone or in combination with selenium could prevent prostate cancer. Patients who were diagnosed with prostate cancer were selected from that study, and the control group consisted of men from that study who were not diagnosed with prostate cancer. **The authors found that increasing quartiles of omega-3 fatty acids resulted in an increasing risk for diagnosis of prostate cancer, and high-grade disease in particular.**

The question is whether the conclusions and the study itself are valid. I think there are a number of concerns about the study design that raise serious questions. First, this was not a prospectively designed trial in which some men were randomized to receive omega-3 fatty acids at different intakes to determine whether the omega-3 fatty acids did result in an increased risk for disease. Making firm conclusions from the study design is impossible. More importantly, there are some questions about the design of the study that raise serious questions about the validity of the data.

The men in the control group were not diagnosed with prostate cancer. However, over 400 sites participated in the SELECT trial, and it wasn't mandated how often patients had a prostate-specific antigen (PSA) test, how that PSA test was managed, whether they had a prostate biopsy, or how the prostate biopsy was done. Furthermore, if a patient had a negative biopsy, there was no standardized procedure for determining whether a second biopsy should be performed. **The bottom line is that the control group is not reliable or valid.** We could have had a study in which all men in the control group had a biopsy to make sure that they didn't have cancer, and it's likely that the inclusion of this control group would have resulted in a bias in terms of how men were assigned to the different categories or groups that they were in.

Another design flaw is that they assigned Gleason 3+4 tumors into the low-risk category and Gleason 4+3 tumors into the high-risk category, when the standard approach is to have Gleason 7 assigned to an intermediate-risk group of patients. Why they did that is unclear, although the senior author suggested that they may have needed more events or more cancers in order to assess the data. Nevertheless, trying to make that claim with Gleason 4+3 in a high-risk group is not valid. Another problem is that this is a single point in time measurement. Blood samples were obtained at the beginning of the SELECT trial when patients were entered, and that is when the measurements were made. There was no standardized method for how men achieved their level of omega-3 fatty acids. Was it diet or was it supplements? Which supplements were used and what dosages were used? All of these problems contribute to an uncertainty and potential bias in the results.

The bottom line is that we cannot determine from this study design whether the intake of omega-3 fatty acids will cause prostate cancer and raise a man's risk for high-grade disease. The media has taken this and sensationalized the risk associated with omega-3 fatty acid intake, but I believe that the attention is overplayed and the concerns about the study design were not mentioned at all. At the end of the day, this study does not prove that intake of omega-3 fatty acids causes prostate cancer or increases a man's risk for high-grade disease. We would need better-designed trials that are prospective and randomized to be able to make such a claim. Until that is done, we will have to weigh the pros and cons of taking omega-3 fatty acids in terms of its other potential health benefits to decide what to do. Whether it causes prostate cancer is not determined by the results of this trial. I look forward to your comments.

You have seen the data and you can make up your mind about taking these supplements.

SECTION THREE

CARDIOVASCULAR

Heart surgeon speaks out on what really causes heart disease

Dr. Dwight Lundell

PreventDisease. Mar 1, 2012

Obviously, this is just one person's unproven opinion.

What are the biggest culprits of chronic inflammation? Quite simply, they are the overload of simple, highly processed carbohydrates (sugar, flour and all the products made from them) and the **excess consumption of omega-6 vegetable oils** like soybean, corn and sunflower that are found in many processed foods.

While we savor the tantalizing taste of a sweet roll, our bodies respond alarmingly as if a foreign invader arrived declaring war. Foods loaded with sugars and simple carbohydrates, or processed with omega-6 oils for long shelf life have been the mainstay of the American diet for six decades. These foods have been slowly poisoning everyone.

While omega-6's are essential -they are part of every cell membrane controlling what goes in and out of the cell -- they must be in the correct balance with omega-3's.

If the balance shifts by consuming excessive omega-6, the cell membrane produces chemicals called cytokines that directly cause inflammation.

Today's mainstream American diet has produced an extreme imbalance of these two fats. The ratio of imbalance ranges from 15:1 to as high as 30:1 in favor of omega-6. That's a tremendous amount of cytokines causing inflammation. In today's food environment, a 3:1 ratio would be optimal and healthy.

There is no escaping the fact that the more we consume prepared and processed foods, the more we trip the inflammation switch little by little each day. The human body cannot process, nor was it designed to consume, foods packed with sugars and soaked in omega-6 oils.

One tablespoon of corn oil contains 7,280 mg of omega-6; soybean contains 6,940 mg. Instead, use olive oil or butter from grass-fed beef.

Animal fats contain less than 20% omega-6 and are much less likely to cause inflammation than the supposedly healthy oils labelled polyunsaturated.

Lundell's guess is about as good (or useless) as any other unproven guess.

Omega-3 supplements fail to help heart

By Bahar Gholipour, Staff Writer - March 17, 2014

Taking supplements of omega-3 fatty acids doesn't seem to reduce a person's risk of heart disease, a new study finds.

The findings are part of a study that was primarily designed to examine the effects of omega-3 supplements and some vitamins on vision health. About 4,200 people ages 50 to 85 with the age-related eye problem macular degeneration participated in the study. Some of the participants were randomly asked to take omega-3 supplements or the eye vitamins lutein and zeaxanthin, while others were given a placebo.

By the end of the five-year study, about 450 participants had suffered a cardiovascular problem, such as heart attack or stroke. **Researchers found no benefit among individuals who had taken omega-3 or eye vitamins; they were as likely to have experienced a heart problem during the study period as people who took a placebo, according to the study published in JAMA (March 17, 2014) in the journal JAMA Internal Medicine**.

The findings add to "a growing body of evidence from clinical trials that have found little cardiovascular benefit from moderate levels of dietary supplementation," the researchers wrote in the journal article.

Omega-3 fatty acids, which can be found in oily fish and are also available in a supplement form, have been the subject of investigation after some studies suggested they could protect a person's cardiovascular system.

However, the **findings have been inconsistent**. Some diet studies have found people who eat fish regularly had a lower risk of heart disease, whereas other clinical studies failed to find a beneficial link between omega-3 intake and heart disease risk.

Nevertheless, **omega-3 supplements have sold more than $25 billion in 2011**, and their market is estimated to grow 15 percent each year, according to market research studies. These supplements are increasingly used for prevention of cardiovascular disease, either with a doctor's prescription or as over-the-counter products, said Dr. Evangelos Rizos from University Hospital of Ioannina, Greece, in an editorial published along with the study.

Many years of research has failed to find conclusive evidence for the benefits of omega-3 supplementation, and doctors should inform their patients about the uncertainty surrounding the benefits of taking omega-3 supplements, Rizos said.

The study only looked at omega-3 intake from supplements and not from fish. There's some evidence that eating seafood rich in omega-3 fatty acids has health benefits, so the National Institutes of Health suggests such foods be part of a heart-healthy diet.

As omega-3 fatty acids can reduce triglycerides, a type of fat found in the blood, **the supplements should be considered only for people who have severely high triglyceride levels, who are an extreme minority in the population**, Rizos said. Similarly, the Food and Drug Administration has approved omega-3 supplementation only for people with this condition.

The new study also found that lutein and zeaxanthin, antioxidants found in green leafy vegetables, didn't have an effect on heart disease risk, despite previous suggestions that these vitamins may lower the risk of heart problems, the researchers said.

Daily fish oil supplement may not help your heart

Get your omega-3s from food, not pills, experts suggest

3-17-14 http://www.webmd.com/vitamins-and-supplements/news/20140317/daily-fish-oil-supplement-may-not-help-your-heart-studies

March 17, 2014 (HealthDay News) -- **People who take fish oil capsules may not be getting the heart-health benefits they desired, according to a pair of new research reports.**

Both studies found that the omega-3 fatty acids in fish oil supplements do not provide any significant protection against heart disease, when compared to other types of dietary fats.

"**Looking at the 17 randomized clinical trials that we combined, the majority of the trials -- especially the more recent and large-scale ones -- showed consistently little or no significant effect on reducing coronary heart disease events**," said Dr. Rajiv Chowdhury, lead author of a comprehensive review of nutrition research related to fats.

Of the range of fats studied, only trans fats showed a clear negative effect on heart health, according to the review published in the March 18, 2014 *Annals of Internal Medicine* by Chowdhury, a cardiovascular epidemiologist at the University of Cambridge, and colleagues. (Chowdhury, Van Horn, AHA, 2014)

Trans fats can still be found in processed foods -- look for the words "hydrogenated" or "partially hydrogenated" in the ingredient list.

Saturated fats, long considered a dietary no-no, appeared to pose no additional risk for heart disease according to recent research, Chowdhury said. **They carried about the same cardiac risk as unsaturated fats, omega-3 fatty acids and omega-6 fatty acids**.

Saturated fats are solid at room temperature. They can be found in butter, lard, cheese and cream, as well as the fatty white areas on cuts of meat. By contrast, unsaturated fats are liquid at room temperature -- think of vegetable cooking oil or olive oil.

A second study also came to the same conclusion regarding omega-3 fatty acids, via a different route. This study had been reviewing the use of omega-3s for eye health, but researchers used their data to look at whether the supplements also helped prevent heart disease.

That study found no reduction in heart attack, stroke or heart failure among almost 1,100 people taking omega-3 supplements, compared to similar numbers of people taking other supplements for eye health or just an inactive placebo. It appeared online March 17, 2014 in *JAMA Internal Medicine*. (Chowdhury, Van Horn, AHA, 2014)

The meta-analysis performed by Chowdhury's team involved data **from 72 studies with more than 600,000 participants from 18 nations.** The team combined study findings to assess the heart health benefits of all types of dietary fat -- saturated fat, unsaturated fat, and the omega-3 and omega-6 fatty acids.

Until now, doctors have said that saturated fats increase "bad" LDL cholesterol, which can cause plaques to form in your arteries and raise your risk of a heart attack or stroke.

At the same time, omega-3 fatty acids were said to improve heart health because it increases your level of "good" HDL cholesterol. Good cholesterol is believed to help the body rid itself of bad cholesterol.

While this is still true, Chowdhury and his team found that neither effect seemed to make much difference for overall cardiac risk.

"Saturated fats are not essentially the main problem when it comes to risk of heart disease," Chowdhury said. "Also, **omega-3 or omega-6 fatty acids have no or little impact on reducing cardiovascular disease outcomes**."

The Council for Responsible Nutrition, a trade association representing the dietary supplement industry, released a statement calling the new report's viewpoint "potentially irresponsible" and accusing it of causing "nutritional guidance whiplash" for consumers.

"There are thousands of studies and decades of recommendations from government, academic, nutritional and medical organizations and experts supporting the important heart health benefits associated with diets high in polyunsaturated fats, low in saturated fats, and avoidance of trans fats," Duffy MacKay, a naturopathic doctor and the council's senior vice president of scientific and regulatory affairs, said in the prepared statement.

MacKay added that dietary recommendations from the American Heart Association and the federal government both emphasize the importance of omega-3 fatty acids in a person's diet.

Omega-3 fatty acids do play an important role in good nutrition, as do other unsaturated fats, study author Chowdhury noted.

"Omega-3 fatty acids are essential nutrients for health," Chowdhury said. "**We need omega-3 fatty acids for numerous normal body functions, such as controlling blood clotting and building cell membranes in the brain.**"

But **people should focus on getting their omega-3 fatty acids from food rather than through supplements**, the researcher said.

Dr. Linda Van Horn, a professor of preventive medicine at Northwestern University Feinberg School of Medicine and a member of the nutrition committee of the American Heart Association (AHA), agreed.

"There is continuing data to support eating fish on a regular basis for heart health and other health benefits like [mental] function," Van Horn said. "**There's no question that eating fish provides tremendous value in reducing risk for cardiovascular disease, but the use of a supplement -- whether it's a fish oil or any other nutrient -- really needs to be handled carefully.**"

People should keep their overall fat intake low because fats contain twice the calories of proteins or carbohydrates, according to federal guidelines.

Van Horn said the AHA's nutrition committee will review these new findings at its next meeting.

"I don't think we take any of these kind of findings lightly, nor would we recommend the benefit of a supplement ever over a heart-healthy diet," she said, noting that the new review is "further elaborating on nutrient data that weren't even available five or 10 years ago."

And, she added, "While there's a tendency for the American public to throw up their hands, the better way to interpret this is, 'How wonderful we have additional data and can look at these questions that previously went unanswered.'"

For his part, MacKay said the new studies will not alter the tips he provides his patients.

"If you want to play an active role in staying heart healthy, the best advice remains the same: Eat a healthy diet rich in polyunsaturated fats such as omega-3s, add omega-3 supplements if you're not eating enough fatty fish, and exercise regularly," MacKay said.

Eating more fish shown to boost good cholesterol levels

3-5-14 A University of Eastern Finland study has found that eating more fatty fish can increase good cholesterol levels.

The study was published in the journal *PLOS ONE* and found participants who increased their fish fatty consumption to three or four fish meals per week had more large HDL (high-density lipoprotein) -- also known as "good cholesterol" -- particles in their blood than those who did not eat fish so frequently.

For the study, **131 participants** with "impaired glucose metabolism and features of the metabolic syndrome" were divided into three groups, the first asked to eat wholegrain products and bilberries as well as three to four weekly servings of fatty fish, the second asked to eat whole grains in addition to their regular eating habits, and the third, a control group, asked to eliminate whole grains and limit their intake of berries and fish. A total of 106 participants completed the trial.

Daily fish intake in the three groups worked out to be 67g, 42g and 16g respectively. Participants who experienced the most positive changes were those eating three to four fish meals per week, and the greater the increase in fish intake, the greater the increase in concentration of large HDL.

Fish consumed for the study included fatty options such as rainbow trout, salmon, vendace and herring. The fish were prepared without additional butter or cream.

Cholesterol is generally divided into "good" and "bad," with good cholesterol capable of removing bad cholesterol from arteries in addition to lowering risk of cardiovascular disease. Bad cholesterol contributes to increased risk of this disease.

"People shouldn't fool themselves into thinking that if their standard lipid levels are OK, there's no need to think about the diet, as things are a lot more complicated than that. Soft vegetable fats and fish are something to prefer in any case," postdoctoral researcher Maria Lankinen says.

Researchers also emphasize the importance of maintaining a heart-healthy diet that's low in red meat and high in fish and other foods that lower bad cholesterol, such as olive oil, whole grains and nuts.

2/3 of people who have heart attacks every year have what doctors consider normal or good levels of LDL vs HDL cholesterol. Food for thought

Clinical evidence is strongest for heart disease and problems that contribute to heart disease, but omega-3 fatty acids may also be used for:

High cholesterol

People who follow a Mediterranean style diet tend to have higher HDL or "good" cholesterol levels, which help promote heart health. Inuit Eskimos, who get high amounts of omega-3 fatty acids from eating fatty fish, also tend to have increased HDL cholesterol and decreased triglycerides (fats in the blood). Several studies have shown that fish oil supplements reduce triglyceride levels. Finally, walnuts (which are rich in alpha linolenic acid or ANA, which converts to omega-3s in the body) have been reported to lower total cholesterol and triglycerides in people with high cholesterol levels.

High blood pressure

Several clinical studies suggest that diets rich in omega-3 fatty acids lower blood pressure in people with hypertension. An analysis of 17 clinical studies using fish oil supplements found that taking 3 or more grams of fish oil daily may reduce blood pressure in people with untreated hypertension. Doses this high, however, should only be taken under the direction of a physician.

Heart disease

The role of omega-3 fatty acids in cardiovascular disease is well established. One of the best ways to help prevent heart disease is to eat a diet low in saturated fat and to eat foods that are rich in monounsaturated and polyunsaturated fats (including omega-3 fatty acids). Clinical evidence suggests that EPA and DHA (eicosapentaenoic acid and docosahexaenoic acid, the two omega-3 fatty acids found in fish oil) help reduce risk factors for heart disease, including high cholesterol and high blood pressure. Fish oil has been shown to lower levels of triglycerides (fats in the blood), and to lower the risk of death, heart attack, stroke, and abnormal heart rhythms in people who have already had a heart attack. Fish oil also appears to help prevent and treat atherosclerosis (hardening of the arteries) by slowing the development of plaque and blood clots, which can clog arteries.

Trans fatty acids - A risk factor for cardiovascular disease

Abstract

Trans fatty acids (TFA) are produced either by hydrogenation of unsaturated oils or by biohydrogenation in the stomach of ruminant animals. Vanaspati ghee and margarine have high contents of TFA. **A number of studies have shown an association of TFA consumption and increased risk of cardiovascular disease (CVD).** This increased risk is because TFA increase the ratio of LDL cholesterol to HDL cholesterol. Food and Agriculture Organization of the United Nations and World Health Organization have come up with the recommendation that the contents of TFA in human dietary fat should be reduced to less than 4%. There is high prevalence of CVD in Pakistan. High consumption of vanaspati ghee which contains 14.2-34.3% of TFA could be one of the factors for this increased burden of CVD in Pakistan. Consumption of dietary fat low in TFA would be helpful in reducing the risk of CVD in South Asia. Denmark by banning the sale of food items with TFA has brought down the number of deaths due to coronary heart disease by nearly 50% over a period of 20 years. **Public awareness about the adverse effects of TFA on human health would be extremely important**. Media can play a very effective role in educating the masses and advocating the policy for the sale of only low TFA food items. (Iqbal, 2014)

n-3 Fatty acids from fish or fish-oil supplements, benefit CVD

n-3 Fatty acids from fish or fish-oil supplements, but not alpha-linolenic acid, benefit cardiovascular disease outcomes in primary- and secondary-prevention studies: a systematic review.

Abstract

Studies on the relation between dietary n-3 fatty acids (FAs) and cardiovascular disease vary in quality, and the results are inconsistent. A systematic review of the literature on the effects of n-3 FAs (consumed as fish or fish oils rich in eicosapentaenoic acid and docosahexaenoic acid or as alpha-linolenic acid) on cardiovascular disease outcomes and adverse events was conducted. Studies from MEDLINE and other sources that were of > or =1 y in duration and that reported estimates of fish or n-3 FA intakes and cardiovascular disease outcomes were included. **Secondary prevention was addressed in 14 randomized controlled trials (RCTs) of fish-oil supplements or of diets high in n-3 FAs and in 1 prospective cohort study. Most trials reported that fish oil significantly reduced all-cause mortality, myocardial infarction, cardiac and sudden death, or stroke. Primary prevention of cardiovascular disease was reported in 1 RCT, in 25 prospective cohort studies, and in 7 case-control studies. No significant effect on overall deaths was reported in 3 RCTs that evaluated the effects of fish oil in patients with implantable cardioverter defibrillators.** Most cohort studies reported that fish consumption was associated with lower rates of all-cause mortality and adverse cardiac outcomes. **The effects on stroke were inconsistent.**

Evidence suggests that increased consumption of n-3 FAs from fish or fish-oil supplements, but not of alpha-linolenic acid, reduces the rates of all-cause mortality, cardiac and sudden death, and possibly stroke. **The evidence for the benefits of fish oil is stronger in secondary- than in primary-prevention settings**. Adverse effects appear to be minor. This is the other side of the coin. (Wang et al, 2006)

Omega-3 dietary supplements and the risk of cardiovascular events: a systematic review.

Abstract

Epidemiologic data suggest that omega-3 fatty acids derived from fish oil reduce cardiovascular disease. The clinical benefit of dietary fish oil supplementation in preventing cardiovascular events in both high and low risk patients is unclear.

OBJECTIVE:

To assess whether dietary supplements of eicosapentaenoic acid (EPA) and docosahexaenoic acid (DHA) decrease cardiovascular events across a spectrum of patients.

DATA SOURCES:

MEDLINE, Embase, the Cochrane Database of Systematic Reviews, and citation review of relevant primary and review articles.

STUDY SELECTION:

Prospective, randomized, placebo-controlled clinical trials that evaluated clinical cardiovascular end points (cardiovascular death, sudden death, and nonfatal cardiovascular events) and all-cause mortality in patients randomized to EPA/DHA or placebo. We only included studies that used dietary supplements of EPA/DHA which were administered for at least 1 year.

DATA EXTRACTION:

Data were abstracted on study design, study size, type and dose of omega-3 supplement, cardiovascular events, all-cause mortality, and duration of follow-up. Studies were grouped according to the risk of cardiovascular events (high risk and moderate risk). Meta-analytic techniques were used to analyze the data.

DATA SYNTHESIS:

We identified **11 studies that included a total of 39,044 patients**. The studies included patients after recent myocardial infarction, those with an implanted cardioverter defibrillator, and patients with heart failure, peripheral vascular disease, and hypercholesterolemia. The average dose of EPA/DHA was 1.8 +/- 1.2 g/day and the mean duration of follow-up was 2.2 +/- 1.2 years. **Dietary supplementation with omega-3 fatty acids significantly reduced the risk of cardiovascular deaths, sudden cardiac death, all-cause mortality, and nonfatal cardiovascular events.** The mortality benefit was largely due to the studies which enrolled high risk patients, while the reduction in nonfatal cardiovascular events was noted in the moderate risk patients (secondary prevention only). **Meta-regression failed to demonstrate a relationship between the daily dose of omega-3 fatty acid and clinical outcome.**

CONCLUSIONS:

Dietary supplementation with omega-3 fatty acids should be considered in the secondary prevention of cardiovascular events. (Marik et al, 2009)

Omega-3 supplements don't lower heart disease risk

By Alice Park @aliceparkny Sept. 12, 2012

If you want to protect your heart, stick to exercise and a healthy diet, and pass on the fish oil pills, says a new study.

For years, doctors and health experts have recommended taking fish oil supplements, rich in omega-3 fatty acids, to lower the risk of heart disease. But **the latest study on the issue — an analysis of previous clinical trials on the effects of omega-3s — shows that the supplements don't lower users' risks of heart attack, stroke, sudden death or death from heart disease or any cause.** Although the rates of these events were lower among those taking omega-3 supplements compared with those not taking them, **the differences were not statistically meaningful**, the authors said.

It's not the first time that the cardiovascular benefits of fish oil have been questioned: another recent analysis of previous research found that the supplements didn't prevent heart attack or stroke in people with heart disease. (Separately, **other research has suggested that that pills have little effect on boosting memory in Alzheimer's patients, reducing symptoms of the disease or improving thinking and verbal skills compared with placebo.**)

In the current analysis, published in the *Journal of the American Medical Association* and led by Dr. Moses Elisaf of the Lipid Disorders Clinic at the University Hospital of Ioannina in Greece, the scientists **reviewed 20 studies** dating back to 1989 that involved 68,680 participants. Volunteers in the studies, most of whom were heart patients, were randomly assigned to take either 1.5 g of omega-3 supplementation or a placebo every day for about two years. They were followed for heart events, including death, heart attack and stroke.

While the omega-3 users showed a 9% lower rate of heart-related death compared with the controls, and an 11% lower rate of heart attack, these differences were too small to attribute to the omega-3 pills.

The findings may lead to some confusion among people — both heart patients and those who are healthy but trying to avoid heart disease — who may be taking omega-3 supplements daily.

While some early studies did show a significant benefit from taking fish oil pills, data from newer clinical trials weakened that effect. That may be because at least one early, important study did not blind participants or researchers, meaning that everyone knew who was taking omega-3s or placebo. Further, inconsistencies between the included trials, such as the dosages of supplement used or preexisting conditions among participants, may have contributed to the discouraging findings.

Much other past data showing benefits of omega-3s also came from studies that did not randomize participants into fish oil and placebo groups, and instead retrospectively compared heart events in people who chose to consume more omega-3 fats than others.

Another reason the current study failed to find a benefit may be that more people are using better treatments for heart disease these days, including cholesterol-lowering statin drugs. Elisaf says he wasn't able to eliminate the potential influence of these medications in lowering rates of heart attack and death from heart disease overall. "We need more data in order to have a clear answer about the role of omega-3 fatty acid supplementation in everyday clinical practice," he says.

The authors acknowledge that additional research may help determine whether omega-3 supplements may still benefit people depending on their individual risk of heart disease, or if their diets are low in foods that are naturally rich in the fatty acids.

Currently the **American Heart Association (AHA)** advises people with high triglyceride levels to eat more fatty fish — the omega-3s in oily fish help boost good cholesterol and lower triglycerides — but to discuss supplementation with their doctor if they can't get enough from their diet. **The organization does not recommend the pills in general as a way to protect the heart.**

Both the AHA and many doctors recommend eating more fish, however: everyone, including healthy people and heart patients, should eat at least two servings of fish per week to benefit from the omega-3 fats. "If people are taking supplements because their physician prescribed them, they should consult with their physician before stopping," says Dr. Donna Arnett, president of the AHA and professor of epidemiology at the University of Alabama at Birmingham. "But I would tell them they should not stop eating fish. **The results of this study are about dietary supplements. So dietary sources of omega-3s may be different than supplements. They should not assume that dietary sources are not useful.**"

Which means that the advice you've been hearing all along remains the same — eat more fish. It's good for your heart.

Read more: http://healthland.time.com/2012/09/12/omega-3-supplements-dont-lower-heart-disease-risk-after-all/#ixzz2Z52mP3rl

Fish Oil for Heart Attack Prevention: Is It a Myth?

A new study finds that **omega-3 fatty acids don't help patients with heart disease avoid future heart-related problems**.

By Alice Park @aliceparkny April 10, 2012

Fish has long been a staple of healthy eating, since it's packed with omega-3 fatty acids and antioxidants that can help protect against heart disease and cancer. In fact, experts are so convinced of the benefits of the omega-3s in fish that health officials recently recommended Americans eat more of it — about 8 ounces, or two to three servings, of fish a week — in its latest revision of the Dietary Guidelines for Americans.

But what about fish oil capsules? Doctors have also believed that taking omega-3s as supplements can offer a similar protective benefit to the heart. But **a new 2012 study published in the *Archives of Internal Medicine* throws the theory into doubt: according to the analysis of 14 controlled trials in which nearly 20,500 patients with a history of heart disease were randomly assigned to take omega-3 supplements or placebo, those taking the fatty acid pills had about the same rates of heart disease, death from heart attacks, congestive heart failure and stroke as those on placebo.**

To date, the studies on omega-3 fatty acids and recurrent heart problems have been **contradictory: some have shown that heart patients taking omega-3 supplements had a lower risk of heart attack and heart-related death than those not taking them, but others have shown no such benefit.** The difference may have to do with how some of the earlier studies were set up, says one of the current study's co-authors, Seung-Kwon Myung from Seoul National University. In some trials, the participants knew they were taking omega-3 supplements, and they might have had a bias toward seeing a benefit because of this knowledge. (Myung did not include these types of unblinded trials in his analysis.) "I think the beneficial effects of omega-3 supplementation shown in those trials are not reliable," says Myung.

Still, Myung's findings don't necessarily mean that omega-3s — the study looked at the fatty acids EPA (eicosapentaenoic acid) and DHA (docosahexaenoic acid) — are useless when it comes to preventive health. Indeed, **the American Heart Association (AHA) recommends that both heart patients and those who don't yet have heart disease eat fatty fish at least two times a week, and if they can't consume that much fish, then to boost their omega-3 intake with supplements.**

According to the American Heart Association (AHA), studies show that omega-3 fatty acids can decrease the risk of abnormal heartbeats, keep triglyceride levels down and inhibit the build up of atherosclerotic plaques in the heart's blood vessels.

It's possible, says Myung, that natural sources of omega-3 fatty acids may be more potent than supplements. "**I recommend heart patients (as well as healthy people) not to take omega-3 fatty acid supplements because there is no evidence of those beneficial effects against cardiovascular disease**," he says. "However, I recommend at least two servings per week of fish because it has been reported that fish consumption has the preventive effect for cardiovascular disease based on the previous observational studies."

It's also possible that Myung and his colleagues failed to see a strong positive effect from omega-3 supplements among people with pre-existing heart disease because these patients may need a higher level of omega-3s to see benefit. The researchers looked at a range of doses of EPA and DHA, but perhaps a scarred, damaged heart that has survived a heart attack or angina is affected differently by omega-3 fatty acids than an intact and healthy heart.

As Harvard researchers Drs. Frank Hu and JoAnn Manson also point out in a commentary accompanying the new study, it's possible too that drugs like statins may mask the benefit from fish oils because the medications are so much more powerful. That may also explain why older trials have tended to show a fish oil benefit, while newer ones have not.

Either way, there's no downside to eating more fish, which happens to be a good source of protein that's far lower in saturated fat than red meat. So while it may not help heart patients avoid another heart event, it probably won't hurt them either.

Read more: http://healthland.time.com/2012/04/10/fish-oil-for-heart-attack-prevention-is-it-a-myth/#ixzz2Z54hOwLL

Omega-3: Fishing Out the Recent Evidence

JoAnn E. Manson, MD, DrPH

June 04, 2013

Dr. JoAnn Manson is Professor of Medicine at Brigham and Women's Hospital and Harvard Medical School. I'd like to talk today about the recent confusing reports on omega-3 fish oil. Is there a way for us to make sense of these recent studies that seem to be at odds with earlier evidence that suggested cardioprotection from omega-3 fatty acids? Have omega-3 fatty acids lost their luster, or are there other explanations for these recent findings?

There are several mechanisms through which omega-3 fatty acids may protect against cardiovascular disease, including reducing inflammation, lowering clotting risk, reducing triglyceride levels, and lowering the risk for irregular heart rhythms. However, **three recent randomized trials in high-risk populations (those with either multiple risk factors or a history of cardiovascular disease) have suggested very**

little benefit from omega-3 fatty acids. (Roncaglioni, Tombesi et al, 2013) (Kotwal et al, 2012) (Rizos et al, 2012) (

Disappointing Results From Omega-3 Fatty Acids Trials

(cardiovascular risk factors) by JoAnn Manson, *Medscape*. Jun 04, 2013

A recent report was published in the *New England Journal of Medicine* in early May 2013. Patients with multiple cardiovascular risk factors were given 1 gram of fish oil per day vs placebo, and it showed no benefit. (Roncaglioni, Tombesi et al, 2013)

Also, other meta-analyses have been published in the past year that looked at all of the randomized trials in aggregate. These are secondary-prevention, randomized trials with high-risk populations. In general, these meta-analyses have shown disappointing results. (Kotwal et al, 2012) (Rizos et al, 2012)

It is very important to keep in mind that these high-risk populations -- secondary-prevention populations -- include many individuals who are already taking multiple heart medications such as statins, aspirin, and ACE inhibitors, which may obscure the effect of omega-3 fatty acids. There may be very little incremental benefit from omega-3 fatty acids in that setting. What can we conclude from these recent findings?

What Should We Recommend to Our Patients?

First, these randomized trials of fish oil do not cast out on the recommendation to have at least 2 servings of dietary fish per week. That is a recommendation from the American Heart Association and many other professional societies, and many studies suggest benefit. Some of the benefit may be because dietary fish is replacing other foods that could increase risk, such as red meat or foods high in saturated fat. Do recommend at least 2 servings of fish per week, particularly the darker fatty fish such as salmon and mackerel.

Second, in patients who are candidates for prescription omega-3 fatty acids, **those who have very high triglyceride levels, these findings do not cast doubt on that indication for use. That would still be an appropriate use**. In patients who are taking fish oil and are doing very well on it and feel strongly that the fish oil is helping their symptoms or are a benefit to them, there is no strong basis from these studies for encouraging them to stop, because **there were no major risks associated with fish oil found in the studies.**

Trials in Primary Prevention and Other Outcomes

We need primary-prevention trials of omega-3 fatty acids in usual-risk general populations. We are doing such a trial, the VITAL (VITamin D and OmegA-3 TriaL) trial, at Brigham and Women's Hospital. (Manson et al, 2012)

It is a nationwide trial with more than 20,000 men and women, testing omega-3 fatty acids in primary prevention. We also need to look at other health outcomes where omega-3 fatty acids may be promising. Many of these outcomes will be looked at in the VITAL trial, including prevention of cognitive decline, depression, autoimmune diseases, diabetes, and eye diseases such as macular degeneration and dry eye syndrome.

But at present, the focus should be on increasing dietary fish intake. (Manson, 3013) (Omega-3: Fishing Out the Recent Evidence. *Medscape*. Jun 04, 2013)

Fish oil doesn't help prevent heart attacks

Published May 09, 2013

Eating fish is good for your heart but taking fish oil capsules does not help people at high risk of heart problems who are already taking medicines to prevent them, a large study in Italy found.

The work makes clearer who does and does not benefit from taking supplements of omega-3 fatty acids, the good oils found in fish such as salmon, tuna and sardines.

Previous studies have suggested that fish oil capsules could lower heart risks in people with heart failure or who have already suffered a heart attack. **The American Heart Association recommends them only for people who have high levels of fats called triglycerides in their blood**, says the group's president, Dr. Donna Arnett of the University of Alabama at Birmingham.

Fish oil capsules failed to prevent flare-ups of atrial fibrillation, a common heart rhythm problem, in a large study in 2010.

The new study was led by the Mario Negri Institute for Pharmacological Research in Milan. It tested 1 gram a day of **fish oil versus dummy capsules** in **12,513 people** throughout Italy. They had not suffered a heart attack but were at high risk of having one because of diabetes, high blood pressure, high cholesterol, smoking, obesity or other conditions. Most already were taking cholesterol-lowering statins, aspirin and other medicines to lower their chances of heart problems.

Researchers at first planned to compare the rate of death, heart attacks and strokes in the two groups, but these were less frequent than anticipated. So they started measuring how long it was before people in either group suffered one of these fates or was hospitalized for heart-related reasons. After five years, the rate was the same - about 12 percent of each group had one of these problems.

"They're very high-risk people and so the level of other treatments was very high," Arnett said. "When you're being aggressively treated for all of your other risk factors, **adding fish oil yielded no additional benefits."**

Results are published in the ***New England Journal of Medicine***. Makers of fish oil supplements helped pay for the study.

Eating fish is touted to help protect against heart disease, and **the Heart Association recommends it at least twice a week.**

"People who choose to eat more fish are more likely to eat heart healthier diets and engage in more physical activity," and studies testing the benefit of supplements may not be able to completely adjust for differences like these, said Alice Lichtenstein, director of the cardiovascular nutrition lab at Tufts University in Boston.

The results do show that **people can't rely on a pill to make up for a bad diet**, she said.

Polyunsaturated fatty acids as antioxidants

Abstract

The susceptibility of fatty acids to oxidation is thought to be directly dependent on their degree of unsaturation. However, some in vitro and in vivo studies suggest that the relation between chemical structure and susceptibility to oxidation is not as straightforward as hypothesized from theoretical viewpoints. Indeed, long chain polyunsaturated fatty acids (LC-PUFAs) might be less oxidizable than others under specific experimental conditions. We investigated the free radical-scavenging potential of PUFA and the production of reactive oxygen/nitrogen (ROS/RNS) species by human aortic endothelial cells (HAECs) supplemented with different fatty acids. **Fatty acid micelles scavenged superoxide in an unsaturation-dependent manner**, up to eicosapentaenoic acid, which was the most effective fatty acid. **Supplementation of HAEC with polyunsaturated fatty acids of the omega 3 series resulted in lower formation of ROS**, as compared with cells supplemented with saturates, monounsaturates, or polyunsaturates of the omega 6 series. This effect was maximal at concentrations of 10muM. The effects of omega 3 fatty acids on reactive species production appear to be stronger when ROS were evaluated, as a milder, albeit significant effect was observed on RNS generation. Based on in vivo data **showing reduced excretion of lipid peroxidation products after omega 3 intake and our data on ROS production and direct superoxide scavenging by LC-PUFAs**, notably those of the omega 3 series, we propose that this series of fatty acid might act as indirect anti- rather than pro-oxidant in vascular endothelial cells, hence diminishing inflammation and, in turn, **the risk of atherosclerosis and cardiovascular disease**. (Richard et al, 2008)

Other sources on omega-3 fish oil failed cardiovascular studies

Review: omega-3 polyunsaturated fatty acid supplements do not reduce major cardiovascular events in adults.

Review: **omega-3 fatty acid supplements provide no protective benefit in cardiovascular disease.** (Halim, Newby, 2912) (Smith, 2012)

Fish Beats Fish Oil Pills

After adjusting for several risk factors, **participants consuming 2 to 4 fish servings a week had a moderate but significant 6% lower risk for cerebrovascular disease compared with those having 1 or fewer fish servings a week.**

Participants eating 5 or more fish servings a week had a 12% lower risk. In a dose-response meta-analysis, an increment of 2 servings per week of any fish was associated with a 4% reduced risk for cerebrovascular disease.

In contrast, **there was no evidence for similar inverse associations with cerebrovascular disease for long-chain omega 3 fatty acids measured as circulating biomarkers in observational studies or fish oil supplements in primary and secondary prevention trials.**

"We expected to find significant associations for fish intake and long-chain omega 3 fatty acids (both biomarkers and intake)," Dr. Franco said. "The beneficial effect of fish intake on cerebrovascular risk is likely to be mediated through the interplay of a wide range of nutrients abundant in fish," he added.

It is possible, the researchers say, that eating more fish curbs the intake of other foods, such as red meat, that may be detrimental to vascular health; or higher fish intake may simply be an indicator of a generally healthier diet or higher socioeconomic status, both associated with better vascular health.

Having 1 or 2 Weekly Servings "Reasonable" Advice

The current findings are "in line with disappointing results" from controlled trials of supplementation with long-chain omega 3 fatty acids for the prevention of CHD, say the coauthors of a commentary published with the study.

"It seems that the additional benefit of supplementation in patients who are optimally managed may be small," write Janette de Goede and Johanna M Geleijnse, PhD, of the Division of Human Nutrition, Wageningen University, the Netherlands.

On the basis of available evidence, it is "reasonable to advise people that eating one or two portions of fish a week could reduce the risk of CHD and stroke," they write.

"Any benefit of long chain omega 3 fatty acid supplementation for the secondary prevention of CHD and stroke is likely to be small," they conclude. "However, it is possible that patients who are less than optimally medically treated or who have additional risk factors (for example, as a result of comorbidities such as diabetes) may benefit." Please remember that some studies have shown an increased risk for type 2 diabetes from fish oil.

Vitamins don't lower heart risks in men: FISH OIL STUDIES

11-5-12 LOS ANGELES (AP) — Multivitamins might help lower the risk for cancer in healthy older men but **do not affect their chances of developing heart disease**, new research suggests.

Two other studies found fish oil didn't work for an irregular heartbeat condition called atrial fibrillation, even though it is thought to help certain people with heart disease or high levels of fats called triglycerides in their blood.

The bottom line: Dietary supplements have varied effects and whether one is right for you may depend on your personal health profile, diet and lifestyle.

"Many people take vitamin supplements as a crutch," said study leader Dr. Howard Sesso of Brigham and Women's Hospital in Boston. **"They're no substitute for a heart-healthy diet, exercising, not smoking, keeping your weight down," especially for lowering heart risks.**

The studies were presented at an American Heart Association conference in Los Angeles.

A separate analysis released in connection with the meeting showed that **at least 1 in 3 baby boomers who are in good shape will eventually develop heart problems or have a stroke.** The upside is that that will happen about seven years later than for their less healthy peers.

The study is "a wake-up call that this disease is very prevalent in the United States and even if you're doing a good job, you're not immune," said Dr. Vincent Bufalino, a Chicago-area cardiologist and spokesman for the American Heart Association.

The findings came in an analysis of five major studies involving nearly **50,000 adults aged 45 and older who were followed for up to 50 years.**

The research was published online by the **Journal of the American Medical Association**, along with the vitamin paper and one fish oil study.

Multivitamins are America's favorite dietary supplement. About one-third of adults take them. Yet **no government agency recommends their routine use for preventing chronic diseases,** and few studies have tested them to see if they can.

A leading preventive medicine task force even recommends against beta-carotene supplements, alone or with other vitamins, to prevent cancer or heart disease because some studies have found them harmful. And vitamin K can affect bleeding and interfere with some commonly used heart drugs.

Sesso's study involved nearly 15,000 healthy male doctors given monthly packets of Centrum Silver or fake multivitamins. After about 11 years, there were no differences between the groups in heart attacks, strokes, chest pain, heart failure or heart-related deaths.

Side effects were fairly similar except for **more rashes among vitamin users.** The National Institutes of Health paid for most of the study. Pfizer Inc. supplied the pills and other companies supplied the packaging.

The same study found that **multivitamins cut the chance of developing cancer by 8 percent — a modest amount and less than what can be achieved from a good diet, exercise and not smoking.**

Multivitamins also may have different results in women or people less healthy than those in this study — only 4 percent smoked, for example.

The fish-oil studies tested prescription-strength omega-3 capsules from several **companies in two different groups of people for preventing atrial fibrillation, a fluttering, irregular heartbeat.**

One study from South America aimed to prevent recurrent episodes in 600 participants who already had the condition. The other sought to prevent it from developing in 1,500 people from the U.S., Italy and Argentina having various types of heart surgery, such as valve replacement. About one third of heart-surgery patients develop atrial fibrillation as a complication.

Both studies found fish oil ineffective.

http://news.yahoo.com/study-vitamins-dont-lower-heart-risks-men-170444420.html

Is This Crowded Fish Bowl of Fish Oil Treatments About to Crack?

By Leo Sun October 16, 2013

AstraZeneca's (NYSE:AZN _) problems, which I discussed in a previous article, are well documented. Generic competition for the antipsychotic Seroquel and the antacid Nexium have taken a bite out of its top line, and the upcoming patent expiration of its cholesterol drug, Crestor, threatens to exacerbate its losses.

To offset these top line declines, AstraZeneca is reaching out into other therapies. An interesting one is **Epanova, a fish oil treatment for very high levels of fatty triglycerides** in the blood. High levels of triglycerides, defined as levels of over 500 mg/dL, can cause high blood pressure, high blood glucose levels, obesity, and low levels of HDL ("good") cholesterol -- leading to the increased risk of heart disease, diabetes, and stroke.

Last month, AstraZeneca announced that the Food and Drug Administration had accepted Epanova for review, with a final decision expected by next May. AstraZeneca acquired Epanova from Omthera Pharmaceuticals, which it acquired earlier this year for $443 million. Decision Resources analyst Paramjit Narang believes that Epanova has blockbuster potential and could hit peak sales of $1 billion.

Could Epanova be one of the new drugs that could help balance out AstraZeneca's drug portfolio, or will this be another pipeline failure to pile on top of its failed rheumatoid arthritis treatment, prostate cancer drug, and experimental antidepressant?

Understanding the fish oil market

The market for fish oil treatments for high triglycerides is a narrow one at the moment, dominated by **GlaxoSmithKline**'s (NYSE: GSK _) Lovaza, which was approved in 2004 and generated revenue of $970 million in 2012. **Lovaza has a key weakness, however -- it raises LDL ("bad") cholesterol levels as it lowers triglycerides**. In addition, a recent decision in Delaware reversed a critical court ruling from 2009 that had blocked Par Pharmaceutical and **Teva Pharmaceutical** (NYSE: TEVA _) from manufacturing generic versions of Lovaza. As a result, Par and Teva could soon start selling generic Lovaza, and cause the price of fish oil treatments to fall.

Amarin (NASDAQ: AMRN _), whose sole marketed product is the competing fish oil treatment Vascepa, is another company to watch. Vascepa, which was approved last July, doesn't increase LDL cholesterol levels like Lovaza and Epanova. Vascepa is also being tested on patients with lower levels of triglycerides (higher than 200 mg/dL but lower than 500 mg/dL), which could expand the market for the drug to an additional 36 million patients. Unfortunately, a recent FDA report prompted Amarin to disclose that the eagerly anticipated results from this trial would not be available until 2016. Shares plunged 20% after the announcement on Oct. 11.

Lovaza and Vascepa are both currently approved for patients with "very high" triglyceride levels higher than 500 mg/dL -- the same market that AstraZeneca is targeting with Epanova.

Although analysts had originally projected peak sales of $1.5 billion for Vascepa, the drug only generated $5.5 million in sales for Amarin last quarter. The major problem is that Amarin lacks a larger pharmaceutical partner to help it market the drug. With a proper partner, Citi Investment Research believes that sales of Vascepa could hit $2.6 billion. However, that figure looks silly considering the challenges it could face from Lovaza and upcoming generic versions.

How does Epanova fit into AstraZeneca's strategy?

In a phase 3 study, Epanova notably lowered levels of non-HDL cholesterol when administered with a cholesterol-lowering statin treatment (such as AstraZeneca's own Crestor). Non-HDL cholesterol consists of LDL and VLDL cholesterol, both "bad" types of cholesterol. When combined with a statin, Epanova reduced levels of VLDL cholesterol by 14% to 22%, based on the dosage, whereas the increase in LDL levels dropped from 5% to 1% on the same dosage. By itself, Epanova raises LDL levels, just like Lovaza.

AstraZeneca believes that with this study, it could win regulatory approval for a fixed-dose combination of Epanova with Crestor, which will lose patent exclusivity in 2016. Crestor is one of AstraZeneca's remaining pillars of revenue, achieving peak sales of $7 billion in 2011 and generating $6.3 billion in sales last year.

Crestor is the last blockbuster statin treatment that is still patent protected. The past decade was considered a golden age for statin-based cholesterol treatments, such as **Pfizer**'s Lipitor and **Merck**'s Zocor. These treatments generated billions of dollars in annual revenue for both companies before their market shares were swallowed up by generic competition.

However, AstraZeneca's attempt to combine a fish oil treatment with a statin could yield unpredictable results, considering statins' long list of side effects, which include muscle and liver damage, digestive problems, elevated blood sugar, and diabetes. However, **AstraZeneca knows that a Crestor-Epanova combo is really its only way to penetrate the fish oil market**, since the market could be saturated with generic Lovaza from Teva and Par by the time the FDA reaches a decision to approve Epanova next May, 2014.

A Foolish final thought

In the opinion of Leo Sun, Epanova or a Crestor-Epanova treatment will not be the game-changing treatment that AstraZeneca hopes it will be.

GlaxoSmithKline's Lovaza will probably never exceed the $1 billion blockbuster threshold, due to Teva and Par's inevitable generic versions. Those generics will flatten pricing across a narrow market. Meanwhile, Amarin's Vascepa might be a safer treatment, but it is neglected by larger companies, and doesn't have the marketing muscle to compete against the likes of GlaxoSmithKline, Teva, and Par. The potential indication of Vascepa for patients with high triglyceride levels is now pushed back to 2016 -- which renders it completely irrelevant as far as investors are concerned.

Therefore, AstraZeneca is diving into a very crowded fish bowl of fish oil treatments, which is on the verge of cracking. Investors should be concerned, and not excited, about the amount of money and time AstraZeneca is investing in this project, which simply appears to be a way to extend the life of Crestor.

HYPERTENSION

Omega-3 does not change blood pressure

The effects of omega-3 on blood pressure and the relationship between serum visfatin level and blood pressure in patients with type II diabetes.

Abstract

BACKGROUND:

Hypertension is a condition normally detected in people with type II diabetes. It eventually leads to cardiovascular diseases in the patient. Visfatin is an adipocytokine which is secreted from adipose tissue and can affect the inflammatory reaction and also serum lipid levels. Additionally, omega-3 inhibits the accumulation of fat and formation of insulin resistance. The current study tried to investigate the effects of omega-3 on blood pressure compared to placebo and the relationship between serum visfatin levels and blood pressure.

METHODS:

A total number of 71 women with type II diabetes were randomly assigned to 2 groups to receive either omega-3 capsules or placebo capsules. In the first step, a questionnaire consisting age, height, weight, waist and hip circumferences, and systolic and diastolic blood pressure was filled out for each subject. Blood samples were then collected for laboratory tests. The next step was to conduct 8 weeks of intervention. All variables, except age, were measured again after the intervention. Hip circumference was considered as the maximum circumference of the buttocks. Waist circumference was measured by placing a tape horizontally across the abdomen at the end of a normal exhalation. Laboratory tests included the assessment of visfatin, glucose, and glycated hemoglobin (HbA1c) concentrations. Lipid profile, i.e. low density lipoprotein (LDL), high density lipoprotein (HDL), triglyceride (TG), and cholesterol, was also assessed. Using SPSS18, data obtained from the study was analyzed by a variety of appropriate statistical tests.

RESULTS:

There was a significant change in mean differences of systolic and diastolic blood pressure. Blood pressure showed a significant reduction in the omega-3 group compared to the placebo group. However, **In type II diabetes, no significant changes were observed in systolic and diastolic blood pressure before and after daily consumption of omega-3 capsules.**

CONCLUSION:

Based on the results of this study, a daily consumption of omega-3 is suggested for patients with type II diabetes. (Hosseinzadeh et al, 2012). **RMH Note: this is contrary to the opinion of others.**

Omega-3 does not block inflammation or oxidative stress in hemodialysis patients

Effects of marine omega-3 fatty acids on serum systemic and vascular inflammation markers and oxidative stress in hemodialysis patients.

Abstract

BACKGROUND AND AIMS:

High concentrations of serum inflammation markers, especially vascular inflammation markers, are an important risk factor for cardiovascular diseases in hemodialysis patients. The present study was designed to investigate the effects of marine omega-3 fatty acids on serum systemic and vascular inflammation markers and oxidative stress in hemodialysis patients.

METHODS:

Thirty-four hemodialysis patients were randomly assigned to either the marine omega-3 fatty acid or the placebo group. Patients in the omega-3 fatty acid group received 2,080 mg marine omega-3 fatty acids daily for 10 weeks, whereas the placebo group received a corresponding placebo. At baseline and the end of week 10, 5 ml blood was collected after a 12- to 14-hour fast.

RESULTS:

Mean serum soluble intercellular adhesion molecule type I (sICAM-1) decreased significantly in the omega-3 fatty acid group at the end of week 10 compared to baseline ($p < 0.05$) and this reduction was significant in comparison with the placebo group ($p < 0.05$). No significant differences were observed between the two groups in mean changes in serum soluble vascular cell adhesion molecule type 1, sE-selectin, sP-selectin, C-reactive protein, interleukin-6, tumor necrosis factor-α, malondialdehyde and total antioxidant capacity.

CONCLUSION:

The results of the present study indicate that, in hemodialysis patients, 2,080 mg marine omega-3 fatty acids can reduce serum sICAM-1, a risk factor for cardiovascular diseases, but **it has no effect on serum systemic inflammation markers and oxidative stress in hemodialysis patients.** (Kooshki et al, 2011)

SECTION FOUR

MENTAL HEALTH

True headlines in 2012 have read, "Soy Provides Women With No Additional Cognitive Benefits" and "Fish Oils Don't Help Ward Off Dementia." **In a 2012 review by the Cochrane Library, researchers found participants taking omega-3 scored no better in standard tests of memory and mental performance than a placebo.** They called the studies "disappointing."

"Disappointing" is the word that have been used repeatedly in describing the numerous failed studies involving antioxidant supplements. Please refer to my section at the end of the book on my "companion books."

What's so special about the Mediterranean diet?

For years the marketing and promotion of dietary supplements that claim to enhance memory have left many people confused and wary. Now recent evidence-based research reported in the Annals of Neurology suggests that **people who closely follow the Mediterranean diet have a 40 percent lower risk of Alzheimer's disease**. The takeaway: **The food you eat, not the pills, can prevent or slow the rate of cognitive decline**. (Johns Hopkins Newsletter, August 2013)

How does stress affect memory?

We all know that living a stress-filled life is unhealthy. Turns out stress is worse for us than we thought. Johns Hopkins researchers have linked high levels of the stress hormone cortisol with poor cognitive performance in older adults. And another study, reported in the journal Neurology, found that **depressed and anxious people are 40 percent more likely to develop mild cognitive impairment**. In this fascinating section, Dr. Rabins provides key "stress erasers" - proactive steps you can take to reduce the stress in your life. Dr. Peter V. Rabins is an acclaimed author and geriatric psychiatrist at Johns Hopkins - and one of the nation's leading experts on the care and management of patients with Alzheimer's disease and other forms of dementia. http://www.johnshopkinshealthalerts.com/

Diets lacking omega-3s lead to anxiety, hyperactivity in teens

Main Category: Nutrition / Diet

July 31, 2013

Diets lacking omega-3 fatty acids - found in foods like wild fish, eggs, and grass-fed livestock - can have worsened effects over consecutive generations, especially affecting teens, according to a University of Pittsburgh study.

Published in *Biological Psychiatry,* the Pitt team found that in a rodent model **second-generation deficiencies of omega-3s caused elevated states of anxiety and hyperactivity in adolescents and affected the teens' memory and cognition**.

"We have always assumed that stress at this age is the main environmental insult that contributes to developing these conditions in at-risk individuals but this study indicates that nutrition is a big factor, too," said Bita Moghaddam, lead author of the paper and professor of neuroscience in the Kenneth P. Dietrich School of Arts and Sciences. "We found that this dietary deficiency can compromise the behavioral health of adolescents, not only because their diet is deficient but because their parents' diet was deficient as well. This is of particular concern because adolescence is a very vulnerable time for developing psychiatric disorders including schizophrenia and addiction."

Performing experiments in rats in Moghaddam's laboratory, **the research team examined a "second generation" of omega-3-deficient diets, mimicking present-day adolescents**. Parents of many of today's teens were born in the 1960s and 1970s, a time period in which omega-3-deficient oils like corn and soy oil became prevalent, and farm animals moved from eating grass to grain. Since omega-3s are present in grass and algae, much of today's grain-fed cattle contain less of these essential fatty acids.

The Pitt team administered a set of behavioral tasks to study the learning and memory, decision making, anxiety, and hyperactivity of both adults and adolescents. Although subjects appeared to be in general good physical health, there were behavioral deficiencies in adolescents that were more pronounced in second-generation subjects with omega-3 deficiencies. Overall, these adolescents were more anxious and hyperactive, learned at a slower rate, and had impaired problem-solving abilities.

"**Our study shows that, while the omega-3 deficiency influences the behavior of both adults and adolescents, the nature of this influence is different between the age groups**," said Moghaddam. "We observed changes in areas of the brain responsible for decision making and habit formation."

The team is now exploring epigenetics as a potential cause. This is a process in which environmental events influence genetic information. Likewise, the team is exploring markers of inflammation in the brain since omega-3 deficiencies causes an increase of omega-6 fats, which are proinflammatory molecules in the brain and other tissues.

"It's remarkable that a relatively common dietary change can have **generational effects**," said Moghaddam. "It indicates that our diet does not merely affect us in the short-term but also can affect our offspring."

University of Pittsburgh. (Moghaddam, 2013) (Bondi et al, 2013)

The cult of omega-3

By Brendan O'Neill

March 1, 2010 **Hardly a week goes by without a new health claim being made of eating oily fish.** But is it really as magical as we are told?

If there were a top 40 of good foods, a chart rundown of the right things to eat, then anything containing omega-3 fatty acids would have been number one for years. **They even have their own international awareness day.**

Omega-3 is the name given to a family of unsaturated fatty acids found mainly in oily fish, such as salmon, herring, sardines and anchovies, and also in eggs, meat, milk and cheese.

There's no evidence that omega-3 reduces the risk of death or heart attack or stroke or anything like that in those of us who have not recently had a heart attack - Dr. Lee Hooper. (Hooper *et al.*, 2006)

The naturally occurring acids of the omega-3 family can allegedly boost our brain power, keep our hearts healthy, strengthen our bones, and much more. You can ingest the fatty acids by eating a lot of the right kind of fish or by taking fish oil supplements - little golden capsules rich in omega-3.

Hardly a week goes by without yet another media report on "The wonders of omega-3 fatty acids" (as a headline in Canada put it).

Last month it was reported omega-3 can protect against psychotic disorders such a schizophrenia. An international team of researchers gave a daily dose to 81 people deemed to be at risk from psychosis and found **it seemed to cut the rate of psychotic illness - including schizophrenia - by 25%. RMH Note: other studies failed to support this result.**

But how much of this is hype, and how much reality? Is there a danger that a largely fish-derived fatty acid is being turned into a modern-day magic potion?

Dietician Evelyn Tribole is a firm believer in their potency.

Packaging tag

"While it can seem that omega-3s do everything but wash your windows, it's important to remember that **they are essential nutrients**", says Ms Tribole, author of **The Ultimate Omega-3 Diet: Maximize the Power of Omega-3s to Supercharge Your Health, Battle Inflammation, and Keep Your Mind Sharp.**

She says **modern forms of food production are reducing the amount of omega-3 in our foods, "contributing to a global omega-3 fat deficiency in the diets of most people**".

"For example, animals that graze on grass have higher omega-3 contents in their meat - and the longer they are out to pasture, the more omega-3s accumulate in their meat. But today the great majority of animals dine on **[corn grain], which is devoid of omega-3s**."

That is bad, she says, because "remarkable and consistent" scientific studies show us omega-3 is good for brain function, mood disorders, heart health and more. And she dismisses the claim that this is just a fad.

"Yes, food and nutrition seem to run in fashionable trends, with followers and believers. In this case, however, there is a lot of good evidence for the benefits of omega-3s."

But **others are skeptical**.

Dr Lee Hooper, lead author of one of the most thorough studies on the apparent benefits of omega-3, published in the British Medical Journal in 2006, urges people not to get "carried away". (Hooper *et al.*, 2006)

The interest in omega-3 has snowballed over the past decade, giving rise to more and more scientific studies, books about how omega-3 can make you **super-healthy**, and government- and corporate-funded omega-3 promotion groups, such as **the Omega-3 International Awareness Day and The Omega-3 Group in Scotland.**

Evidence wanting

Over the past 10 years, about 12,500 scientific studies on the benefits of omega-3 have been published, both reflecting and reinforcing the fashion for consuming this apparent super-food. **Today, everything from loaves of bread to frozen fish fingers come with a "RICH IN OMEGA-3" tag**.

Yet the "systematic review" carried out by Dr Hooper's team shows the claims are often as fishy as the omega-3-rich foods themselves. (Hooper *et al.*, 2004) (Hooper *et al.*, 2006)

"According to the evidence we have so far, omega-3 does not seem to help for cancer prevention or treatment; with children's learning or behavior; with cognitive function; or in preventing cognitive decline with age or mental health problems, including bipolar disease, schizophrenia."

Similarly, there's "no evidence that the fatty acids assist with cystic fibrosis, allergies, asthma, ulcerative colitis, Crohn's disease, or kidney disease".

Dr Hooper's study found evidence omega-3 improves children's learning abilities and behavior to be "very poor".

On the plus side, "omega-3 probably does help with arthritis, pain and stiffness," Dr. Hooper says. **And it definitely seems useful for people recovering from a heart attack.**

It's beneficial for those who have had a heart attack because **research shows that the "long-chain fatty acids" in the omega-3 family get into the membranes of our cells, helping to "improve the heart's electrical activity" and reduce blood pressure**, among other things.

Trendy nutrient

Crucially, though, **this doesn't mean those who have not had a heart attack can reduce their risk of having one by consuming omega-3,** says Dr Hooper.

"There's no evidence that omega-3 reduces the risk of death or heart attack or stroke or anything like that in those of us who have not recently had a heart attack," Dr. Hooper says.

Dr Hooper says **her aim is not to generate a backlash against a trendy nutrient, but simply to get to the truth about its limited benefits**.

But if so many of the claims are just hype, how did it get to that stage? Why are so many benefits laid at the door of omega-3?

Dr Hooper says believes **the fashion for omega-3 betrays our herd-instinct** - how, "as a group", we periodically get overexcited about certain foodstuffs. There always seems to be some "new food panacea" to our problems, she says.

Another doctor, Michael Fitzpatrick, says the omega-3 fad is just the flipside of the anti-junk food campaign. Just as we see certain kinds of "junk food" as "morally and constitutionally corruptive", we tend to elevate other foods as **"saviors of human health".**

So much so, says Dr Fitzpatrick, GP and author of *The Tyranny of Health*, that today **there is almost a "cult of omega-3".**

TIME.com: Omega-3s as study aid?

Prostate cancer is the most common cancer in men, and while the latest statistics show that most men will eventually develop prostate cancer if they live long enough, only a specific type of cancer, known as high-grade, carries high risk of serious health problems.

While a quarter of a million Americans are diagnosed with prostate cancer each year, only about 30,000 of those cases are fatal, and almost all of them involve high-grade cancer. The latest research found that the association between omega-3s and prostate cancer held for both high- and low-grade prostate cancers.

It's not that omega-3s are harmful, but that the fatty acids may have more complex effects on the body than previously thought.

"We have this tendency to talk about good foods and bad foods, good nutrients and bad nutrients," says Doctor Theodore Brasky, a research assistant professor at The Ohio State University Comprehensive Cancer Center and the study's head author.

The **nutrients commonly found in fish fight potentially damaging inflammation, but they may also increase oxidative damage to the DNA in cells**, similar to the effects of stress, that can create fertile ground for cancers to grow.

TIME.com: Omega-3 supplements do not lower heart disease risk

The study measured omega-3 blood levels in the participating men, and did not include information on the volunteers' eating habits, so researchers could not differentiate between the effects of fatty acids from fish from those of supplements.

However, the overwhelming majority of the participants did not take fish oil supplements.

Based on the results, Brasky says that men with a family history of prostate cancer should discuss with their doctor whether fish oil supplements are safe for them, since these pills tend to contain concentrated doses of omega-3 — **supplements contain between 30% to 60% of a serving of fish, and if a fish oil supplement is taken everyday, that adds up to a lot of daily fish oil**. Brasky also suggested that men cut down on their fatty fish intake, though not eliminate it entirely.

Andrew Vickers, a statistician specializing in prostate cancer at Memorial Sloan-Kettering Cancer Center, agrees, saying that **fish oil supplements may pose a relatively higher risk for prostate cancer than fish in the diet**.

"The problem comes when you take components of a diet and put it in a pill," Vickers says.

TIME.com: Omega-3s may not protect brain health

Most health experts recommend that people try to eat a healthy, balanced diet to protect against diseases and most cancers, and turn to supplements only if that's not possible, since supplements may provide only partial benefits.

That's why **the American Cancer Society does not currently recommend that men take fish oil supplements**, according to Marjorie McCullough, the society's strategic director of nutritional epidemiology.

Brasky's work isn't the first to suggest that omega-3 fatty acids may have both positive and negative effects on the body.

In a September 2012 article in the Journal of the American Medical Association, researchers found that omega-3 supplements were not associated with lower risks of stroke or cardiac death.

Those results were confirmed by another study in the New England Journal of Medicine that showed omega-3 supplements did not reduce risk of dying from a heart event among a group of people at high risk of heart disease.

Researchers involved in those studies, however, acknowledged that they were not able to account for the effect of other medications to treat heart problems, such as cholesterol-lowering drugs and blood pressure medications, in keeping death rates down. In the same way, more research will have to tease apart how other nutrients in a balanced diet — including antioxidants — work together to influence the effect of individual nutrients like omega-3 fatty acids.

Omega-3 fatty acids are highly concentrated in the brain

Omega-3 fatty acids are highly concentrated in the brain and supplements had appeared to be important for cognitive (brain memory and performance) and behavioral function. Allegedly, infants who do not get enough omega-3 fatty acids from their mothers during pregnancy are at risk for developing vision and nerve problems. Symptoms of omega-3 fatty acid deficiency include fatigue, poor memory, dry skin, heart problems, mood swings or depression, and poor circulation.

Large population studies had suggested that getting omega-3 fatty acids in the diet, primarily from fish, helps protect against stroke caused by plaque buildup and blood clots in the arteries that lead to the brain. Eating at least 2 servings of fish per week was thought to reduce the risk of stroke by as much as 50%. But, more recent studies debunked the notion that fish oil prevented strokes.

However, **high doses of fish oil and omega-3 fatty acids may increase the risk of bleeding.**

People who eat more than 3 grams of omega-3 fatty acids per day (equivalent to 3 servings of fish per day) may have higher risk for hemorrhagic stroke, a potentially fatal type of stroke in which an artery in the brain leaks or ruptures.

Source: Omega-3 fatty acids | University of Maryland Medical Center http://umm.edu/health/medical/altmed/supplement/omega3-fatty-acids#ixzz2h9a77C2y

ALZHEIMER'S DISEASE

Omega-3s cross blood-brain barrier in Alzheimer's patients

(December 5, 2013. Medical News Today)

The blood-brain barrier protects the brain from harmful chemicals in the blood, but it also blocks drugs from reaching it. However, researchers have suggested that omega-3 fatty acid supplements can cross this barrier in Alzheimer's patients, influencing markers for the disease and inflammation.

The researchers, from the Karolinska Institutet in Sweden, have published their research in the ***Journal of Internal Medicine***.

They note that **omega-3s, along with other polyunsaturated fatty acids, accumulate in the central nervous system (CNS) throughout gestation**.

Although the prevailing belief is that these **fatty acids are repeatedly replaced throughout life**, the team says little is known about how this happens and whether diet changes can impact transportation of these acids across the blood-brain barrier.

According to the researchers, several diseases can change the fatty acid characteristics of the CNS. They cite **Alzheimer's disease patients, who normally have lower concentrations of an omega-3 called docosahexaenoic acid (DHA).**

Lead author Dr. Yvonne Freund-Levi says: "Earlier population studies indicate that omega-3 can protect against Alzheimer's disease, which makes it interesting to study the effects of dietary supplements containing this group of fatty acids in patients who have already developed the disease."

As part of a larger study - the OmegAD project, which follows 204 patients with Alzheimer's - the researchers assessed whether omega-3 supplements change the CNS fatty acid profile.

Researchers observed higher levels of fatty acids in the CNS of Alzheimer's patients who took omega-3 supplements, which suggests these acids crossed the blood-brain barrier.

A total of **33 individuals** took part in this recent study. Of these, 18 received an omega-3 supplement each day for 6 months, while 15 received a placebo during this time.

By the end of the study, the omega-3 group had higher levels of DHA and EPA (eicosapentaenoic acid, which is another omega-3) in their cerebrospinal fluid and blood, whereas the placebo group did not show any change.

Additionally, the researchers observed that the DHA levels corresponded with the degree of change in Alzheimer's disease and markers of inflammation in the cerebrospinal fluid.

The researchers say these observed changes suggest transfer of the fatty acids across the blood-brain barrier.

Prof. Jan Palmblad, another study author, notes that it was previously observed in animals that "DHA dietary supplements can lead to an increase in DHA concentrations in the CNS."

Previous attempts to treat Alzheimer's disease in humans using traditional anti-inflammatory drugs have not produced memory function improvements, the researchers note. But now that they have observed increased DHA concentrations in the central nervous system of humans, they are hopeful about future treatments for the disease.

"However," adds Prof. Palmblad, "much work remains to be done before we know how these fatty acids can be used in the treatment of Alzheimer's disease to halt memory loss."

Medical News Today recently reported on a study that suggested exercise is beneficial for dementia patients.

Fish Oil Fail: Omega-3s May Not Protect Brain

Fish Oil Fail: Omega-3s May Not Protect Brain Health After All

A meta-analysis finds that taking omega-3 supplements may not do much to preserve memory, but here's why the finding isn't the last word.

By Alexandra Sifferlin @acsifferlin June 13, 2012

Despite the widely touted benefits of omega-3 fatty acids for preserving cognitive function and memory, **a new review by the *Cochrane Library* finds that those effects may be overstated: healthy elderly people taking omega-3 supplements did no better on tests of thinking and verbal skills than those taking placebo.** http://summaries.cochrane.org/CD005379/fish-oils-for-the-prevention-of-dementia-in-older-people. Accessed 5-8-14.

A number of previous studies have associated omega-3 consumption with better brain health and a lower risk of Alzheimer's disease. **One recent study by Columbia University researchers found that people who ate diets higher in omega-3s had lower blood levels of beta amyloid**, the telltale protein that gums up brains in Alzheimer's patients.

In another 2012 study published in the journal *Neurology* in February, researchers showed that people with the highest levels of omega-3s in their blood had bigger brain volumes and performed better on tests of visual memory and abstract reasoning, compared with those with the lowest levels.

Much of this previous data has been observational, however.

So, for the *Cochrane* review, researchers looked specifically at so-called "gold standard" studies, those that randomly assigned people to take either omega-3s or a placebo and then tracked the participants over time. The authors of the review, from the London School of Hygiene & Tropical Medicine, included three studies involving a total of **3,536 people** over the age of 60, which lasted between six and 40 months. All the participants started the studies in good cognitive health.

In two studies, Cochrane researchers compared the effects of omega-3 (fish oil) capsules versus placebo capsules containing

olive or sunflower oil. In the third study, participants used either omega-3-fortified margarine or a regular margarine spread. In the end, the 2012 data showed that participants who got extra omega-3s performed no better on standard tests of mental abilities, memory or verbal fluency than those who took placebos.

The 2012 results of the available studies show no benefit for cognitive function with omega-3 PUFA supplementation among cognitively healthy older people. See more at: http://summaries.cochrane.org/CD005379/fish-oils-for-the-prevention-of-dementia-in-older-people#sthash.m6oXtAP4.dpuf. http://summaries.cochrane.org/CD005379/fish-oils-for-the-prevention-of-dementia-in-older-people. Accessed 5-8-14.

"Our analysis suggests that there is currently no evidence that omega-3 fatty acid supplements provide a benefit for memory or concentration in later life," says study co-author Alan Dangour, a nutritionist at the London School of Hygiene & Tropical Medicine. "We hope that people will use this new evidence to help inform their decisions on dietary supplement use."

Still, it's possible that the cognitive benefits of omega-3s may take longer than a few years — longer than the studies included in the review lasted — to show up. Cognitive decline and dementia may take several years to develop, and researchers saw very little mental decline in any of the study participants, so further research is needed to find out the longer-term effects of omega-3 supplementation.

It's also possible that taking omega-3 supplements may help only those who are low in the fatty acid to start with, while offering less benefit for those who already get enough through their regular diets.

None of this is to say that a diet naturally high in omega-3s — from fish, for example — isn't good for your health. The authors recommend that people eat two portions of fish a week, including one portion of oily fish. "The evidence of health benefits from the consumption of omega-3 fatty acids is strongest for heart health, but there may also be other health benefits," says Dangour.

What's good for the heart is also good for the brain, researchers say, so there are plenty of lifestyle changes you can make to help protect your cognitive health as you age: get regular exercise, eat well and keep your weight and blood pressure down.

Omega-3s Fail to Keep Aging Brains Sharp

Tia Ghose, September 25, 2013

Omega-3 fatty acids may not help keep the aging brain sharp, at least in older women, new research suggests.

Contrary to earlier studies, new research led by University of Iowa investigators suggests that omega-3 fatty acids may not benefit thinking skills. The study was published in the Sept. 25 online issue of *Neurology*, the medical journal of the American Academy of Neurology.

The study, published Sept. 25, 2013 in the journal **Neurology**, found that **there were no differences in the cognitive skills of older women who had high blood levels of the fatty acids compared with those whose levels were lower.**

"**Our study of omega-3 blood levels and cognitive function did not find a protective association in older, postmenopausal women**," study co-author Eric Ammann, a doctoral researcher in epidemiology at the University of Iowa, wrote in an email to LiveScience

Along with randomized trials also showing no effect, the findings suggest that omega-3s may not be the brain booster they were once thought to be, Ammann said.

The study involved 2,157 women age 65 to 80 who were enrolled in the Women's Health Initiative clinical trials of hormone therapy. The women were given annual tests of thinking and memory skills for an average of six years. Blood tests were taken to measure the amount of omega-3s in the participants' blood before the start of the study.

The researchers found no difference in cognitive skills between the women with high and low levels of omega-3s in the blood at the time of the first memory tests. There was also no difference between the two groups in how fast their thinking skills declined over time. (Ammann et al, 2013)

Brain booster?

Early studies found that **people who consumed more fish and nuts tended to have sharper minds and better memories than**

those who didn't. And **other studies found that omega-3 fatty acids reduce inflammation**, which is a risk factor for heart disease.

But a recent randomized trial found that people taking omega-3 supplements did not have a lower risk for cognitive decline or improvements in memory.

Ammann and his colleagues measured the blood levels of omega-3s in **2,157 women** ages 65 and older. The women completed a series of cognitive tests over five years, aimed at measuring their working memory, verbal skills and spatial ability.

The team found no differences over the course of the study in the cognitive function or decline of older women with high versus low levels of the fatty acid. That suggests the omega-3s were not providing a brain boost for the women, the researchers said. (Ammann et al, 2013)

While past studies suggested that people who eat more omega-3 rich foods do tend to have better brain function, "this might not be cause-and-effect," Ammann said.

"People who eat lots of fish or nuts, or who take omega-3 supplements, tend to be more affluent and health-conscious than those who don't," he said. Women in the study with higher levels of blood omega-3s also tended to eat more fish.

"They are also less likely to smoke, more likely to exercise, and have a lower body mass index," all factors that are separately tied to better brain health and health overall, Ammann said.

Omega-3 does not fight cognitive decline

September 27, 2013

There have been many studies advocating how omega-3 fatty acids can benefit our health. But a new study suggests that high levels of omega-3 are of no benefit to cognitive decline in older women.

Omega-3 polyunsaturated fatty acids (PUFAs) are types of fats commonly found in plant and marine life. Of particular interest to nutritionists and health care professionals are two types of omega-3 acids - DHA (docosahexaenoic acid) and EPA (eicosapentaenoic acid) - due to their rumored health benefits.

The acids are thought to play an important role in reducing inflammation throughout the body. And studies have shown numerous other health benefits, including the potential to prevent or delay cognitive decline. But researchers from the University of Iowa suggest otherwise.

Their study, published in 2013 in the journal ***Neurology*, involved 2,157 women** aged between 65 and 80, who were enrolled in the Women's Health Initiative clinical trials of hormone therapy. (Ammann et al, 2013)

The research team took blood tests from all women before the beginning of the study, in order to measure the amount of omega-3 present in their blood.

The study showed that **women who ate omega-3s did not perform better on memory tests, compared with women who had low levels of the fatty acids in their blood**.

The women were required to complete thinking and memory skills tests annually over an average of 6 years.

The study revealed that there was no difference in results between women who had high levels of omega-3 in their blood at the time the first memory tests were completed and women who had low levels of omega-3 in their blood.

Additionally, the results showed that **there was no difference in how fast thinking skills declined over time between women who had high or low levels of omega-3 in their blood.**

Despite findings, change of diet 'not recommended'

These results are contrary to earlier studies. Last year, *Medical News Today* reported on a study suggesting that increasing consumption of omega-3 may improve the memory of young adults.

More recently, researchers from Loyola University Stritch School of Medicine suggested that omega-3 may help prevent alcohol-related dementia.

Eric Ammann, of the University of Iowa and study author, told *Medical News Today*:

"**We found that omega-3 levels were not associated with cognitive changes over the course of the study, or with cognitive function at baseline**. Identifying interventions that might delay congitive decline is an important goal, so a finding of no association is somewhat of a disappointment. But it's imortant that people have a clear idea of what works and what doesn't." (Ammann et al, 2013)

However, Ammann adds that the researchers do not recommend people change their diet based on these results:

"Our study was observational and should not be viewed as a definitive answer on the relationship between omega-3s and cognitive function. In making health-related decisions about diet and supplements, we would advise people to consider the total body of evidence and to consult with their healthcare providers." (Ammann et al, 2013)

Ammann told *Medical News Today* that it is likely more randomized trials of omega-3 supplements will be done, which will provide more definitive information on the relationship between omega-3s and cognitive function in older adults.

"In addition," he notes, "longitudinal studies that track people's dietary practices in middle age and later years may provide richer data on the effects of diet on long-term health outcomes."

Doug Brown, director of research at the Alzheimer's Society, notes this is not the first study to suggest that omega-3 does not protect against cognitive decline, but he says the results of this study are inconclusive.

"It's important to note that the study looked at cognitive decline due to aging and not specifically at dementia, which is caused by diseases of the brain," he adds.

"Don't avoid your favorite fish supper or a handful of cashews on account of this research. The best thing people can do to try and reduce their risk of developing dementia is to eat a healthy, varied diet and take regular exercise."

Some believe that the omega-3 fatty acids found in nuts are different from the omega-3 fatty acids found in fish, the nuts containing alpha-linolenic acid at a very high proportion, compared to fish which contain very little alpha-linolenic and much more DHA and EPA than nuts.

Omega-3s may *not* prevent cognitive decline

Fish And Nuts May Not Boost Your Thinking Skills After All, But Here's Why You Should Still Eat Them

By Susan Scutti | Sep 25, 2013

Two new studies, one conducted in the U.S. and the other in Spain, came to similar conclusions but unfortunately that's not good news: both suggest that omega-3 fatty acids may *not* prevent cognitive decline. Despite this unhappy result, the researchers still recommend each of us continue to include fish and nuts in our diets.

What Are Omega-3s?

Omega-3 fatty acids, also known as polyunsaturated fatty acids, are necessary to maintain your health but the body does not produce them on its own. In fact, those who are deficient in omega-3 fatty acid develop symptoms, including fatigue, poor memory, dry skin, heart problems, mood swings, depression, and poor circulation. Eating correctly is one way to get the appropriate amount each day. High amounts of omega-3s can be found in fatty fish and some nuts, including salmon, tuna, halibut, seafood, algae, walnuts, and butternuts.

Omega-3 fatty acids are highly concentrated in the brain and appear to be crucial for cognitive function (memory and performance) as well as behavioral function. Scientists have found that mothers who do not provide enough omega-3 fatty acids to their fetus during pregnancy may be at risk of delivering a baby who has or develops vision and nerve problems. Omega-3 fatty acids **may** reduce inflammation and help lower risk of chronic diseases, such as cancer, arthritis, and even heart disease. For these reasons, the American Heart Association recommends eating fish at least two times a week.

American Study

Researchers at the University of Iowa conducted a study involving **2,157 participants**, all women between the ages of 65 and 80 who were enrolled in the Women's Health Initiative clinical trials of hormone therapy. Before the start of the study, researchers analyzed results of blood tests to measure the amount of omega-3s. Then, the women were given annual tests of thinking and memory skills for an average of six years. Among these women, some showed high levels of omega-3s in their blood, while others showed low levels, but **the researchers found no difference in memory test scores at the time of the first test.** Additionally, **no differences emerged in how quickly their thinking skills declined over time.** (Ammann et al, 2013)

"There has been a lot of interest in omega-3s as a way to prevent or delay cognitive decline, but **unfortunately our study did not find a protective effect in older women**," study author Eric Ammann, of the University of Iowa, stated in a press release. "However, we do not recommend that people change their diet based on these results. We know that fish and nuts can be healthy alternatives to red meat and full-fat dairy products, which are high in saturated fats."

Spanish Study

In their efforts to update and summarize any evidence related to the effect of diet and nutritional factors on the risk of Alzheimer's disease and cognitive aging, researchers conducted **a search of Medline and Web of Knowledge** for epidemiological and clinical studies published between Jan. 2000 and Feb. 2013. One criteria for inclusion in their study was use of combinations of the following keywords: "Alzheimer's disease," "mild cognitive impairment," "cognitive function," "dietary factors," "omega-3," "antioxidants," "B vitamins," "dietary patterns," and "Mediterranean diet."

What did they find? **Data from randomized controlled trials did not show a consistent effect, even if data from observational studies pointed to a protective role for certain nutrients, such as omega-3 fatty acids, antioxidants, B vitamins, and a Mediterranean diet. In other words, true scientific evidence is lacking.**

"Whether confounding factors such as age, disease stage, other dietary components, cooking processes, and other methodological issues explain the divergent results remains to be established," the authors wrote in their study.

Although many hoped a diet rich in omega-3 fatty acids might be a way of preventing Alzheimer's disease, unfortunately the research fails to provide evidence supporting such claims. Despite such disheartening results, the fact remains that omega-3s are clearly important to developing brains as discovered in a recent study conducted by British researchers; and omega-3s remain important for ongoing brain function in adults. While continuing to eat our fish and nuts, we can all search for some other ways to save our brains.

(Otaegui-Arrazola et al, 2013) (Ammann et al, 2012) (Ammann et al, 2013)

Fish Oil May Protect Against Alcohol-Related Dementia

September 18, 2013

Exposure to a compound found in fish oil may protect against the development of dementia in heavy drinkers, new research suggests.

A study presented at the recent Congress of the European Society for Biomedical Research on Alcohol in Warsaw, Poland, examined rat brain cells exposed to alcohol levels equivalent to 4 times the legal driving limit.

Results showed that the **cell cultures that were also exposed to omega-3 docosahexanenoic acid (DHA) showed approximately 90% less neuroinflammation and 90% less neuronal brain cell death compared with the cells that were not exposed to the fish oil compound.**

"We hypothesized that omega-3 fatty acids, specifically DHA (which has been shown to neuroprotect from other acquired brain insults in the laboratory and to some degree in human studies) would suppress or prevent the neuronal degeneration due to binge alcohol exposure," **principal investigator Michael A. Collins, PhD**, professor in the Department of Molecular Pharmacology and Therapeutics at the Stritch School of Medicine at Loyola University, Chicago, Illinois, told *Medscape Medical News*.

"And basically, that is what we found," he added.

Relevant to humans

Dr. Collins noted that although **this was an animal study** designed to measure neurodegeneration and related phenomena, and not a study specifically of dementia, "since brain degeneration underlies persistent or permanent dementia, **the results were extrapolated to what might happen in humans."**

And although he noted in a release that further studies are now needed, "fish oil has the potential of helping preserve brain integrity in abusers. At the very least, it wouldn't hurt them."

In 2011, Dr. Collins and colleagues published a meta-analysis of 143 studies showing that consuming up to 2 alcoholic drinks a day for men and 1 drink a day for women appeared to reduce the risk for dementia and cognitive impairment.

However, "too much alcohol overwhelms the cells," they noted in a release.

"Our previous work and that of others had **linked neurodegeneration to 'neuroinflammatory'-like mechanisms that include oxidative stress (oxygen and nitrogen free radicals).** The oxidative stress, we suspected, resulted in part from alcohol-induced excessive release of unsaturated fatty acids from brain membranes," explained Dr. Collins.

In the current study, the researchers exposed brain cell cultures from adult rats to heavy amounts of alcohol and then compared half the cells, which were further exposed to omega-3 DHA, with the other nonexposed half.

"Our results indicate excessive arachidonic acid (AA) mobilization due to increased phospholipase A2 (PLA2) levels/activity, and this appears related to elevations in astroglial aquaporin-4 (AQP4) and brain edema," write the investigators.

In other words, excessive drinking can cause higher levels of PLA2 activity, leading to excessive production of AA (a polyunsaturated omega-6 fatty acid), which in turn leads to increased AQP4/neuroinflammation and swelling of the brain.

However, inhibiting AQP4 was found to be neuroprotective to the cells.

Adding omega-3 DHA to the cell cultures not only significantly decreased the release of AA and the elevated levels of PLA2 and AQP4 but also decreased ADP-ribose polymerase-1 (PARP1) elevations and overall neurodamage.

Dr. Collins reported that the investigators are planning now to conduct studies that replicate the findings in intact adult rats exposed to binge-drinking levels of alcohol and that elucidate how DHA exerts its protection in the brain.

However, he stressed that **helping heavy drinkers to cut back the amounts they consume or to quit altogether is the best way to protect their brains**.

"We don't want people to think it's okay to take a few fish oil capsules and then continue to go on abusing alcohol," he said. (14th Congress, 2013)

Fish oil could prevent alcohol-related dementia

Sep 11, 2013

Omega-3 fish oil could help protect against alcohol-related dementia, according to a study presented at the 14th Congress of the European Society for Biomedical Research on Alcoholism in Warsaw, Poland.

The study, conducted by researchers from Loyola University Chicago Stritch School of Medicine, analyzed brain cell cultures of rats who had been exposed to large quantities of alcohol.

In a previous study carried out by the same research team, it was discovered that moderate social drinking, defined as two alcoholic drinks a day for men and one for women, could reduce the risk of neuronal degeneration, a condition that frequently underlies dementia.

The research showed that small amounts of alcohol could improve the fitness of brain cells, by "toughening them up" to cope with stress later in life that could lead to dementia. However, high amounts of alcohol were found to "overwhelm" the cells, leading to inflammation and cell death.

For this most recent study, the researchers assessed hippocampal and cortical brain cultures from rats that had been exposed to large quantities of alcohol - the equivalent to a human being four times over the legal alcohol limit for driving.

The cells were then compared with brain cells that had been exposed to the fish oil - omega-3 docosahexaenoic acid (DHA) - alongside the same large quantity of alcohol.

Results showed that the brain cells exposed to the combination of fish oil and alcohol showed as much as 95% less neuroinflammation and neuronal death in the brain cells, compared with the brain cells that were exposed to alcohol alone.

Michael Collins, of Loyola University Chicago and study author, explained the findings to *Medical News Today*:

Prof. Collins adds that the research team hopes to study whether fish oil supplements could prevent the binge alcohol-induced neurodegeneration and functional memory impairments in adult rats in the future.

"This could lead to human studies with fish oil, which is remarkably nontoxic as far as I know," he adds.

Although the researchers say this study shows that fish oil has the potential to help preserve brain integrity in alcohol abusers, Prof. Collins says the best way to protect the brain is to stop drinking or cut down to moderate amounts:

According to the Alzheimer's Society, a condition similar to alcohol-related dementia - often referred to as Wernicke-Korsakoff's syndrome - is diagnosed in about 1 in 8 people with alcoholism. Though it is not a dementia, the syndrome is accompanied by short-term memory loss due to thiamine deficiency, which can be brought on by excessive drinking. Studies have shown that the condition is most common in men between the ages of 45 and 65 with a long history of alcohol misuse.

Omega-3 fish oil has been linked to numerous other health benefits. **Research published in the *BMJ* this year suggested that consuming at least 1-2 portions of oily fish a week could reduce the risk of breast cancer by 14%.**

However, other research has shown omega-3 could have a negative effect on health. A study conducted by US researchers this year revealed that **males with high blood concentrations of omega-3 fatty acids** are at a higher risk of developing prostate cancer. (Whiteman, 2013)

STROKES

Fish, not supplements, may reduce strokes

Eating Oily Fish May Help Protect Against Stroke

Megan Brooks - Nov 01, 2012

Eating at least 2 servings of oily fish a week is moderately but significantly associated with a reduced risk for stroke, but **taking fish oil supplements does not seem to have the same effect, suggest results of a large meta-analysis of relevant research**.

"Consumption of fish and long-chain omega 3 fatty acids has been associated with a reduced risk of coronary heart disease [CHD] and sudden cardiac death," Oscar H. Franco, MD, PhD, professor of preventive medicine, Erasmus MC, University Medical Center, Rotterdam, the Netherlands, told *Medscape Medical News*. "However, observational and experimental evidence supporting a similar benefit for cerebrovascular disease remain conflicting," he said.

To help clarify the value of fish intake on stroke risk, Dr. Franco and colleagues **performed a systematic review and meta-analysis of 26 prospective cohort studies and 12 randomized controlled trials involving a total of 794,000 participants and 34,817 cerebrovascular outcomes.**

"Observational findings in this meta-analysis show that consumption of both fish and long chain omega 3 fatty acids may modestly reduce the risk of stroke, whereas **results were significant only for fish intake,"** he concluded.

They report their findings in an article published online **October 30 in *BMJ*.**

Omega-3 intake improves memory in young adults

10-31-12

Healthy young adults can improve their working memory by increasing their Omega-3 fatty acids intake.

The finding came from a study, the first of its kind, from a team at the University of Pittsburgh and was published in ***PLOS One***.

There have been several studies indicating that omega-3 essential fatty acids, found in foods such as grass-fed livestock and wild fish, are critical for the human body to function. **One report indicated omega-3 fatty acids can lower a person's chance of developing colon cancer. Another study indicated that they can protect men against heart failure.**

However, until now, there had been no research on their impact on the working memory of healthy young adults. Bita Moghaddam, project investigator and professor of neuroscience, said:

"Before seeing this data, I would have said it was impossible to move young healthy individuals above their cognitive best. We found that members of this population can enhance their working memory performance even further, despite their already being at the top of their cognitive game."

The experts examined healthy young males and females ages 18 to 25 from all ethnicities who heightened their Omega-3 intake with supplements for 6 months. Their progress was recorded through phone calls and outpatient procedures.

Before starting off on the supplements, all subjects had their blood samples analyzed and underwent positron emission tomography (PET) imaging, in order to observe how their tissues and organs were functioning.

A working memory test, known as "n-back test", was then given to the participants, in which they were provided a series of letters and numbers. They had to remember what number/letter had been revealed one, two, and three times prior.

Moghaddam explained: "What was particularly interesting about the pre-supplementation n-back test was that it

correlated positively with plasma Omega-3. This means that the Omega-3s they were getting from their diet already positively correlated with their working memory."

The subjects completed the same series of outpatient procedures after they finished taking Lovaza, an Omega-3 supplement approved by the Food and Drug Administration, for six months. **Results of this last stage, from the working memory test and blood samples, showed an improvement in working memory.**

"So many of the previous studies have been done with the elderly or people with medical conditions, leaving this unique population of young adults unaddressed," revealed Matthew Muldoon, associate professor of medicine at Pitt. "But what about our highest-functioning periods? Can we help the brain achieve its full potential by adapting our healthy behaviors in our young adult life? We found that we absolutely can."

Although the main goal of the research was to recognize the effects of Omega-3s on young adults, the scientists also wanted to observe the brain mechanism linked to regulating Omega-3.

Prior research on rodents suggested that eliminating Omega-3 from the diet can lower dopamine storage - the neurotransmitter linked to mood and working memory - and reduce density in the striatal vesicular monoamine transporter type 2 (VMAT2) - a protein linked to decision making.

This made the team believe that cognitive performance was raised by the increase of VMAT2 protein. However, PET imaging showed that this was not true.

Rajesh Narendarn, research leader and associate professor of radiology, concluded:

> "It is really interesting that diets enriched with Omega-3 fatty acid can enhance cognition in highly functional young individuals. Nevertheless, it was a bit disappointing that our imaging studies were unable to clarify the mechanisms by which it enhances working memory."

Ongoing trials in the Moghaddam lab on animals demonstrate that **brain mechanisms that are impacted by Omega-3s may be affected differently in young adults and adolescents than in older adults.**

Keeping this in mind, the experts are further analyzing the influence of Omega-3 fatty acids in younger people to determine the mechanism that affects cognition.

Written by Sarah Glynn

What Can You Tell Patients? No doubt many of your patients are among those **Americans who spent $1.1 billion on omega-3 supplements in 2011—an increase of 5.4% from 2010, according to estimates from the *Nutrition Business Journal*.** This is a good opportunity to remind patients not to rely solely on supplements to prevent cardiovascular disease. As the meta-analysis did not reveal any adverse effects from the consumption of omega-3s, **they should be considered one component of a healthy lifestyle alongside smoking cessation, exercise, and eating lots of whole grains and vegetables.** And as we've learned from studies of antioxidant supplements, consumption of foods rich in vitamins and minerals—in this case, oily fishes, walnuts, and flax seed oil, may confer health benefits that supplements cannot.

Iron, omega-3s tied to different effects on kids' brains

11-8-12 For children with low stores of two brain-power nutrients, supplements may have different, and complex, effects, a new clinical trial suggests.

Iron deficiency is the most common nutritional deficiency worldwide, affecting about 2 billion people, according to the World Health Organization.

Poor children in developing countries are at particular risk for shortfalls in iron, as well as other nutrients, including the omega-3 fats found largely in oily fish.

So the new study looked at the effects of giving **321 schoolchildren** in South Africa either supplements containing iron, omega-3s or both. All of the kids had low levels of both nutrients, which are vital for children's growth and healthy brain development.

After about eight months, researchers found varied changes in the kids' memory and learning abilities.

In general, **children given iron showed improvements on tests of memory and learning.** That was especially true if they had outright anemia - a disorder wherein the **blood's oxygen-carrying capacity** is reduced, causing problems like fatigue and difficulty with concentration and memory. Please remember that iron is a prooxidant.

For example, on a memory test, anemic kids given iron were able to recall an extra two words out of 12.

In contrast, a new study looked at the effects of giving **321 schoolchildren** in South Africa either supplements containing iron, omega-3s or both and **there was no overall benefit linked to omega-3 supplements. And when the researchers zeroed in on kids with anemia, those who used omega-3s did worse than before on one test of memory.** (Baumgartner et al, 2012)

Then there were the children with clear iron deficiency, but not anemia. Of those kids, girls who got omega-3s fared worse, while boys Improved their test scores.

What it all means for kids with nutritional deficiencies is unclear, according to lead researcher Jeannine Baumgartner, of North-West University in Potchefstroom, South Africa.

One limitation of the study, she said in an email, is that the number of children in each group her team analyzed was small. There were 67 kids with anemia, for example.

Thus, "the results need to be interpreted cautiously," Baumgartner told Reuters Health in an email.

There are still a lot of questions, according to Baumgartner, whose group's findings are published in the **American Journal of Clinical Nutrition**.

The children in this study were 6 to 11 years old. But, Baumgartner said, animal research suggests brain deficits that take shape early in life might not be reversible.

"The question arises whether supplementation during school age might be too late to achieve beneficial effects on cognitive performance," she said.

Still, the omega-3 findings are consistent with some recent animal research. Baumgartner said her team found that **in rats deficient in**

both iron and omega-3s, giving either supplement alone seemed to worsen the animals' memory performance. The picture was better, though, when the rats were given both iron and omega-3s.

In children, things are more complicated. Other nutritional deficiencies, as well as exposure to toxins like lead and the general effects of poverty could all dampen kids' brain development, Baumgartner pointed out.

"We believe that more research is needed to investigate the biological and functional links between nutrients essential for brain development and cognitive functioning," she said.

Since this study focused on impoverished children with low iron, and possibly other nutritional deficiencies, the results cannot be extended to children in general, according to Baumgartner.

In the U.S., recommendations call for babies to get an iron test during the first year of life to check for deficiencies. For healthy kids older than six months, the recommended iron intake varies from 7 to 15 mg of iron per day, depending on their age and sex.

There is a risk from getting too much iron and experts tell parents to ask their doctor before giving children iron supplements.

The current study was partly funded by Unilever, which makes omega-3-enriched spreads. Paul Lohmann GmbH provided the iron supplements, and Burgerstein AG provided the omega-3s. (Baumgartner et al, 2012)

Conclusions: In children with poor iron and n−3 FA status, iron supplementation improved verbal and nonverbal learning and memory, particularly in children with anemia. In contrast, **DHA/EPA supplementation had no benefits on cognition and impaired working memory in anemic children and long-term memory and retrieval in girls with ID** (iron deficiency). The trial was registered at clinicaltrials.gov as NCT01092377. (Baumgartner et al, 2012)

DEPRESSION

Studies have found mixed results as to whether taking omega-3 fatty acids can help depression symptoms. Several studies have found that people who took omega-3 fatty acids in addition to prescription antidepressants had a greater improvement in symptoms than those who took antidepressants alone.

Other studies show that omega-3 fatty acid intake helps protect against postpartum depression, among other benefits.

However, other studies have found no benefit.

Studies are also mixed on whether omega-3 fatty acids alone have any effect on depression.

The efficacy of n-3 fatty acids DHA and EPA (fish oil) for perinatal depression

Abstract

Depressive symptoms are common during pregnancy and the postpartum period. Although essential n-3 PUFA may have beneficial effects on depression, it remains unclear whether they are also effective for perinatal depression. The purpose of the present study was to assess the efficacy of n-3 supplementation for perinatal depression, by performing a meta-analysis on currently available data. After a thorough literature search, we included **seven randomized controlled trials in the meta-analysis, all with EPA and/or DHA supplementation. Most studies were judged to be of low-to-moderate quality**, mainly due to small sample sizes and failure to adhere to Consolidated Standards of Reporting Trials guidelines. Some studies were not primarily designed to address perinatal depression. A total of **309 women on n-3 fatty acid supplementation were compared with 303 women on placebo treatment**. n-3

Fish oil supplementation was not found to be significantly more effective in perinatal depression than placebo at post-treatment with a pooled effect size using a fixed-effects model. (Jans et al, 2010)

Heterogeneity was low-to-moderate (I2 = 30 %). In a subgroup analysis of three small studies of pregnant women with major depression, there was some indication of effectiveness. **In conclusion, the question of whether EPA and DHA administration is effective in the prevention or treatment of perinatal depression cannot be answered yet**. Future research should focus on women who are clinically depressed (or at risk). The quality of research in this area needs to improve. (Jans et al, 2010)

EPA may be more efficacious than DHA in treating depression

EPA but not DHA appears to be responsible for the efficacy of omega-3 long chain polyunsaturated fatty acid supplementation in depression: evidence from a meta-analysis of randomized controlled trials.

Abstract

BACKGROUND:

Epidemiologic and case-control data suggest that increased dietary intake of omega-3 long-chain polyunsaturated fatty acids (omega3 LC-PUFAs) may be of benefit in depression. However, **the results of randomized controlled trials are mixed and controversy exists as to whether either eicosapentaenoic acid (EPA) or docosahexaenoic acid (DHA) or both are responsible for the reported benefits.**

OBJECTIVE:

The aim of the current study was to provide an updated meta-analysis of all double-blind, placebo-controlled, randomized controlled trials examining the effect of omega3 LC-PUFA supplementation in which depressive symptoms were a reported outcome. The study also aimed to specifically test the differential effectiveness of EPA versus DHA through meta-regression and subgroup analyses.

DESIGN:

Studies were selected using the PubMed database on the basis of the following criteria: (1) randomized design; (2) placebo controlled; (3)

use of an omega3 LC-PUFA preparation containing DHA, EPA, or both where the relative amounts of each fatty acid could be quantified; and (4) reporting sufficient statistics on scores of a recognizable measure of depressive symptoms.

RESULTS:

Two hundred forty-one studies were identified, of which 28 met the above inclusion criteria and were therefore included in the subsequent meta-analysis. Using a random effects model, overall standardized mean depression scores were reduced in response to omega3 LC-PUFA supplementation as compared with placebo. However, significant heterogeneity and **evidence of publication bias were present**. Meta-regression studies showed a significant effect of higher levels of baseline depression and lower supplement DHAEPA ratio on therapeutic efficacy. Subgroup analyses showed significant effects for: (1) diagnostic category (bipolar disorder and major depression showing significant improvement with omega3 LC-PUFA supplementation versus mild-to-moderate depression, **chronic fatigue and non-clinical populations not showing significant improvement**); (2) therapeutic as opposed to preventive intervention; (3) adjunctive treatment as opposed to monotherapy; and (4) supplement type. **Symptoms of depression were not significantly reduced in 3 studies using pure DHA or in 4 studies using supplements containing greater than 50% DHA**. In contrast, **symptoms of depression were significantly reduced in 13 studies using supplements containing greater than 50% EPA and in 8 studies using pure ethyl-EPA**. However, further meta-regression studies showed significant inverse associations between efficacy and study methodological quality, study sample size, and duration, thus limiting the confidence of these findings. Thus, **study results are mixed and conflicted.**

CONCLUSIONS:

The current meta-analysis provides evidence that **EPA may be more efficacious than DHA in treating depression**. However, owing to the identified limitations of the included studies, larger, well-designed, randomized controlled trials of sufficient duration are needed to confirm these findings. (Martins, 2009) a meta-analysis of randomized controlled trials.

EPA and DHA did not prevent depression during pregnancy or postpartum

The Mothers, Omega-3, and Mental Health Study: a double-blind, randomized controlled trial.

Abstract

OBJECTIVES:

Maternal deficiency of the omega-3 fatty acid, docosahexaenoic acid (DHA), has been associated with perinatal depression, but there is evidence that supplementation with eicosapentaenoic acid (EPA) may be more effective than DHA in treating depressive symptoms. This trial tested the relative effects of EPA- and DHA-rich fish oils on prevention of depressive symptoms among pregnant women at an increased risk of depression.

STUDY DESIGN:

We enrolled **126 pregnant women at risk for depression** (Edinburgh Postnatal Depression Scale score 9-19 or a history of depression) in early pregnancy and **randomly assigned** them to receive EPA-rich fish oil (1060 mg EPA plus 274 mg DHA), DHA-rich fish oil (900 mg DHA plus 180 mg EPA), or soy oil placebo. Subjects completed the Beck Depression Inventory (BDI) and Mini-International Neuropsychiatric Interview at enrollment, 26-28 weeks, 34-36 weeks, and at 6-8 weeks' postpartum. Serum fatty acids were analyzed at entry and at 34-36 weeks' gestation.

RESULTS:

One hundred eighteen women completed the trial. **There were no differences between groups in BDI scores or other depression endpoints at any of the 3 time points after supplementation.** The EPA- and DHA-rich fish oil groups exhibited significantly increased postsupplementation concentrations of serum EPA and serum DHA respectively. Serum DHA- concentrations at 34-36 weeks were inversely related to BDI scores in late pregnancy.

CONCLUSION:

EPA-rich fish oil and DHA-rich fish oil supplementation did not prevent depressive symptoms during pregnancy or postpartum.

(Mozurkewich et al, 2013) a double-blind, randomized controlled trial.

Trial evidence that examines the effects of n–3 PUFAs on depressed mood is limited and is difficult to summarize and evaluate because of considerable heterogeneity. **The evidence available provides little support for the use of n–3 PUFAs to improve depressed mood.** (Appleton et al, 2006)

These data do reinforce the results of other studies of ϖ3-FA in unipolar depression patients (Marangell et al, 2003) and in obsessive-compulsive disorder patients (Fux et al, 2004) where placebo-controlled crossover trials found **that EPA is virtually ineffective**.

Omega-3 fatty acids for depression

Systematic review and meta-analysis.

Abstract

We conducted a meta-analysis of randomized, placebo-controlled trials of omega-3 fatty acid (FA) treatment of major depressive disorder (MDD) in order to determine efficacy and to examine sources of heterogeneity between trials. PubMed (1965-May 2010) was searched for randomized, placebo-controlled trials of omega-3 FAs for MDD. Our primary outcome measure was standardized mean difference in a clinical measure of depression severity. In stratified meta-analysis, we examined the effects of trial duration, trial methodological quality, baseline depression severity, diagnostic indication, dose of eicosapentaenoic acid (EPA) and docosahexaenoic acid (DHA) in omega-3 preparations, and whether omega-3 FA was given as monotherapy or augmentation. **In 13 randomized, placebo-controlled trials examining the efficacy of omega-3 FAs involving 731 participants, meta-analysis demonstrated no significant benefit of omega-3 FA treatment compared with placebo. Meta-analysis demonstrated significant heterogeneity and publication bias.** Nearly all evidence of omega-3 benefit was removed after adjusting for publication bias using the trim-and-fill method. Secondary analyses suggested a trend toward increased efficacy of omega-3 FAs in trials of lower methodological quality, trials of shorter duration, trials which utilized completers rather than intention-to-treat analysis, and trials in which study participants had greater baseline depression severity. **Current published trials suggest a small, non-significant benefit of omega-3 FAs for major depression. Nearly all of the treatment efficacy observed in the published literature may be attributable to publication bias.** (Bloch, Hannestad, 2012)

Omega-3 Fatty acids in depressive disorders

A comprehensive meta-analysis of randomized clinical trials

Abstract

BACKGROUND:

Despite omega-3 polyunsaturated fatty acids (PUFA) supplementation in depressed patients have been suggested to improve depressive symptomatology, previous findings are not univocal.

OBJECTIVES:

To conduct an updated meta-analysis of randomized controlled trials (RCTs) of omega-3 PUFA treatment of depressive disorders, taking into account the clinical differences among patients included in the studies.

METHODS:

A search on MEDLINE, EMBASE, PsycInfo, and the Cochrane Database of RCTs using omega-3 PUFA on patients with depressive symptoms published up to August 2013 was performed. Standardized mean difference in clinical measure of depression severity was primary outcome. Type of omega-3 used (particularly eicosapentaenoic acid [EPA] and docosahexaenoic acid [DHA]) and omega-3 as mono- or adjuvant therapy was also examined. Meta-regression analyses assessed the effects of study size, baseline depression severity, trial duration, dose of omega-3, and age of patients.

RESULTS:

Meta-analysis of 11 and 8 trials conducted respectively on patients with a DSM-defined diagnosis of major depressive disorder (MDD) and patients with depressive symptomatology but no diagnosis of MDD **demonstrated significant clinical benefit of omega-3 PUFA treatment** compared to placebo. Use of mainly EPA within the preparation, rather than DHA, influenced final clinical efficacy. Significant clinical efficacy had the use of omega-3 PUFA as adjuvant rather than mono-therapy. No relation between efficacy and study size, baseline depression severity, trial duration, age of patients, and study quality was found. **Omega-3 PUFA resulted effective in RCTs on patients with bipolar disorder**, whereas **no evidence was found for those exploring their efficacy (of omega-3 Fatty acids) on depressive symptoms in young populations, perinatal depression, primary disease other than depression and healthy subjects**. (Grosso et al, 2014)

CONCLUSIONS:

The use of omega-3 PUFA is effective in patients with diagnosis of MDD and on depressive patients without diagnosis of MDD. (Grosso et al, 2014)

BIPOLAR DISORDERS

In a clinical study of 30 people with bipolar disorder, those who took fish oil in addition to standard prescription treatments for bipolar disorder for 4 months experienced fewer mood swings and relapse than those who received placebo. But another 4 month long clinical study treating people with bipolar depression and rapid cycling bipolar disorder <u>did not find that EPA helped reduce symptoms</u>.

(Stoll et al, 1999)

Omega-3 PUFA resulted effective in RCTs on patients with bipolar disorder. (Grosso et al, 2014)

Fish oil pills don't improve kids' braininess

9-29-11

Despite some evidence that taking fish oil pills during pregnancy can help children's brain development, a new study suggests that **fish oil supplements make no difference in measures of intellect when the kids are six years old**. The findings support the results of an earlier **Norwegian study** that **also found no differences in IQ among seven-year-olds whose mothers did or did not take fish oil supplements while pregnant and breastfeeding.**

Fatty acids, such as docosahexaenoic acid (DHA), that are found in fish and other foods are considered to be important for the developing fetus.

The question, however, has been whether adding more of these fats to mothers' diets through supplements will further benefit the baby.

In the current experiment, researchers asked expectant mothers during the second half of their pregnancies to take fish oil, fish oil plus a folate supplement, folate alone or a pill that did not contain any supplements.

Nearly seven years later, the team, led by Dr. Cristina Campoy at the University of Granada in Spain, gave intelligence tests to **154** children from this group.

The kids performed similarly on the tests, regardless of what type of pill their mothers had taken during pregnancy.

The results, published in the **American Journal of Clinical Nutrition**, do not mean that fatty acids like DHA are not important.

In fact, the researchers found that the children of women who had high levels of DHA in their red blood cells around the time they gave birth scored above average on the intelligence tests at age six.

These mothers, however, were not necessarily given fish oil supplements. Rather, the **result could reflect mothers' intake of DHA from various sources over a longer period of time**, and might mean that long term fatty acid intake "is more beneficial than receiving supplementation alone during pregnancy," the authors wrote in their study.

A recent study in Australia also found that docosahexaenoic acid (DHA) supplements did not help the visual development of babies (see Reuters Health story of May 26, 2011).

The current study did not measure the diets of the children, something that could have influenced the results, said Dr. Ingrid Helland at Oslo University Hospital, who led the earlier Norwegian research.

"It might be that subtle beneficial effects of (prenatal fish oil) supplementation are being overshadowed by other factors (genetics, social stimulation, nutrition etc)," Helland wrote in an email to Reuters Health.

She is not totally giving up on the idea that taking fish oil might be beneficial.

"If a friend would ask me if she should take supplements or not, I would recommend supplementation, but emphasize that **we still do not have any scientific proof that it benefits the child," said Helland.** SOURCE: http://bit.ly/nW3xdX American Journal of Clinical Nutrition, online August 17, 2011.

SECTION FIVE

ARTHRITIS

Rheumatoid arthritis is an autoimmune condition where the body's own immune cells start "attacking" the joints of the body, causing pain and inflammation. The small joints of the hands and feet are most commonly first affected.

Something's Fishy in Rheumatoid Arthritis

Jonathan Kay, MD

December 20, 2013

Patients often come to my office interested in alternative treatments -- complementary and alternative medications. **One of these is fish oil, which many patients are taking for cardiovascular purposes.** Omega-3 fatty acids can suppress the production of proinflammatory eicosanoids and were studied in the 1980s and early 1990s as potential treatments for established rheumatoid arthritis. **Fish oil showed minimal benefit in the treatment of established rheumatoid arthritis, and the doses required were enough to make a patient smell somewhat fishy.**

In September, 2013 an interesting study was published online in ***Annals of the Rheumatic Diseases*** **by Proudman and colleagues from Australia** (Proudman et al, 2013) a randomized, double-blind controlled trial. It compared high-dose with low-dose fish oil (5.5 g/day compared with 400 mg/day) in patients with early rheumatoid arthritis of less than 1-year duration and who used fish oil as an adjunctive treatment to triple therapy. They employed a treat-to-target strategy in which triple therapy was escalated, with the dose of methotrexate being increased gradually and then ultimately switching to leflunomide therapy and, if necessary, biologic agents. **The requirement of a patient switching to leflunomide was considered failure of adjunctive fish oil therapy.**

Interestingly, **a statistically significantly smaller proportion of patients on high-dose fish oil ended up on leflunomide compared with those taking low-dose fish oil. Patients also seemed to do better in terms of achieving Disease Activity Score remission on fish oil compared with triple therapy or standard nonbiologic therapy alone.**

This approach to using fish oil as an adjunctive treatment rather than as a primary treatment in patients with early rheumatoid arthritis may be very appropriate in the therapeutic armamentarium that we now have for rheumatoid arthritis. Not only may it benefit patients and allow for less aggressive treatment with nonbiologic disease-modifying antirheumatic drugs, but it may also have cardiovascular benefits. Those will need to be determined in future studies. However, this initial study by Proudman and colleagues is very interesting and deserves notice. (Something's Fishy in rheumatoid arthritis. Medscape. Dec 29, 2013)

Fish oil does not appear to slow progression of RA

Most clinical studies examining omega-3 fatty acid supplements for arthritis have focused on rheumatoid arthritis (RA), an autoimmune disease that causes inflammation in the joints. A number of small studies have found that fish oil helps reduce symptoms of RA, including joint pain and morning stiffness. One study suggests that people with RA who take fish oil may be able to lower their dose of non-steroidal anti-inflammatory drugs (NSAIDs). However, **unlike prescription medications, fish oil does not appear to slow progression of RA, only to treat the symptoms. Joint damage still occurs.**

Laboratory studies suggest that diets rich in omega-3 fatty acids (and low in the inflammatory omega-6 fatty acids) may help people with osteoarthritis, although more study is needed. **New Zealand green lipped mussel (Perna canaliculus), another potential source of**

omega-3 fatty acids, has been reported to reduce joint stiffness and pain, increase grip strength, and improve walking pace in a small group of people with osteoarthritis. For some people, symptoms got worse before they improved.

An analysis of **17 randomized, controlled clinical trials** looked at the pain relieving effects of omega-3 fatty acid supplements in people with RA or joint pain caused by inflammatory bowel disease (IBS) and painful menstruation (dysmenorrhea).The results suggest that **omega-3 fatty acids, along with conventional therapies such as NSAIDs, may help relieve joint pain associated with these conditions.**

Source: Omega-3 fatty acids | University of Maryland Medical Center http://umm.edu/health/medical/altmed/supplement/omega3-fatty- acids#ixzz2h9ZiV18L.

Eating oily fish 'halves rheumatoid arthritis risk'

8-14-13 Eating at least one portion of oily fish, such as salmon or mackerel, a week can halve the risk of developing rheumatoid arthritis, experts believe.

The findings come from a study of more than **32,000 Swedish women** and they offer another reason to follow the established dietary advice of regularly consuming fish for good health. (Giuseppe et al, 2013)

A fishy diet is beneficial because it is rich in omega-3, say researchers.

Omega-3 is said to protect both the heart and the brain, but that has basically been debunked.

It appears to be a good anti-inflammatory agent, which would explain how it might combat arthritis, say researchers in the journal **Annals of the Rheumatic Diseases**.

Oily fish

- Includes herring, mackerel, pilchard, salmon, sardine, trout and fresh tuna
- Rich in long-chain omega-3 fatty acids and vitamin D

- Some white fish and shellfish also contain omega-3 but not as much as oily fish
- A healthy diet should include at least two portions of fish a week, including one of oily fish
- A portion of oily fish is around 140g when cooked
- Pregnant women and those who want to conceive in the future should eat no more than two portions of oily fish a week because it can contain low levels of pollutants that can build up in the body

Source: NHS Choices

In the study, which spanned a decade, women who consistently ate any type of fish at least once a week cut their risk of developing rheumatoid arthritis by nearly a third.

And those who ate at least one portion of oily fish or four servings of other fish each week halved their risk.

'Substantial changes in diets'

The study did not look at fish oil supplements, but experts say these may also be beneficial. Prof Alan Silman, medical director of Arthritis Research UK, said: "**We've known for some time that there is good evidence that, in people with active arthritis, taking fish oils can reduce the level of inflammation.**"

He said the study suggests that taking high levels of fish oils can prevent inflammation from starting in the joint. "One of the challenges is that this can mean quite substantial changes in people's diets."

Rheumatoid arthritis affects more than 580,000 people in England and Wales. As the disease progresses, the immune system attacks the joints, making them stiff, swollen and painful.

Analysis by Bazian.

Edited by NHS Choices. **Oily fish may reduce risk of rheumatoid arthritis**

Tue, 13 Aug 2013

In this cohort study the researchers wanted to know if there is an association between dietary long-chain n-3 polyunsaturated fatty acids (n-3 PUFAs) and the risk of developing rheumatoid arthritis. **But cohort studies cannot show causation.**

We can't conclude from the results of this study that n-3 PUFAs are directly responsible for the reduction in risk seen. This is because it is possible that there are other factors (confounders) responsible for the association seen.

For example, it is possible that people who eat a healthier diet that includes more fatty acids also have other healthier lifestyle behaviors that may also reduce their risk of developing certain conditions, such as a healthier diet overall and taking more regular exercise.

This story was generally well reported by the media, but The Guardian and the Daily Express headline writers could have been a little more precise. They both talk about "arthritis", which is an umbrella term that covers a range of conditions that cause joint pain and swelling. The study in question looked at rheumatoid arthritis, which is one of the less common types of arthritis.

Behind The Headlines - Health News from NHS Choices

Oily fish may reduce risk of rheumatoid arthritis

Tue, 13 Aug 2013 13:33:00 EST

"Eating fish could halve risk of arthritis" is the encouraging news in The Guardian, as a Swedish study found that women who regularly ate high levels of oily fish were less likely to develop rheumatoid arthritis.

Researchers asked women about their diet at two time points a decade apart to assess their intake of long-chain n-3 polyunsaturated fatty acids (omega-3 fatty acids).

The researchers then **followed up the women six years** after their diet was last assessed to see if they had developed rheumatoid arthritis.

They found that **women whose dietary intake of omega-3 fatty acids consistently exceeded 0.21g per day at both time points had a 52% decreased risk of rheumatoid arthritis** compared with women who consistently reported a dietary intake of 0.21g per day or less.

This corresponds to at least one serving of oily fish a week, or four servings a week of lean fish, such as cod.

However, **the way this study was carried out means that it can't prove that eating fish directly prevented women developing rheumatoid arthritis**. Despite this, there are many health benefits from regularly eating oily fish, including a reduced risk of cardiovascular disease.

Where did the story come from?

The study was carried out by researchers from the Karolinska Institutet and Karolinska University Hospital, Sweden. It was funded by the Swedish Research Council and Committee for Research Infrastructure and the Karolinska Institutet, a medical university.

The study was published in the peer-reviewed Annals of the Rheumatic Diseases.

This story was generally well reported by the media, but The Guardian and the Daily Express headline writers could have been a little more precise. They both talk about **"arthritis", which is an umbrella term that covers a range of conditions that cause joint pain and swelling.** The study in question looked at rheumatoid arthritis, which is one of the less common types of arthritis.

What did the research involve?

The researchers studied **32,232 women** born between 1914 and 1948 who were living in a region of Sweden.

The women completed questionnaires on height, weight, the number of children they had, educational level, smoking history, physical activity and the use of dietary supplements.

Women who were diagnosed with non-rheumatoid arthritic conditions, had extreme energy intake, died before January 1 or took fish oil supplements were not eligible for the study.

The women completed a **food frequency questionnaire** at two time points: 1987 and 1997. The researchers calculated dietary intake of n-3 PUFAs by multiplying the frequency of food consumption (mainly fish and seafood) by the nutrient content of age-specific portion sizes.

New cases of rheumatoid arthritis were identified using two registers: the Swedish Rheumatology Register and the Outpatient Register of the Swedish National Board of Health and Welfare. The researchers were interested in cases that developed between January 1 2003 and December 31 2010. This was so women who had arthritis at the start of the study would not be wrongly identified as new cases.

The researchers looked at whether there was a link between the risk of developing rheumatoid arthritis and n-3 PUFAs and fish intake. They adjusted for the following confounders:

- cigarette smoking
- alcohol intake
- use of aspirin
- energy intake

What were the basic results?

Of the 32,232 women included in the study, 205 developed rheumatoid arthritis during the period January 1 2003 to December 31 2010, an average follow-up of seven-and-a-half years.

Dietary intake of n-3 PUFAs was divided into fifths (quintiles). Women in the bottom quintiles ate 0.21g per day or less of n-3 PUFAs, according to the food frequency questionnaire in 1997.

An intake of n-3 PUFAs of more than 0.21g per day (reported on the food frequency questionnaire in 1997) was associated with a 35% decreased risk of developing rheumatoid arthritis compared with a lower intake.

The researchers calculated that **28% of rheumatoid arthritis cases could be avoided if everyone had an intake of more than 0.21g n-3 PUFAs per day**.

They also found that higher dietary intakes of n-3 PUFAs further reduced the risk of rheumatoid arthritis until an intake of 0.35g per day was reached. After this level, no additional benefit was seen with a higher intake.

When women consistently reported an intake exceeding 0.21g per day (both in 1987 and 1997), this was associated with a 52% (95% CI 29-67%) decreased risk of rheumatoid arthritis compared with women who consistently reported a dietary intake of 0.21g per day or less.

The researchers also found that **women who reported eating at least one serving of fish (either oily or lean) per week in both 1987 and 1997 had a 29% decreased risk of rheumatoid arthritis** compared with women who ate less than one serving per week.

RMH Note: It is curious that "lean" fish would also be capable of causing a 29% reduced risk of RA, if the active anti-rheumatoid ingredient is omega-3s.

Conclusion

This is a well-designed cohort study that found an association between an increased dietary intake of long-chain n-3 polyunsaturated fatty acids and a reduced risk of rheumatoid arthritis in a cohort of middle-aged and older women in Sweden.

This study has many strengths, including:

- it was prospective, meaning that information was collected as the study was being performed
- it used a large sample of women taken from the general population
- diet was assessed at two time points, both long before rheumatoid arthritis was diagnosed

But **because this is a cohort study, we cannot conclude from its results that dietary long-chain n-3 polyunsaturated fatty acids are directly responsible for the reduction in risk seen.**

This is because of the confounding factors that could also potentially be responsible for the association seen.

Although the researchers adjusted their analyses for the lifestyle factors of smoking and alcohol intake, which are associated with the risk of rheumatoid arthritis, **it is possible that people who eat a healthier diet that includes more fatty acids could also have other healthy lifestyle behaviors.** This could include having a healthier diet overall (such as a diet with plenty of fruit and vegetables and low in saturated fats) and taking more regular exercise.

In addition, this study provides no information about whether dietary intake of long-chain n-3 polyunsaturated fatty acids is associated with a reduced risk of rheumatoid arthritis in men or younger women. Further studies are required to confirm whether long-chain n-3 polyunsaturated fatty acids really do reduce your risk of developing rheumatoid arthritis.

However, it is currently recommended that people should aim to eat at least two portions of fish a week, including one portion of oily fish. Babies, children and women who are pregnant, breastfeeding or planning to have children should have no more than two portions of oily fish a week.

Eating this amount of fish would provide more than 0.21g of long-chain n-3 polyunsaturated fatty acids, which was the level associated with a reduction in the risk of developing rheumatoid arthritis.

EXERCISE

Omega-3 effects on exercise

Omega-3 does not attenuate exercise-induced oxidative stress

Abstract

The purpose of this randomized study was to measure the influence of 6 weeks of LCPUFA (600 mg EPA and 400 mg DHA per day) supplementation alone or in association with 30 mg vitamin E, 60 mg vitamin C and 6 mg β-carotene on resting and exercise-induced lipid peroxidation in judoists (n = 36). Blood samples were collected at rest before (T (1)) and after the supplementation period, in preexercise (T (2)) and postexercise (T (3)) conditions, for analysis of α-tocopherol, retinol, lag phase (Lp) before free radical-induced oxidation, maximum rate of oxidation (R (max)) during the propagating chain reaction, maximum amount of conjugated dienes (CD(max)) accumulated after the propagation phase, and nitric oxide, malondialdehyde and lipoperoxide (POOL) concentrations. Dietary data were collected using a 7-day diet record. **There were no significant differences among treatment groups with respect to habitual intakes of energy from fat, carbohydrate, or protein**. At T (1), there were no significant differences among treatment groups with respect to lipid peroxidation, lag phase, and levels of α-tocopherol or retinol. **The consumption of an n-3 LC PUFA supplement increased oxidative stress at rest and did not attenuate the exercise-induced oxidative stress**. The addition of antioxidants did not prevent the formation of oxidation products at rest. On the contrary, **it seems that the combination of antioxidants added to the n-3 LCPUFA supplement led to a decrease in, CD(max), R (max), and POOL and MDA concentrations after a judo training session**. (Filaire et al, 2011)

Omega-3s do not alter immunity, inflammation or increase exercise performance

Abstract

The purpose of this study was to test the influence of 2.4 g/d fish oil n-3 polyunsaturated fatty acids (n-3 PUFA) over 6 wk on exercise performance, inflammation, and immune measures in 23 trained cyclists before and after a 3-d period of intense exercise. Participants were randomized to n-3 PUFA (n = 11; 2,000 mg eicosapentaenoic acid [EPA], 400 mg docosahexaenoic acid [DHA]) or placebo (n = 12) groups. They ingested supplements under double-blind methods for 6 wk before and during a 3-d period in which they cycled for 3 hr/d at ~57% W(max) with 10-km time trials inserted during the final 15 min of each 3-hr bout. Blood and saliva samples were collected before and after the 6-wk supplementation period, immediately after the 3-hr exercise bout on the third day, and 14 hr postexercise and analyzed for various immune-function and inflammation parameters. **Supplementation with n-3 PUFA resulted in a significant increase in plasma EPA and DHA but had no effect on 10-km time-trial performance**;

preexercise outcome measures; exercise-induced increases in plasma cytokines, myeloperoxidase, blood total leukocytes, serum C-reactive protein, and creatine kinase; or the decrease in the salivary IgA:protein ratio. In conclusion, **6 wk supplementation with a large daily dose of n-3 PUFAs increased plasma EPA and DHA but had no effect on exercise performance** or in countering measures of inflammation and immunity before or after a 3-d period of 9 hr of heavy exertion. (Nieman et al, 2009)

Omega-3s increase oxidative stress in Judo athletes

Effect of 6 Weeks of n-3 Fatty-Acid Supplementation on Oxidative Stress in Judo Athletes

The aim of this investigation was to assess the effects of **6 wk of eicosapentanoic acid (EPA) and docosahexanoic acid (DHA) supplementation** on resting and exercise-induced lipid peroxidation and antioxidant status in judoists. Subjects were **randomly assigned** to receive a placebo or a capsule of polyunsaturated fatty acids (PUFAs; 600 mg EPA and 400 mg DHA). Blood samples were collected in pre-exercise and postexercise conditions (judo-training session), both before and after the supplementation period. The following parameters were analyzed: α-tocopherol, retinol, lag phase, maximum rate of oxidation (Rmax) during the propagating chain reaction, maximum amount of conjugated dienes (CDmax) accumulated after the propagation phase, nitric oxide (NO) and malondyaldehide (MDA) concentrations, salivary glutathione peroxidase activity, and the lipid profile. Dietary data were collected using a 7-day dietary record. A significant interaction effect between supplementation and time ($p < .01$) on triglycerides was noted, with values significantly lower in the **n-3 long-chain-PUFA (LCPUFA)** group after supplementation than in the placebo group. Significant interaction effects between supplementation and time on resting MDA concentrations and Rmax were found ($p = .03$ and $p = .04$, respectively), with elevated values in the n-3 LCPUFA group after supplementation and no change in the placebo group's levels. **The authors observed a significantly greater NO and oxidative-stress increase with exercise (MDA, Rmax, CDmax, and NO) in the n-3 LCPUFA group than with placebo.** No main or interaction effects were found for retinol and α-tocopherol. These results indicate that **supplementation with n-3 LCPUFAs significantly increased oxidative stress at rest and after a judo-training session.** (Flaire et al, 2010)

RMH Note: Contrary to predictions, this means that the antioxidant omega-3 does not decrease EMODs as predicted (an antioxidant would decrease oxidative stress). Instead, it increases EMOD (ROS) production (oxidation). (McAnulty et al, 2010)

Omega-3s increase oxidative stress in Judo athletes

Effect of 6 Weeks of n-3 Fatty-Acid Supplementation on Oxidative Stress in Judo Athletes

Abstract

PURPOSE:

n-3 fatty acids are known to exert multiple beneficial effects including anti-inflammatory actions that may diminish oxidative stress. Supplementation with antioxidant vitamins has been proposed to counteract oxidative stress and improve antioxidant status. Therefore, this project investigated the effects of daily supplementation in 48 trained cyclists over 6 wk and during 3 d of continuous exercise on F2-isoprostanes (oxidative stress), plasma n-3 fatty acids, and antioxidant status (oxygen radical absorption capacity and ferric-reducing antioxidant potential).

METHODS:

Cyclists were randomized into n-3 fatty acids (N3) (n = 11) (2000 mg of eicosapentaenoic acid and 400 mg of docosahexaenoic acid), a vitamin-mineral (VM) complex (n = 12) emphasizing vitamins C (2000 mg), E (800 IU), A (3000 IU), and selenium (200 microg), a VM and n-3 fatty acid combination (VN3) (n = 13), or placebo (P) (n = 12). Blood was collected at baseline and preexercise and postexercise. A 4 x 3 repeated-measures ANOVA was performed to test main effects.

RESULTS:

After exercise, F2-isoprostanes were higher in N3. Eicosapentaenoic acid and docosahexaenoic acid plasma values were higher after supplementation in both n-3 supplemented groups. Oxygen radical absorption capacity declined similarly among all groups after exercise. Ferric-reducing antioxidant potential exhibited significant interaction and significantly increased after exercise in VN3 and VM.

CONCLUSIONS:

This study indicates that **supplementation with n-3 fatty acids alone significantly increases F2-isoprostanes after exhaustive exercise.** Lastly, **antioxidant supplementation augments plasma antioxidant status and modestly attenuates but does not prevent the significant n-3 fatty acid associated increase in F2-isoprostanes postexercise.** (McAnulty et al, 2011)

Combining flavonoids, antioxidants and n-3 fatty acids reduces post exercise EMODs

Abstract

Consumption of plant flavonoids, antioxidants, and n-3 fatty acids is proposed to have many potential health benefits derived primarily through antioxidant and anti-inflammatory activities. This study examined the effects of **1,000 mg quercetin + 1,000 mg vitamin C (QC); 1,000 mg quercetin, 1,000 mg vitamin C, 400 mg isoquercetin, 30 mg epigallocatechin gallate, and 400 mg n-3 fatty acids (QFO);** or placebo (P), taken each day for 2 wk before and during 3 d of cycling at 57% W(max) for 3 hr, on plasma antioxidant capacity (ferricreducing ability of plasma [FRAP], oxygen-radical absorbance capacity [ORAC]), plasma oxidative stress (F(2)-isoprostanes), and plasma quercetin and vitamin C levels. Thirty-nine athletes were recruited and randomized to QC, QFO, or P. Blood was collected at baseline, after 2 wk supplementation, immediately postexercise, and 14 hr postexercise. Statistical design used a 3 (groups) × 4 (times) repeated-measures ANOVA with post hoc analyses. Plasma quercetin was significantly elevated in QC and QFO compared with P. Plasma F(2)-isoprostanes, FRAP, and vitamin C were significantly elevated and ORAC significantly decreased immediately postexercise, but no difference was noted in the overall pattern of change. Post hoc analyses revealed that the QC and QFO groups did not exhibit a significant increase in F(2)-isoprostanes from baseline to immediately postexercise compared with P. This study indicates that **combining flavonoids and antioxidants with n-3 fatty acids is effective in reducing the immediate postexercise increase in F(2)-isoprostanes.** Moreover, this effect occurs independently of changes in plasma antioxidant capacity. (McAnulty, AOX, 2011)

Omega-3s and quercetin reduce Al-induced oxidative stress

Abstract

Exposure to high levels of aluminum (Al) leads to neurodegeneration, which may be mediated through over-generation of free radicals. So, in the present study, we investigated the ability of both quercetin and omega 3 to ameliorate adverse effects of Al on brain antioxidants by monitoring the main brain antioxidant enzymes on molecular and cellular levels. The obtained results indicated that Al induced oxidative stress through induction of free radical production and inhibition of activity and expression of the antioxidant enzymes catalase (CAT), glutathione reductase (GR), and glutathione peroxidase (GPx); and at the same time induced superoxide dismutase (SOD) activity and gene expression. Both **quercetin (QE) and omega 3 have the ability to overcome Al-induced oxidative stress**, manifested by the significant reduction in free radical concentration and induction of the activity and gene expression of the brain antioxidant enzymes. (Ali et al, 2014)

Vitamins C and E attenuated exercise VO(2) max

Abstract

Antioxidant supplementations are commonly used as an ergogenic aid for physical exercise despite its limited evidence. The study aimed to investigate the effects of a polyphenol mixture and vitamins on exercise endurance capacity. Seventy regularly exercising male participants were randomly assigned to receive oligomerized lychee fruit extract, **a mixture of vitamin C (800 mg) and E (320 IU),** or a placebo for 30 consecutive days. The study results showed that oligomerized lychee fruit extract significantly elevated the submaximal running time. The adjusted mean change was 3.87 min (95% CI: 1.29, 6.46) for oligomerized lychee fruit extract, 1.33 (-1.23, 3.89) for the vitamins, and 1.60 (-1.36, 4.56) for the placebo. Oligomerized lychee fruit extract significantly increased the anaerobic threshold by 7.4% (1.8, 13.0). On the other hand, **vitamins significantly "attenuated (tapered or narrowed)" VO(2)max by -3.11 ml/kg/m.** Their effects on plasma free radical amount, however, were similar. Our results suggest that a polyphenol-containing supplement and typical antioxidants may have different mechanisms of action and that the endurance-promoting effect of oligomerized lychee fruit extract may not directly come from the scavenging of free radicals but may be attributed to other non-antioxidant properties of polyphenols, which requires further investigation. (Kang et al, 2012)

Vitamins C and E block post-exercise muscle repair

Abstract

In this **double-blind, randomized**, controlled trial, we investigated the effects of vitamin C and E supplementation on endurance training adaptations in humans. Fifty-four young men and women were randomly allocated to receive either 1000 mg of vitamin C and 235 mg of vitamin E or a placebo daily for 11 weeks. During supplementation, the participants completed an endurance training programme consisting of three to four sessions per week (primarily of running), divided into high-intensity interval sessions [4-6 × 4-6 min; >90% of maximal heart rate (HRmax)] and steady state continuous sessions (30-60 min; 70-90% of HRmax). Maximal oxygen uptake (VO2 max), submaximal running and a 20 m shuttle run test were assessed and blood samples and muscle biopsies were collected, before and after the intervention. Participants in the **vitamin C and E** group increased their VO2 max and performance in the 20 m shuttle test (10 ± 11%) to the same degree as those in the placebo group. However, the mitochondrial marker cytochrome c oxidase subunit IV (COX4) and cytosolic peroxisome proliferator-activated receptor-γ coactivator 1 α (PGC-1α) increased in the m. vastus lateralis in the placebo group by 59 ± 97% and 19 ± 51%, respectively, but not in the vitamin C and E group. Furthermore, mRNA levels of CDC42 and mitogen-activated protein kinase 1 (MAPK1) in the trained muscle were lower in the vitamin C and E group than in the placebo group. **Daily vitamin C and E supplementation attenuated increases in markers of mitochondrial biogenesis following endurance training.** However, no clear interactions were detected for improvements in VO2 max and running performance. Consequently, **vitamin C and E supplementation hampered cellular adaptations in the exercised muscles**, and although this did not translate to the performance tests applied in this study, **we advocate caution when considering antioxidant supplementation combined with endurance exercise**. (Paulsen et al, 2014)

Antioxidants reduce post-exercise muscle repair

Antioxidant supplementation reduces skeletal muscle mitochondrial biogenesis.

Abstract

PURPOSE:

Exercise increases the production of reactive oxygen species (ROS) in skeletal muscle, and athletes often consume antioxidant supplements in the belief they will attenuate ROS-related muscle damage and fatigue during exercise. However, exercise-induced ROS may regulate beneficial skeletal muscle adaptations, such as increased mitochondrial biogenesis. We therefore investigated the effects of long-term antioxidant supplementation with vitamin E and α-lipoic acid on changes in markers of mitochondrial biogenesis in the skeletal muscle of exercise-trained and sedentary rats.

METHODS:

Male Wistar rats were divided into four groups: 1) sedentary control diet, 2) sedentary antioxidant diet, 3) exercise control diet, and 4) exercise antioxidant diet. Animals ran on a treadmill 4 d · wk at ~ 70%VO2max for up to 90 min · d for 14 wk.

RESULTS:

Consistent with the augmentation of skeletal muscle mitochondrial biogenesis and antioxidant defenses, after training there were significant increases in peroxisome proliferator-activated receptor γ coactivator 1α (PGC-1α) messenger RNA (mRNA) and protein, cytochrome C oxidase subunit IV (COX IV) and cytochrome C protein abundance, citrate synthase activity, Nfe2l2, and SOD2 protein. **Antioxidant supplementation reduced PGC-1α mRNA, PGC-1α and COX IV protein, and citrate synthase enzyme activity ($P < 0.05$) in both sedentary and exercise-trained rats**.

CONCLUSIONS:

Vitamin E and α-lipoic acid supplementation suppresses skeletal muscle mitochondrial biogenesis, regardless of training status. (Strobel et al, 2011)

MACULAR DEGENERATION(AMD)

Omega-3 effect on macular degeneration (AMD)

AREDS2: The Bottom Line on Supplements for AMD

Julia A. Haller, MD, Joseph I. Maguire, MD - Jun 12, 2013

Commentary: This was a presentation by Julia Haller, Ophthalmologist-in-Chief at Wills Eye Institute here in Philadelphia and her colleague, Dr. Joseph Maguire of their retina service, who serves as the principal investigator on the AREDS2 (Age-Related Eye Disease Study 2) trial, the results of which were recently released.

Their commentary is a collaboration between Wills Eye Institute and Medscape.

Joe, we are here to talk about the results of the AREDS2 study. What is the bottom line?

Joseph I. Maguire, MD: The first AREDS trial was initiated to see whether nutritional supplements could reduce the risk for progression to advanced age-related macular degeneration (AMD) as people mature through life. The original results were released in 2001 and showed that a combination of vitamins C and E with zinc and copper, as well as vitamin A in the form of beta-carotene, reduce by 25% the risk of developing high-risk macular degeneration over time.

The **AREDS2** trial asked whether we could augment that benefit by adding to the supplement. The first addition was **omega-3 fatty acids (fish oil)**, and the second was a combination of 2 carotenoids, lutein and zeaxanthin, which are prevalent in leafy green vegetables and highly colored fruits and vegetables.

Dr. Haller: This was a complicated study with lots of different groups and randomizations. What are you telling your patients now?

Dr. Maguire: Correct. A lot of different subgroups were included. The take-home message is twofold: **First, omega-3 fatty acids did not confer additional benefit to reducing the risk for progression to high-risk AMD over time**; and second, **lutein and zeaxanthin**

did add to the benefit, but only in the lowest-quintile group of folks who may not have been getting as much lutein and zeaxanthin in their usual diet compared with the other groups. Because there were so many subgroups, it seemed that the folks who took lutein and zeaxanthin instead of beta-carotene had more of a benefit. We theorized that beta-carotene may have inhibited the absorption of lutein and zeaxanthin in those folks.

Dr. Haller: In other words, the people who were taking all of the supplements, including beta-carotene, effectively got less lutein and zeaxanthin.

Dr. Maguire: Effectively, yes. Finally, we know from previous studies that beta-carotene increases the risk for cancer in active smokers or people who have had lung cancer previously. In AREDS2, folks who were previous smokers also had a higher risk for lung cancer.

Dr. Haller: It may be a risk from the beta-carotene.

Dr. Maguire: Exactly. **The study concluded that omega-3 fatty acids are not necessary to enhance the vitamin supplement, but that lutein and zeaxanthin could be substituted for beta-carotene.**

Dr. Haller: That is what I am telling my patients about new dietary supplements. What is the buzz in your clinic? Are patients interested in supplements? Are they asking about nutritional factors that may be involved with their AMD?

Dr. Maguire: They always are. **Omega-3 fatty acids have been shown to be beneficial in cardiac disease, stroke prevention, et cetera, so it is a bit of a disappointment that it did not help in AMD.** Patients are very informed about that. Of course, people are more interested in healthy diets these days, and the carotenoids lutein and zeaxanthin, which are present in very high concentrations in vegetables and fruit were a **positive, although a mild one**.

Dr. Haller: What do you say when patients ask, "Where do I get this supplement, Dr. Maguire? Can I buy it at the store?"

Dr. Maguire: You will see a big shift in the vitamins at the pharmacy now. There is not a commercially available supplement that includes all of these elements. It takes a while for the industry to revamp things and get it onto the shelves. An AREDS2 vitamin supplement is commercially available, but that has fish oil in it and it is a little bit more expensive. It has all of the other components though. You can take one of the products that has lutein in it instead of the beta-carotene, which we previously directed our smoking patients to take, but it does not include the zeaxanthin just yet.

Dr. Haller: This is good news for people with macular degeneration. There is no other treatment for the dry macular degeneration. It is exciting news that **there is the potential of as much as a 15%-20% increase in their protection against advanced AMD with an adjustment of their drugs.**

Dr. Maguire: I think so, too.

Dr. Haller: Thank you, Joe. It is a pleasure to be here with Dr. Maguire from Wills Eye Institute in Philadelphia, in collaboration with Medscape. Thank you.

Antioxidants, Omega-3 Fail to Halt Macular Degeneration

Damian McNamara May 07, 2013

Antioxidant and omega-3 supplements do not reduce the risk for advanced macular degeneration, according to results from the highly anticipated Age-Related Eye Disease Study (AREDS2).

Although the primary results are disappointing, important clinical messages emerged during its presentation here at the Association for Research in Vision and Ophthalmology 2013 Annual Meeting. The results were published online **May 5, 2013 in the *JAMA: The Journal of the American Medical Association*** to coincide with their presentation.

The new data point to ways to change the nutritional formulation from the initial AREDS trial to reduce potential risks without sacrificing benefit for people at high risk for advanced age-related macular degeneration (*Arch Ophthalmol.* 2001;119:1417-1436).

"**AREDS resulted in a formulation of vitamin C, beta carotene, zinc, and vitamin E that reduced the risk of progression of**

advanced disease by 25%" at 5 years, Emily Chew, MD, from the National Eye Institute in Bethesda, Maryland, told *Medscape Medical News*. "We wanted to see if we could tweak it a bit by adding components to it."

Bolstered by promising evidence from animal and observational studies, Dr. Chew and her team sought to determine if the addition of the carotenoids lutein and zeaxanthin and/or the omega-3 fatty acids docosahexaenoic acid (DHA) and eicosapentaenoic acid (EPA) could further forestall progression to advanced macular degeneration.

It didn't work. "In the overall analysis, using 3 treatment groups, we found no significant difference in rates of macular degeneration," Dr. Chew said. In fact, **risk was not significantly reduced with any treatment, compared with placebo**, over a median of 4.9 years of follow-up.

A total **4,203 participants were randomized** to placebo with no additional supplementation or to 1 of 3 treatment groups. The first group received a tablet of 10 mg lutein plus 2 mg zeaxanthin — both antioxidants found in green leafy vegetables. The second group received a gel cap with 350 mg DHA plus 650 mg EPA. The third group received both the tablet and gel cap on a daily basis.

When asked by *Medscape Medical News* to comment on the findings, Abdhish Bhavsar, MD, said, "**I was quite surprised to see that AREDS2 did not show any difference between the primary outcome treatment groups**. However, the study involved a very complex clinical trial design and tried to answer some difficult questions on lutein plus zeaxanthin and DHA plus EPA." Dr. Bhavsar, a retinal surgeon, is director of clinical research at the Retina Center in Minneapolis, Minnesota, and national clinical spokesperson for the American Academy of Ophthalmology.

Although no significant additional overall benefit emerged, **a subanalysis showed that lutein plus zeaxanthin supplementation might help some patients.** When stratified by dietary intake of these antioxidants at baseline, participants in the lowest quintile who took the supplements showed a 26% risk reduction against progression to advanced macular degeneration.

"That is not exactly small," Dr. Chew said. "People who are not eating enough show a benefit."

Silver Lining

Another **secondary analysis** of the data yielded **a 10% risk reduction in progression to advanced macular degeneration in patients who took lutein plus zeaxanthin**, compared with those who did not. "So this appears to have an effect," Dr. Chew said.

"Secondary-level analyses seem to point in the direction that lutein and zeaxanthin are associated with a reduction in progression to advanced and neovascular age-related macular degeneration," Dr. Bhavsar said. "Thus, at the present time — although based on secondary analyses — it seems that the best medical evidence points to considering lutein and zeaxanthin in addition to the AREDS formula."

The best medical evidence points to considering lutein and zeaxanthin in addition to the AREDS formula.

The researchers also performed a **secondary randomization of 3,036 participants** to evaluate refinements in the initial formulation — specifically, daily supplementation with lower zinc levels, without beta carotene, or both.

Dr. Chew and colleagues responded to concerns from nutritionists that **the amount of zinc in AREDS exceeds the absorbable amount.** They assessed the potential removal of beta carotene to reduce the risk for lung cancer in smokers that has been seen in other randomized controlled trials (*J Natl Cancer Inst.* 1996;88:1550-1559) and (*Am J Clin Nutr.* 1995;62:1427S-1430S).

Lowering zinc dose did not significantly alter progression to advanced macular degeneration, nor did the removal of the beta carotene. A recommendation to change the zinc dose, therefore, was not made based on the findings.

For this reason, smokers were randomized to 1 of 2 formulations without beta carotene in AREDS2. In the second randomization component of AREDS2, more lung cancers still occurred in the beta carotene group than in the no beta carotene group (2.0% vs 0.9%). The vast majority of participants (91%) who developed lung cancer were former smokers, "so former smokers are at risk for lung cancer with beta carotene," Dr. Chew said.

"The bottom line is that we have enough data to suggest we can remove the beta carotene in the AREDS formulation and

substitute it with the lutein and zeaxanthin," she pointed out. "This way there is one formulation for people to take whether they have ever smoked or not."

Researchers enrolled participants in AREDS2 from October 2006 to September 2008 at 82 clinical sites. All were 50 to 85 years of age (mean, 73 years) and at high risk for progression to advanced macular degeneration because of bilateral large drusen or large drusen in one eye and advanced macular degeneration in the other.

Low rates of loss to follow-up (3%) and good adherence to the treatment regimen are strengths of the study. Generalizability of results is a potential limitation, as is the inability to determine if the null findings are attributable to lack of efficacy of the supplements, inadequate dose, inadequate duration, or a combination of these.

The study found that while **omega-3 fatty acids had no effect on the formulation**, lutein and zeaxanthin together appeared to be a safe and effective alternative to beta-carotene. (AREDS2, 2013)

AREDS failed but not a failure

Association for Research in Vision and Ophthalmology 2013 Annual Meeting. Presented May 5, 2013.

The AREDS2 trial failed to prove what many patients and clinicians hoped that it would prove, but it should not be viewed as a "failure," because it produced high-quality clinical data. Identifying ineffective treatments is an integral part of the larger process of finding the most effective treatment. Although carotenoids and omega-3 fatty acids are not the long-awaited answer to delaying the progression of AMD, we are edging closer to a cure because we now know the true effects of these supplements.

Sardi's extreme views are fishy

Orthomolecular Medicine News Service, December 11, 2013

Something's Fishy About Macular Degeneration Fish Oil Studies

by Bill Sardi

(OMNS Dec 11, 2013) Just seven months ago National Eye Institute researchers claimed fish oil "doesn't seem to help macular degeneration," a sight-robbing eye disease that plagues adults in their senior years. (http://www.sciencedaily.com/releases/2013/05/130513152403.htm)

So how could another newly published study produce exactly opposite results? In fact, fish oil didn't just slow down the insidious progression of this eye disease, it restored vision to every patient placed on high-dose fish oil. It was therapeutic and curative, not just preventive.

The study I'm referring to is likely to be dismissed.The study group was small - only 25 patients. **There was no inactive placebo pill given to another group of patients for comparison, a requirement for scientific validity. RMH Note: Ergo, this was NOT a scientific study, but it does represent the extreme views of some authors.** And it's also possible (but not plausible) that all the patients in the study were abjectly deficient in omega-3 fish oils, producing an atypical effect. But the study group was based in the Mediterranean where fish consumption is high. And it's not likely any placebo effect was involved.

The study is so convincing, especially when combined with all of the positive fish oil studies conducted over the last decade (see chart below), eye physicians would now be derelict in their duty not to recommend every long-living senior adult to consume more fish, or better yet - take concentrated fish oil capsules, if they want to maintain their sight throughout their retirement years.

Compilation fish oil/age-related dry macular degeneration studies

PharmNutrition Dec 2013: Invalid scientific study showed 100% improvement

Ophthalmology Aug 2013: No visual acuity improvement

J Amer Med Assn May 2013: Visual improvements were not significant

Olive oil shown to halve risk to develop advanced AMD in another study (Archives Ophthalmology 127: 674, May 2009)

Growing evidence

The study I'm referring to was just published in the PharmNutrition journal. (Georgiou et al, 2013) (Georgiou T, Neokleous A, Nicolaou D, Sears B. Pilot study for treating dry age-related macular degeneration (AMD) with high-dose omega-3 fatty acids. PharmaNutrition, Available online 18 October 2013. http://dx.doi.org/10.1016/j.phanu.2013.10.001)

It raises many questions, particularly why has it taken so long to discover high-dose fish oil can restore lost sight to many Americans. The data pointing to fish oil as a dietary agent that can stave off vision loss with advancing age has been growing for over a decade.

Except for one "fishy" study, all other human clinical fish oil studies published over the past 13 years indicate fish oil slows down or prevents macular degeneration, a sight-robbing condition that affects central vision used for reading, driving and face recognition.

The latest published study was more momentous than prior studies as it didn't just show fish oil slows down the progression of the disease; it actually began to restore vision to patients within days of starting a daily regimen of high-dose fish oil capsules.

Slowing macular degeneration down is one thing, but reversing it is another. There is no cure for the common form of the disease, called dry macular degeneration. **Antioxidant dietary supplements recommended for this disease slow down its progression by maybe 10 percent at best. RMH Note: Probably Not.**

Macular degeneration patients began experiencing improvement in visual acuity from the get-go. After six months a third of the patients could see letters that were three lines smaller on the eye chart. Another third saw two lines better and the remaining third a single line of improvement.

100% of patients with macular degeneration experienced improved vision when the normal course of the disease is insidiously progressive loss of central vision.

High dose

The dose of fish oil was the highest used in any study so far — 5000 milligrams (3400 mg EPA, 1600 mg DHA), or a bit less than two tablespoons a day. That much fish oil is likely to be costly for retirees on fixed incomes, around two dollars a day. A six-month course would certainly be worth the investment, especially when some seniors might be able to renew their driver's license or resume activities that help them stay independent.

The one "fishy" negative study was reported in the Journal of the American Medical Association in May of this year. (AREDS2, 2013) (The Age-Related Eye Disease Study 2 (AREDS2) Research Group. Lutein + Zeaxanthin and Omega-3 Fatty Acids for Age-Related Macular Degeneration: The Age-Related Eye Disease Study 2 (AREDS2) Randomized Clinical Trial. JAMA. 2013;309(19):2005-2015)

National Eye Institute researchers said fish oil "doesn't seem to help age-related macular degeneration."

That study compared a low dose of omega-3 fish oil with an antioxidant formula providing lutein, zeaxanthin, zinc and copper (no true placebo group or inactive pill was used). The dose of fish oils in the treatment group was much lower than prior studies.

Some skeptical researchers I have consulted express concerns over the fact this study was conducted largely among well-nourished subjects who likely eat a lot of fish in their diet. I'm informed that the comparison group consumed up to 720 milligrams of fish oil from their daily diet. Also some study subjects in the comparison group may have been supplementing with folic acid which raises blood levels of omega-3 oils. (Das, 2008) (Das UN. Folic acid and polyunsaturated fatty acids improve cognitive function and prevent depression, dementia, and Alzheimer's disease--but how and why? Prostaglandins Leukot Essent Fatty Acids. 2008 Jan;78(1):11-9)

Researchers concede that "study results may not be generalizable, because the study population is a highly selected group of highly educated and well-nourished people." Was the study rigged to fail?

(Bill Sardi is a well-known nutritional medicine writer and is the founder of Knowledge of Health, Inc. http://knowledgeofhealth.com/ Copyright (C) 2013 Bill Sardi.)

SECTION SIX

DANGERS

Adverse events are mild to moderate

BACKGROUND: Omega-3 (n-3) fatty acid supplementation is becoming increasingly popular. However given its antithrombotic properties the potential for severe adverse events (SAE) such as bleeding has safety implications, particularly in an older adult population. A systematic review of randomized control trials (RCT) was conducted to explore the potential for SAE and non-severe adverse events (non-SAE) associated with n-3 supplementation in older adults.

METHODS: A comprehensive search strategy using Medline and a variety of other electronic sources was conducted. Studies investigating the oral administration of n-3 fish oil containing eicosapentaenoic acid (EPA), docosahexaenoic acid (DHA) or both against a placebo were sourced. The primary outcome of interest included reported SAE associated with n-3 supplementation. Chi-square analyses were conducted on the pooled aggregate of AEs.

RESULTS: Of the 398 citations initially retrieved, a total of 10 studies involving 994 older adults aged >=60 years were included in the review. Daily fish oil doses ranged from 0.03 g to 1.86 g EPA and/or DHA with study durations ranging from 6 to 52 weeks. No SAE were reported and there were no significant differences in the total AE rate between groups. Non-SAE relating to **gastrointestinal (GI) disturbances were the most commonly reported** however there was no significant increase in the proportion of GI disturbances reported in participants randomized to the n-3 intervention.

CONCLUSIONS: The potential for AEs appear mild-moderate at worst and are unlikely to be of clinical significance. The use of n-3 fatty acids and the potential for SAE should however be further researched to investigate whether this evidence is consistent at higher doses and in other populations. These results also highlight that well-documented data outlining the potential for SAE following n-3 supplementation are limited nor adequately reported to draw definitive conclusions concerning the safety associated with n-3 supplementation. A more rigorous and systematic approach for monitoring and recording AE data in clinical settings that involve n-3 supplementation is required. (Villane et al, 2013)

GENERAL DISCUSSION BY OTHERS

Omega-3: Fishing Out the Recent Evidence

JoAnn E. Manson, MD, DrPH 6-4-13

Dr. JoAnn Manson, Professor of Medicine at Brigham and Women's Hospital and Harvard Medical School. talked about the recent confusing reports on omega-3 fish oil. Is there a way for us to make sense of these **recent studies that seem to be at odds with earlier evidence that suggested cardioprotection from omega-3 fatty acids?** Have omegas-3 fatty acids lost their luster, or are there other explanations for these recent findings?

There are several mechanisms through which omega-3 fatty acids may protect against cardiovascular disease, including reducing inflammation, lowering clotting risk, reducing triglyceride levels, and lowering the risk for irregular heart rhythms. However, the **recent randomized trials in high-risk populations (those with either multiple risk factors or a history of cardiovascular disease) have suggested very little benefit from omega-3 fatty acids.** (Roncaglioni et al, 2013) (Kotwal et al, 2012) (Rizos et al, 2012)

Disappointing Results From Omega-3 Fatty Acids Trials

A recent report was published in the *New England Journal of Medicine* in early May. (Roncaglioni et al, 2013)

Patients with multiple cardiovascular risk factors were given 1 gram of fish oil per day vs placebo, and it showed no benefit.

Also, other meta-analyses have been published in the past year that looked at all of the randomized trials in aggregate. (Kotwal et al, 2012) (Rizos et al, 2012). **These are secondary-prevention, randomized trials with high-risk populations. In general, these meta-analyses have shown disappointing results.**

It is very important to keep in mind that these high-risk populations -- secondary-prevention populations -- include many individuals who are already taking multiple heart medications such as statins, aspirin, and ACE inhibitors, which may obscure the effect of omega-3 fatty acids. There may be very little incremental benefit from omega-3 fatty acids in that setting. What can we conclude from these recent findings?

What Should We Recommend to Our Patients?

First, **these randomized trials of fish oil do not cast out on the recommendation to have at least 2 servings of dietary fish per week. That is a recommendation from the American Heart Association and many other professional societies, and many studies suggest benefit.** Some of the benefit may be because dietary fish is replacing other foods that could increase risk, such as red meat or foods high in saturated fat. Do recommend at least 2 servings of fish per week, particularly the darker fatty fish such as salmon and mackerel.

Second, in patients who are candidates for prescription omega-3 fatty acids, those who have very high triglyceride levels, these findings do not cast doubt on that indication for use. That would still be an appropriate use. In patients who are taking fish oil and are doing very well on it and feel strongly that the fish oil is helping their symptoms or are a benefit to them, there is no strong basis from these studies for encouraging them to stop, because **there were no major risks associated with fish oil found in the studies**.

CVD Benefits in Fish Oil: Is EPA the Pearl?

Carol Peckham, Howard S. Weintraub, MD Jun 05, 2013

NEJM Study on Use of Fish Oil Prevention of CVD

Editor's Note: A recent study in the New England Journal of Medicine (NEJM) reported that **there is no cardiovascular protective benefit from fish oil supplements in high-risk patients (those with multiple cardiovascular risk factors or atherosclerotic vascular disease but not myocardial infarction**). (Roncaglioni et al, 2013)

Some meta-analyses have also reported a lack of effect, (Kotwal et al, 2012) (Rizos et al, 2012) **although other trials have reported 20% to 50% reductions in total mortality and sudden death using doses of 0.85 to 4.0 g/day, with treatment durations from 12 to 42 months.** (Jacobson, 2006)

The current study used 1 g/day and the results were reported after 1 year. For a perspective on this study, Medscape interviewed **Howard Weintraub**, Clinical Director of the Center for the Prevention of Cardiovascular Disease at New York University School of Medicine, New York University Medical Center.

Medscape: Do you think the NEJM study definitively proves the case against use of fish oil supplements in preventing cardiovascular disease?

Dr. Weintraub: Other fish oil studies more or less came to the same conclusions, although the NEJM study was prospective, placebo-randomized, and large, with 12,513 patients. One was published in the *Journal of the American College of Cardiology* a year or so ago. (Mozaffarian, Wu, 2011)

Another was a review we did at New York University, published in 2010. (Weitz et al, 2010). It had some interesting data about the use of fish oils, but **we couldn't support the idea that you should give these agents to everybody for prevention of cardiovascular events.**

However, to make a broad, sweeping comment about fish oil on the basis of this one study may be premature. First, you want to recognize the use of 1 g rather than 4 g of fish oil. Next, the population that was studied was not hypertriglyceridemic. You also want to look at the fish oil that was used. Namely, some literature raises interest about the ratios of the different components of fish oil, namely eicosapentaenoic acid (EPA) and docosahexaenoic acid (DHA). Also, if you go to different stores -- a nutrition store or Costco -- you're at different ends of the spectrum. **You may not only find very different ratios of EPA to DHA, but you also may have differences in purity or the presence of either fluorocarbons or mercury.**

I think that taking fish oil in a daily dose of 1 g in the expectation of preventing cardiovascular morbidity and mortality or major events has been done mostly in Europe and is not practiced much here. It's rare to see somebody in this country who had either cardiac events or stents who is using fish oil just for that indication. There is some evidence in the literature for it, but **the current prescriptions in the United States for fish oil are 4 g given for hypertriglyceridemia**. I have not used fish oil for prevention of cardiovascular morbidity or mortality. Hence, as long as I haven't used it for this indication, this study doesn't have any impact on the way I use fish oil and won't put a nail in the coffin, or a nail in the lid.

Medscape: Are there studies on non-fish oil agents that might be more promising in preventing cardiovascular events?

Dr. Weintraub: There have been a number of recent disappointing studies on agents other than fish oil for preventing cardiovascular events. The current state of confusion about reducing cardiovascular risk is not helped by results from studies like **AIM-HIGH** (Boden et al, AIM-HIGH, 2011) and **THRIVE** (HPS2-THRIVE, 2013), in which **the addition of niacin [to a statin] provided no protection**, although it might not have been expected to, based upon the baseline lipids of the population. Other studies, such as **FIELD** (Keech et al, 2005), looked at fibrates, and **ACCORD** (Gerstein et al, ACCORD, 2011) studied the effect of intensive glucose lowering on cardiovascular outcomes. (Boden et al, AIM-HIGH, 2011)

None of these studies showed any benefit with non-statin agents for protecting against cardiovascular events or helped physicians in making decisions about how to treat patients.

Looking at EPA

Medscape: So, is fish oil then also out of the question for cardiovascular protection?

Dr. Weintraub: If you were to put 50 cardiologists and endocrinologists in the same room and ask them to name 1 study in which another medicine was added to a statin and there were meaningful significant reductions in cardiovascular events, they would probably look around and not be sure. I would say that **one such study is JELIS, which was conducted in Japan and added fish oil to a statin for patients with high cholesterol (6.5 mmol/L or greater).** (Itakura et al, JELIS, 2012) (Yokoyama et al, JELIS, 2007) (Jacobson, 2007)

It's important to note that **the study used only EPA**, with a purity of something like 94% or 96%. At a mean follow-up of 4.6 years, they observed a 19% relative reduction in major coronary events in those on EPA, although the effect on triglycerides in that trial was not dramatic. **Unstable angina and nonfatal coronary events were significantly reduced. Sudden cardiac death and coronary death did not differ between groups.** Granted, nobody on our side of the pond thinks that trials populated exclusively with Asian participants would necessarily indicate the same results in people in Europe or the United States, but I think it's an interesting phenomenon.

A small US company has made its own version of EPA, icosapent ethyl (Vascepa®; Amarin Pharma), which has been approved. **They conducted 2 studies: ANCHOR** (Ballanytyne et al, ANCHOR, 2012) **and MARINE, which allowed the FDA to approve icosapent ethyl for the same indication as the other approved fish oil (Lovaza®; GlaxoSmithKline), a combination of EPA and DHA, with a ratio of about 4:3.** (Bays et al, MARINE, 2012)

The MARINE study looked at people with triglyceride levels over 500 mg/dL, which represents about 1% to 2% of the US population, and the ANCHOR study looked at those with triglyceride levels between 200 and 500 mg/dL, which reflects a larger proportion -- about 20% -- of the US population. **One interesting observation was that using a statin along with EPA achieved much greater triglyceride reductions than using EPA without a statin, and the stronger the statin, the better the effect.** So, the interaction between EPA and statins is intriguing. Fish oils may not be dead in the water for this reason alone.

The good news is that we're going to have to wait only 2 to 4 years for answers to the question of whether EPA is beneficial in high-risk patients. An event trial with at least 50% currently recruited is looking at the concomitant addition of icosapent ethyl to therapy in individuals with documented cardiovascular disease and/or diabetes.

I certainly haven't seen any studies in major journals on any comparative difference between the DHA/EPA combinations and the EPA-only agents. However, **if you look at the FDA's Pharmaceutical Inspectorate (PI) for Lovaza, and in most of the data that the company has compiled, there is an average net increase in LDL cholesterol**. Obviously this can turn some people off. **We almost get the same kind of information that was out there with rosiglitazone, when, if you remember, LDL was increased in many of its studies.** So, whether this mattered or not, certainly LDL is one of the few things in the lipid world that we have relative agreement on, that it is bad for you. There are some very interesting theories floating around, but I think that being LDL neutral and reducing inflammatory markers and triglycerides, as is indicated in the MARINE and ANCHOR studies on EPA, may be the difference in how these fish oil drugs behave.

Medscape: What about lifestyle changes? Triglycerides are usually associated with obesity, right?

Dr. Weintraub: Granted, in many cases, lifestyle is the problem in patients with high triglycerides, so you ask the patient for a little help. Sometimes you get it and sometimes you don't. Controlling sugar, watching their diet -- all the things that they can do to lose weight is the most effective approach. **You can get a 20% reduction in triglycerides after dropping a few pounds**, but that's one of the hardest things to do. Other behaviors help: stopping drinking and watching the kind of carbs you're eating. But do we just completely ignore a patient if his triglycerides are still 400? We're just going to turn our heads and walk away? I don't think that's a clever idea. When triglycerides are very high, things do not go well, so you also want medicines that work. However, you don't want to use 4 drugs to get it down. Therefore, I don't think that fish oil as a class is gone.

Medscape: So, if a patient comes in without high triglycerides and he's taking fish oil on his own, do you tell him to stop?

Dr. Weintraub: If you pool a bunch of cardiologists, internists, and even primary physicians and ask, "Do you use fish oil?" they'd probably say, "Well, you know, if someone wants to use it, it's okay." So, if you're on fish oil and you're tolerating it, then continue. However, **would you instigate, provoke, or insist upon fish oil being used to prevent cardiovascular-related mortality and morbidity?**

The answer is probably no. If you're wondering whether you need it, the answer is also no.

On the other hand, **we don't have enough information in the dyslipidemic population, and particularly in people with triglycerides over 500, to say that fish oils are dead. That's where we are now.**

Omega-3s did not change insulin sensitivity

In summary, this study examined the effects of fish oil (FO) treatment on adipose tissue inflammation in obese subjects with the metabolic syndrome. Although **there were no changes in insulin sensitivity**, adipose tissue macrophages were decreased and adipose capillaries increased in the FO-treated subjects, along with a decrease in adipose and plasma MCP-1. Relatively few additional changes in gene expression were detected; although there was evidence suggesting that subjects with the greatest degree of adipose inflammation responded most strongly to the FO treatment. These results suggest that FO treatment has direct beneficial effects on the adipose phenotype and that a more prolonged treatment may lead to improved metabolic function. (Spencer et al, 2013)

Omega-3 PUFA as Biomarkers

Plasma Levels Predict Mortality, CV Events in CHS Analysis

Steve Stiles Apr 03, 2013

The highest levels of plasma phospholipid omega-3 polyunsaturated fatty acids (PUFA), as measured in >2500 older adults initially without coronary heart disease or a history of stroke, **predicted the lowest mortality in the observational, prospective Cardiovascular Health Study** (CHS).

In comparisons of the highest quintile of omega-3 PUFA levels vs the lowest quintile, all-cause mortality fell by 27%, with most of the benefit due to a reduction in cardiovascular death. The rate of arrhythmic death, in particular, fell by nearly one-half.

Such cardiovascular-outcome effects are consistent with abundant evidence from laboratory and clinical studies that omega-3 PUFA intake may benefit heart rate, blood pressure, myocardial contractile function and electrical stability, and endothelial, autonomic, and hemostatic function, write the study's authors, led by **Dr Dariush Mozaffarian** (Harvard School of Public Health, Boston, MA). **Their analysis was published in the April 2, 2013 issue of the *Annals of Internal Medicine*.** (Mozaffarian et al, CHS, 2013)

The CHS longitudinal data allowed **the group not only to link plasma omega-3 PUFA levels with survival**, Mozaffarian told **heart*wire***, it allowed them to estimate the benefit: in this population, **starting at age 65, he said, about 2.2 extra years for people in the highest compared with the lowest plasma-level quintile**.

Outcomes also varied by individual omega-3 PUFAs. For a number of end points, importantly heart-disease mortality and arrhythmic mortality, **there was a pattern of greater benefit from highest levels of docosahexaenoicacid (DHA) vs highest levels of eicosapentaenoic acid (EPA) and an even greater benefit from highest levels of total omega-3 PUFA.**

For the end point of heart-disease death, "DHA seems to have stronger association" than EPA, according to Mozaffarian; the effect, he noted, appears to be dominated by a difference in arrhythmic death. But EPA at the highest levels vs the lowest levels showed **a weakly significant** trend (p=0.04) of benefit for nonfatal MI, **while DHA and total omega-3 PUFA were unquestionably nonsignificant**. Still, he said, **given the "borderline" p value for EPA, "maybe none of them are significantly associated" with respect to nonfatal MI.**

That outcomes varied by type of omega-3 PUFA has implications for dietary recommendations as well as therapeutic preparations of omega-3 PUFA.

"I think that our results support DHA, in particular, being important for heart-disease death and **leaves open the question of whether EPA . . . [has] additional benefit**." Consuming both together is probably wise, as there appear to be "complementary effects," Mozaffarian said. Based on the current analysis, "**If you're going to consume omega-3s, you should at least be sure you're getting DHA. EPA alone might not have the same benefit; I think that's fair to say.**"

As previously covered by **heart*wire***, the CHS enrolled 5201 adults aged ≥65 years in four US communities, two in the East and one in California from 1989 to 1990, plus 687 additional African Americans from 1992 to 1993. The current analysis includes 2692 without CHD, stroke, or heart failure at baseline who were not taking fish-oil supplements and in whom levels of plasma phospholipid omega-3 PUFA were measured in 1992–1993. Their mean age at baseline was 74 years, 64% were women, and 88% were white; they were followed until 2000.

The adjusted hazard ratio (HR) for total mortality was 0.83 for the highest quintile of EPA vs the lowest quintile, 0.80 for DHA, and 0.73 for total omega-3 PUFA. Decreases in HR for total heart-disease mortality were significant only for DHA and total omega-3 PUFA. The same was true for arrhythmic death: DHA and total omega-3 PUFA.

Acknowledging that "this is an observational study--it doesn't prove cause and effect," Mozaffarian said that **it at least supports high plasma levels of omega-3 PUFAs as directly affecting survival.** "If there was confounding--if it was just that people were more educated or had healthy lifestyles--you'd expect that higher [omega-3 PUFA plasma levels] would relate very similarly to a lower risk of every kind of death: [including] respiratory death, infectious death, cancer death, and stroke death. But the bulk of the association seems to be from heart-disease death, and [especially] heart disease death from arrhythmia."

As for the possible advantage high plasma DHA levels may have over high EPA levels with respect to total and heart-disease mortality, which would conceivably conflict with the higher elevations in LDL cholesterol observed with DHA vs EPA supplementation, **Mozaffarian said he doesn't see a paradox**.

"The LDL-raising effect of omega-3s is very modest." If there is any such effect, he said, "it's to make the particles larger and fluffier and therefore potentially less atherogenic." According to Mozaffarian, "it's just hype" to say that an omega-3 PUFA supplement that delivers only EPA should be preferred over a mixed EPA/DHA supplement because of a difference in LDL effects.

In addition to **many brands of nonprescription mixed EPA/DHA supplements on the market, in the US** there is the prescription-only mixed formulation **Lovaza** (GlaxoSmithKline); and just last year, the **FDA** approved the synthetic EPA-only preparation Vascepa (Amarin), which contains **ethyl eicosapentaenoic acid**.

Fish oil doesn't help prevent heart attacks - NEJM

5-9-13 **Fish oil doesn't help prevent heart attacks. Eating fish is good for your heart but taking fish oil capsules does not help people at high risk of heart problems who are already taking medicines to prevent them. Fish oil supplements in high risk patients does not prevent heart attacks.**

Fish oil capsules failed to prevent flare-ups of atrial fibrillation, a common heart rhythm problem, in a large study in 2010.

The new study was led by the Mario Negri Institute for Pharmacological Research in Milan. It tested 1 **gram a day of fish oil versus dummy capsules in 12,513 people throughout Italy. They had not suffered a heart attack but were at high risk of having one because of diabetes, high blood pressure, high cholesterol, smoking, obesity or other conditions.** Most already were taking cholesterol-lowering statins, aspirin and other medicines to lower their chances of heart problems.

"They're very high-risk people and so the level of other treatments was very high," Arnett said. "When you're being aggressively treated for all of your other risk factors, **adding fish oil yielded no additional benefits."**

Results are published in **5-9-13 New England Journal of Medicine**.

Eating fish is good for your heart but taking fish oil capsules does not help people at high risk of heart problems who are already taking medicines to prevent them, a large study in Italy found. The work, published in the Thursday, May 9, 2013 New England Journal of Medicine, makes clearer who does and does not benefit from taking supplements of omega-3 fatty acids.

Results of recent outcomes trials of long-chain omega-3 fatty acids, fibrates, and niacin have been disappointing, failing to show additional reductions in adverse cardiovascular events when combined with statins. (Bradberry, Hilleman, 2013)

Canola oil and omega-3s (fish oil)

Some of the following was excerpted from THE GREAT CANOLA SCAM Part 2 By Sally Fallon and Mary G. Enig

Animal studies on **Low Erucic Acid Rapeseed (LEAR)** oil were performed when the oil was first developed and have continued to the present. The results challenge not only the health claims made for canola oil, but also the theoretical underpinnings of the diet-heart hypothesis.

The first published studies on the new oil were performed in 1978 at the Unilever research facility in the Netherlands. (Vles et al, 1978)

The industry was naturally interested to know whether the new LEAR oil caused heart lesions in test animals. In earlier studies, **animals fed high-erucic-acid rape seed oil showed growth retardation and undesirable changes in various organs, especially the heart, a discovery that touched off the so-called "erucic acid crisis"** and spurred plant geneticists to develop new versions of the seed. (Vles et al, 1978)

The results of the LEAR study were mixed. **Rats genetically selected to be prone to heart lesions developed more lesions on the LEAR oil and the flax oil, than those on olive oil or sunflower oil, leading researchers to speculate that the omega-3 fatty acids (not erucic acid) in LEAR and flax oil might be the culprit.** But rats genetically selected to be resistant to heart lesions showed no significant difference between the four oils tested and LEAR oil did not cause heart problems in mice, in contrast to high-erucic oil which induced severe cardiac necrosis.

In 1979, researchers at the Canadian Institute for Food Science and Technology pooled the results of 23 experiments involving rats at four independent laboratories. All looked at the effects of LEAR and other oils on the incidence of heart lesions. They found that **saturated fats (palmitic and stearic acids) were protective against heart lesions but that high levels of omega-3 fatty acids correlated with high levels of lesions.** They found a lesser correlation with heart lesions and erucic acid. (Trenholm et al, 1979)

Studies carried out at the Health Research and Toxicology Research Divisions in Ottawa, Canada discovered that **rats bred to have high blood pressure and proneness to stroke had shortened life-spans when fed canola oil as the sole source of fat.** (Ratnayake et al, 2000) The results of a later study suggested that **the culprit was the sterol compounds** in the oil, which "make the cell membrane more rigid" and contribute to the shortened life-span of the animals. (Wallsundera et al, 2000)

Such diets have been **presented with great marketing prowess**, but in actuality they appear to be "payola for the food companies and con-ola for the public."

Patient use of dietary supplements: a clinician's perspective

New FDA regulations require dietary-supplement manufacturers to evaluate the identity, purity, strength, and composition of their products. However, these regulations are not designed to demonstrate product efficacy and safety, and dietary-supplement manufacturers are not required to submit efficacy and safety data to the FDA prior to marketing. Product contamination and/or mislabeling may undermine the integrity of dietary-supplement formulations. CONCLUSIONS: **The use of dietary supplements may be associated with adverse events**. Although there are new regulatory requirements for dietary supplements, these products will not require FDA approval or submission of efficacy and safety data prior to marketing under the new regulation. A limitation to the literature used for this review is the lack of prospective, randomized clinical trials on the safety and efficacy of dietary supplements. Clinicians should be aware of all the dietary supplements that their patients consume, and help their patients make informed decisions appropriate to their medical care. (Sadovsky et al, 2008)

Omega-3s do not change laboratory indicators in ulcerative colitis patients

Abstract

OBJECTIVE:

The potential pathogenicity of free radicals may have a pivotal role in ulcerative colitis. Fish oil omega-3 fatty acids exert anti-inflammatory effects on patients with ulcerative colitis (UC), but the precise mechanism of the action of fish oil on oxidative stress is still controversial. The aim of the present work was to verify the blood oxidative stress in patients with UC and determine whether the association of sulfasalazine to fish oil omega-3 fatty acids is more effective than isolated use of sulfasalazine to reduce the oxidative stress.

METHODS:

Nine patients (seven female and two male; mean age = 40 +/- 11 y) with mild or moderate active UC were studied in a randomized crossover design. In addition to their usual medication (2 g/d of sulfasalazine), they received fish oil omega-3 fatty acids (4.5 g/d) or placebo for 2-mo treatment periods that were separated by 2 mo, when they only received sulfasalazine. Nine healthy individuals served as control subjects to study the oxidative stress status. Disease activity was assessed by laboratory indicators (C-reactive protein, alpha1-acid glycoprotein, alpha1-antitrypsin, erythrocyte sedimentation rate, albumin, hemoglobin, and platelet count), sigmoidoscopy, and histology scores. Analysis of oxidative stress was assessed by plasma chemiluminescence and erythrocyte lipid peroxidation, both induced by tert butyl hydroperoxide (t-BuOOH) and by plasma malondialdehyde. Antioxidant status was assayed by total plasma antioxidant capacity (TRAP) and microsomal lipid peroxidation inhibition (LPI). Superoxide dismutase (SOD) and catalase erythrocyte enzymatic activities were also determined.

RESULTS:

No significant changes were observed in any laboratory indicator or in the sigmoidoscopy or histology scores, with the exception of erythrocyte sedimentation rate, which decreased with both treatments. Oxidative stress was demonstrated by significant decreases in TRAP and LPI levels, increased chemiluminescence induced by t-BuOOH, and higher SOD activity in patients with UC. Treatment with fish oil omega-3 fatty acids reverted the chemiluminescence induced by t-BuOOH and LPI to baseline levels but that did not occur when patients received only sulfasalazine. Levels of plasma malondialdehyde, erythrocyte lipid peroxidation, and catalase were not different from those in the control group.

CONCLUSIONS:

The results indicated that **plasma oxidative stress occurs in patients with UC, and there was a significant decrease when the patients used sulfasalazine plus fish oil omega-3 fatty acids.** However, **there was no improvement in most laboratory indi-**

cators, sigmoidoscopy, and histology scores. The results suggested that omega-3 fatty acids may act as free radical scavengers protecting the patients against the overall effect of oxidative stress. (Barbosa et al, 2003)

Omega-3 fails to help ventilator patients

Abstract

The omega-3 (n-3) fatty acids docosahexaenoic acid and eicosapentaenoic acid, along with γ-linolenic acid and antioxidants, may modulate systemic inflammatory response and improve oxygenation and outcomes in patients with acute lung injury.

OBJECTIVE:

To determine if dietary supplementation of these substances to patients with acute lung injury would increase ventilator-free days to study day 28.

DESIGN, SETTING, AND PARTICIPANTS:

The OMEGA study, a randomized, double-blind, placebo-controlled, multicenter trial conducted from January 2, 2008, through February 21, 2009. Participants were 272 adults within 48 hours of developing acute lung injury requiring mechanical ventilation whose physicians intended to start enteral nutrition at 44 hospitals in the National Heart, Lung, and Blood Institute ARDS Clinical Trials Network. All participants had complete follow-up.

INTERVENTIONS:

Twice-daily enteral supplementation of n-3 fatty acids, γ-linolenic acid, and antioxidants compared with an isocaloric control. Enteral nutrition, directed by a protocol, was delivered separately from the study supplement.

MAIN OUTCOME MEASURE:

Ventilator-free days to study day 28.

RESULTS:

The study was stopped early for futility after 143 and 129 patients were enrolled in the n-3 and control groups. Despite an 8-fold increase in plasma eicosapentaenoic acid levels, patients receiving the n-3 supplement had fewer ventilator-free days and intensive care unit-free days. Patients in the n-3 group also had fewer nonpulmonary organ failure-free days. **Sixty-day hospital mortality was 26.6% in the n-3 group vs 16.3% in the control group, and adjusted 60-day mortality was 25.1% and 17.6% in the n-3 and control groups, respectively**. Use of the n-3 supplement resulted in more days with diarrhea.

CONCLUSIONS:

Twice-daily enteral supplementation of n-3 fatty acids, □-linolenic acid, and antioxidants did not improve the primary end point of ventilator-free days or other clinical outcomes in patients with acute lung injury and may be harmful. (Rice et al, 2011)

SECTION SEVEN

A 2013 VIEWPOINT FROM MEDLINEPLUS:

http://www.nlm.nih.gov/medlineplus/druginfo/natural/993.html

This article is included to also give a well rounded overview of literature on the subject of omega-3 fish oils. Please note the high number of "conflicted evidence or results" following various disease entities. Also, some of the conclusions presented here have already been debunked by subsequent or more current scientific studies.

What is it?

Fish that are especially rich in the beneficial oils known as omega-3 fatty acids include mackerel, tuna, salmon, sturgeon, mullet, bluefish, anchovy, sardines, herring, trout, and menhaden. They provide about **1 gram of omega-3 fatty acids in about 3.5 ounces of fish**.

Fish oil supplements often contain small amounts of vitamin E to prevent spoilage. They might also be combined with calcium, iron, or vitamins A, B1, B2, B3, C, or D.

The scientific evidence suggests that fish oil really does lower high triglycerides. **Ironically, taking too much fish oil can actually increase the risk of stroke.**

When fish oil is obtained by eating fish, the way the fish is prepared seems to make a difference. Eating broiled or baked fish appears to reduce the risk of heart disease, but **eating fried fish or fish sandwiches not only cancels out the benefits of fish oil, but may actually increase heart disease risk**.

How effective is it?

Natural Medicines Comprehensive Database rates effectiveness based on scientific evidence according to the following scale: Effective, Likely Effective, Possibly Effective, Possibly Ineffective, Likely Ineffective, Ineffective, and Insufficient Evidence to Rate.

The effectiveness ratings for **FISH OIL** are as follows:

Effective for...

- **High triglycerides**. High triglycerides are associated with heart disease and untreated diabetes. Sometimes they also prescribe drugs such as gemfibrozil (Lopid) for use in addition to these lifestyle changes. Now researchers believe that fish oil, though not as effective as gemfibrozil, can reduce triglyceride levels by 20% to 50%. One particular fish oil supplement called Lovaza has been approved by the FDA to lower triglycerides. Lovaza contains 465 milligrams of EP and 375 milligrams of DHA in 1-gram capsules.

Likely effective for...

- **Heart disease**. Research suggests that consuming fish oil by eating fish can be effective for keeping people with healthy hearts free of heart disease. People who already have heart disease might also be able to lower their risk of dying from heart disease by eating fish or taking a fish oil supplement. However, for people who already take heart medications such as a "statin," adding on fish oil might not offer any additional benefit. **DEBUNKED.**

Possibly effective for...

- **Rheumatoid arthritis**. Fish oil alone, or in combination with the drug naproxen (Naprosyn), seems to help people with rheumatoid arthritis get over morning stiffness faster. People who take fish oil can sometimes reduce their use of pain medications such as nonsteroidal anti-inflammatory drugs (NSAIDs).

- **Menstrual pain (dysmenorrhea)**. Taking fish oil alone or in combination with vitamin B12 seems to improve painful periods and reduce the need for pain medications such as nonsteroidal anti-inflammatory drugs (NSAIDs).

- **Attention deficit-hyperactivity disorder (ADHD) in children.** Taking fish oil seems to improve thinking skills and behavior in 8 to 12 year-old children with ADHD.

- **Raynaud's syndrome.** There's some evidence that taking fish oil can improve cold tolerance in some people with the usual form of Raynaud's syndrome. But people with Raynaud's syndrome caused by a condition called progressive systemic sclerosis don't seem to benefit from fish oil supplements.

- **Stroke.** Moderate fish consumption (once or twice a week) seems to lower the risk of having a stroke by as much as 27%. **DEBUNKED.** However, eating fish doesn't lower stroke risk in people who are already taking aspirin for prevention. On the other hand, **very high fish consumption (more than 46 grams of fish per day) seems to increase stroke risk, perhaps even double it**.

- **Weak bones (osteoporosis).** Taking fish oil alone or in combination with calcium and evening primrose oil **seems** to slow bone loss rate and increase bone density at the thigh bone (femur) and spine in elderly people with osteoporosis.

- **Hardening of the arteries (atherosclerosis)**. Fish oil seems to slow or slightly reverse the progress of atherosclerosis in the arteries serving the heart (coronary arteries), but not in the arteries that bring blood up the neck to the head (carotid arteries). **DEBUNKED.**

- **Kidney problems**. Long-term use (two years) of fish oil 4-8 grams daily can slow the loss of kidney function in high-risk patients with a kidney disease called IgA nephropathy.

- **Bipolar disorder**. Taking fish oil with the usual treatments for bipolar disorder seems to improve symptoms of depression and increase the length of time between episodes of depression. **DEBUNKED.** But fish oil doesn't seem to improve manic symptoms in people with bipolar disorder.

- **Weight loss**. Preliminary research also shows that taking a specific fish oil supplement 6 grams daily (Hi-DHA, NuMega), providing 260 mg DHA/gram and 60 mg EPA/gram, significantly decreases body fat when combined with exercise.

- **Endometrial cancer.** There is some evidence that women who regularly eat about two servings of fatty fish per week have a reduced risk of developing endometrial cancer.

- **Age-related eye disease (age-related macular degeneration, AMD).** There is some evidence that people who eat fish more than once per week have a lower risk of developing age-related macular degeneration. **DEBUNKED, AREDS2.**

- **Reducing the risk of blood vessel re-blockage after heart bypass surgery or "balloon" catheterization (balloon angioplasty).** Fish oil appears to decrease the rate of re-blockage up to 26% when given for one month before the procedure and continued for one month thereafter. When taken for less than one month before angioplasty, fish oil doesn't help protect the blood vessel against closing down. **DEBUNKED.**

- **High blood pressure and kidney problems after heart transplant.** Taking fish oil seems to preserve kidney function and reduce the long-term continuous rise in blood pressure after heart transplantation.

- **Damage to the kidneys and high blood pressure caused by taking a drug called cyclosporine.** Cyclosporine is a medication that reduces the chance of organ rejection after an organ transplant. Fish oil **might help** reduce some of the unwanted side effects of treatment with this drug.

- **Developmental coordination disorder.** A combination of fish oil (80%) and evening primrose oil (20%) seems to improve reading, spelling, and behavior when given to children age 5-12 years with developmental coordination disorder. However, **it doesn't seem to improve motor skills**.

- **Preventing blockage of grafts used in kidney dialysis.** Taking fish oil orally seems to help prevent clot formation in hemodialysis grafts.

- **Psoriasis.** There is some evidence that administering fish oil intravenously (by IV) can decrease severe psoriasis symptoms. But **taking fish oil by mouth doesn't seem to have any effect on psoriasis.**

- **High cholesterol.** There is interest in using fish oil in combination with "statin" drugs for some people with high cholesterol.

Scientists think fish oil may lower cholesterol by keeping it from being absorbed in the intestine. There is some evidence that using vitamin B12 along with fish oil might boost their ability to lower cholesterol.

- **Coronary artery bypass surgery.** Taking fish oil **seems** to prevent coronary artery bypass grafts from re-closing following coronary artery bypass surgery.
- **Cancer-related weight loss.** Taking a high dose (7.5 grams per day) of fish oil seems to slow weight loss in some cancer patients.
- **Asthma.** Some research suggests fish oil may lower the occurrence of asthma in infants and children when taken by women late in pregnancy. However, **fish oil treatment doesn't seem to provide the same benefit for adults.**

Possibly ineffective for...

- Chest pain (angina).
- Gum infection (gingivitis).
- Liver disease.
- Leg pain due to blood flow problems (claudication).
- Preventing migraine headaches.
- Preventing muscle soreness caused by physical exercise.
- Breast pain.
- Skin rashes caused by allergic reactions.
- Stomach ulcers.

Likely ineffective for...

- **Type 2 diabetes.** Taking fish oil **doesn't seem to lower blood sugar in people with type 2 diabetes.** However, fish oil can provide some other benefits for people with diabetes, such as lowering blood fats called triglycerides.

Insufficient evidence to rate effectiveness for...

- **Allergies**. Some research suggests that mothers who take fish oil supplements during the late stages of pregnancy may lower the occurrence of allergies in their children.
- **Alzheimer's disease**. There is some preliminary evidence that fish oil may help prevent Alzheimer's disease. But **it doesn't seem to help prevent a decline in thinking skills for most people who already have mild-to-moderate Alzheimer's disease**.
- **Atopic dermatitis**. Mothers who take fish oil supplements during pregnancy might reduce the occurrence and severity of atopic dermatitis in babies and children who are at risk for this condition. But **fish oil doesn't seem to be effective for treating atopic dermatitis**.
- **Atrial fibrillation**. Research studies into the effects of fish oil on atrial fibrillation have produced **conflicting results**.
- **Depression**. There is inconsistent information about the effect of taking fish oil on depression. Some research shows that taking fish oil along with an antidepressant might help improve symptoms. But other research shows that **taking fish oil does not improve symptoms**.
- **Dry eye syndrome**. Some research links eating more fish with a lower risk of getting dry eye syndrome in women. Some preliminary clinical research also suggests that taking a specific product containing fish oil plus flaxseed oil (TheraTears Nutrition) might reduce symptoms of dry eye and increase tear production.
- **Cancer**. Research studies into the effects of fish oil on cancer prevention have produced **conflicting results**.
- **Cataracts**. There is **some evidence** that eating fish three times a week can modestly lower the risk of developing cataracts.
- **Chronic fatigue syndrome (CFS)**. There is some **conflicting evidence** about the use of a product (Efamol Marine) that combines fish oil and evening primrose oil to reduce the symptoms CFS.
- **Chronic kidney disease**. Preliminary evidence shows that fish oil **might have** benefit for some people with chronic kidney disease who are receiving dialysis treatments.

- **Thinking skills (cognitive function).** Research studies into the effects of fish oil on cognitive function have produced **conflicting results**.

- **Crohn's disease.** Research studies into the effects of fish oil on Crohn's disease have produced **conflicting results**.

- **Prediabetes.** Early studies suggest that fish oil **may help prevent** prediabetes from advancing to type 2 diabetes.

- **Infant development.** There is some evidence that mothers who take 4 grams of fish oil daily during the last half of pregnancy **may improve** their baby's cognitive development by some measures, **but not others (conflicting results)**. At age 2.5 years, these children seem to have better hand and eye coordination, but reasoning, social, motor, and **speech skills are not significantly improved**.

- **Ulcerative colitis.** Research studies into the effects of fish oil on ulcerative colitis have produced **conflicting results**.

- **Pregnancy complications.** There is some evidence that taking fish oil during the last ten weeks of pregnancy can help prevent premature delivery. However, **fish oil doesn't seem to help prevent high blood pressure during pregnancy**.

- **Prematurity.** Baby formula that has been fortified with fatty acids from fish oil and borage **seems to** improve growth and the development of the nervous system in premature infants, especially boys.

- **Salicylate intolerance.** Some limited research suggests that taking fish oil **might improve** symptoms of salicylate intolerance such as asthma attacks and itching.

- **Schizophrenia.** There is one report of fish oil improving schizophrenia in a pregnant woman but other studies have produced **conflicting results**.

- **Systemic lupus erythematosus (SLE).** Research shows **conflicting results**. Some studies suggest that fish oil helps the symptoms of SLE, while others show no effect.

- **Irregular heartbeat affecting the ventricles (ventricular arrhythmias).** Research studies into the effect of fish oil on ventricular arrhythmias have produced **conflicting results**.

- **Improving night vision in children with a disorder called dyslexia**. Children with dyslexia who take fish oil **seem to be** significantly better able to adapt to the dark.

How does it work?

A lot of the benefit of fish oil **seems to come from the omega-3 fatty acids** that it contains.

Omega-3 fatty acids reduce pain and swelling. These fatty acids also prevent the blood from clotting easily.

Are there safety concerns?

Fish oil is **LIKELY SAFE** for most people, including pregnant and breast-feeding women, when taken in low doses (3 grams or less per day). There are some safety concerns when fish oil is taken in high doses. **Taking more than 3 grams per day might keep blood from clotting and can increase the chance of bleeding**.

High doses of fish oil **might also reduce the immune system's activity, reducing the body's ability to fight infection**. This is a special concern for people taking medications to reduce their immune system's activity (organ transplant patients, for example) and the elderly.

Fish oil can cause side effects including belching, bad breath, heartburn, nausea, loose stools, rash, and nosebleeds. Taking fish oil supplements with meals or freezing them can often decrease these side effects.

Consuming large amounts of fish oil from some DIETARY sources is **POSSIBLY UNSAFE**. Some fish meats (especially shark, king mackerel, and farm-raised salmon) can be contaminated with mercury and other industrial and environmental chemicals.

Special precautions & warnings:

Liver disease: Fish oil might increase the risk of bleeding.

Fish or seafood allergy: Some people who are allergic to seafood such as fish might also be allergic to fish oil supplements.

Bipolar disorder: Taking fish **oil might increase some of the symptoms of this condition**.

Depression: Taking fish oil **might increase some of the symptoms of this condition**.

Diabetes: There is some concern that taking **high doses of fish oil might make the control of blood sugar more difficult.**

High blood pressure: Fish oil **can lower blood pressure and might cause blood pressure to drop too low** in people who are being treated with blood pressure-lowering medications.

HIV/AIDS and other conditions in which the immune system response is lowered: Higher doses of fish oil can **lower the body's immune system response.** This would likely be a problem for people whose immune system is already weak.

An implanted defibrillator (a surgically placed device to prevent irregular heartbeat): Some, but not all, research suggests that fish oil **might increase the risk of irregular heartbeat in patients with an implanted defibrillator**.

Familial adenomatous polyposis: There is some concern that fish oil **might further increase the risk of getting cancer in people with this condition.**

Are there interactions with medications?

Birth control pills (Contraceptive drugs)

There is some evidence that birth control pills might interfere with the triglyceride-lowering effects of fish oil.

Some of these drugs include ethinyl estradiol and levonorgestrel (Triphasil), ethinyl estradiol and norethindrone (Ortho-Novum 1/35, Ortho-Novum 7/7/7), and others.

Medications for high blood pressure (Antihypertensive drugs)

Using fish oil with drugs that lower blood pressure **can increase the effects of these drugs and may lower blood pressure too much.**

Some medications for high blood pressure include captopril (Capoten), enalapril (Vasotec), losartan (Cozaar), valsartan (Diovan), diltiazem

(Cardizem), amlodipine (Norvasc), hydrochlorothiazide (HydroDIURIL), furosemide (Lasix), and many others.

Orlistat (Xenical, Alli)

Orlistat (Xenical, Alli) might keep the beneficial fatty acids in fish oil from being absorbed by the body. Taking fish oil and orlistat (Xenical, Alli) at least 2 hours apart may keep this from happening.

Medications that slow blood clotting (Anticoagulant / Antiplatelet drugs)

Using fish oil with medications that slow clotting may cause bleeding.

Some of these drugs include aspirin, clopidogrel (Plavix), dalteparin (Fragmin), dipyridamole (Persantine), enoxaparin (Lovenox), heparin, ticlopidine (Ticlid), warfarin (Coumadin), and others.

Are there interactions with herbs and supplements?

Herbs and supplements that might slow blood clotting

High doses of fish oil seem to slow blood clotting. Taking fish oil with other herbs that slow clotting might cause bleeding in some people. These herbs include angelica, clove, danshen, garlic, ginger, ginkgo, Panax ginseng, red clover, turmeric, willow, and others.

Vitamin E

Fish oil can reduce vitamin E levels.

Are there interactions with foods?

There are no known interactions with foods.

What dose is used?

The following doses have been studied in scientific research:

BY MOUTH:

- For high triglycerides: 1-4 grams/day of fish oil.
- For high blood pressure: Either 4 grams of fish oil or fish oil providing 2.04 grams of EPA and 1.4 grams of DHA per day.
- For atrial fibrillation (one of the chambers of the heart doesn't empty properly and this increases the risk of blood clot formation leading to stroke): Eating tuna or baked or broiled fish providing omega-3 fatty acids (fish oil) one or more times per week seems to reduce the risk of atrial fibrillation in patients aged 65 or older compared to consuming fish once per month or less. But there is no benefit from eating fried fish or a fish sandwich.
- For kidney problems related to using cyclosporine to prevent organ transplant rejection: 12 grams/day containing 2.2 grams EPA and 1.4 grams DHA.
- For reducing the overall risk of death and risk of sudden death in patients with coronary heart disease: Fish oil providing 0.3-6 grams of EPA with 0.6 to 3.7 grams of DHA.
- For asthma in children: Fish oil providing 17-26.8 mg/kg EPA and 7.3-11.5 mg/kg DHA for reducing symptoms. Maternal ingestion of fish oil 4 grams daily, providing 32% EPA and 23% DHA with tocopherol, during late-phase pregnancy has been used for preventing the development of asthma in children.
- For preventing childhood allergies: Maternal ingestion of fish oil 4 grams daily, providing 32% EPA and 23% DHA with tocopherol, during late-phase pregnancy.
- For preventing childhood atopic dermatitis: Maternal ingestion of fish oil 4 grams daily, providing 32% EPA and 23% DHA with tocopherol, during late-phase pregnancy.
- For treating asthma: 17-26.8 mg/kg EPA and 7.3-11.5 mg/kg DHA.

- For preventing and reversing the progression of hardening of the arteries: 6 grams/day of fish oil for the first three months, followed by 3 grams/day thereafter.

- For rheumatoid arthritis: Fish oil providing 3.8 grams/day of EPA and 2 grams/day DHA.

- For attention deficit-hyperactivity disorder (ADHD):A specific supplement containing fish oil 400 mg and evening primrose oil 100 mg (Eye Q, Novasel) six capsules daily.

- For preventing miscarriage in women with antiphospholipid antibody syndrome and a history of past miscarriage: 5.1 grams fish oil with a 1.5 EPA:DHA ratio.

- For painful menstrual periods: A daily dose of EPA 1080 mg and DHA 720 mg.

- For Raynaud's syndrome: A daily dose of 3.96 grams EPA and 2.64 grams DHA.

- For weight loss: A daily serving of 2-7 ounces of fish containing approximately 3.65 grams omega-3 fatty acids (0.66 gram from EPA and 0.60 gram from DHA).

- For slowing weight loss in patients with cancer: 7.5 grams/day of fish oil providing EPA 4.7 grams and DHA 2.8 grams.

- For improving movement disorders in children with poor coordination (dyspraxia): Fish oil providing DHA 480 mg combined with 35 mg arachidonic acid and 96 mg gamma-alpha linoleic acid from evening primrose oil, 24 mg thyme oil, and 80 mg vitamin E (Efalex).

- For developmental coordination disorder in children: Fish oil providing EPA 558 mg and DHA 174 in 3 divided doses.

- For depression along with conventional antidepressants: Fish oil 9.6 grams/day.

- To prevent full psychosis from developing in people with mild symptoms: Fish oil 1.2 grams/day.

- For keeping veins open after coronary bypass surgery: 4 grams/day of fish oil containing EPA 2.04 grams and DHA 1.3 grams.

- For preventing the collapse of arteries opened by "balloon" therapy (PTCA): 6 grams/day of fish oil starting one month before PTCA and continuing one month after PTCA, followed by 3 grams of fish oil daily thereafter for six months.

- For reducing and preventing the long-term continuous rise in blood pressure and to preserve kidney function after heart transplantation: 4 grams/day of fish oil (46.5% EPA and 37.8% DHA).

- For preventing clotting after placement of a tube for dialysis: 6 grams/day of fish oil.

- For preserving kidney function in patients with severe IgA nephropathy: 4-8 grams/day of fish oil has been used.

- For combined high triglycerides and high cholesterol: Fish oil providing EPA 1800-2160 mg and DHA 1200-1440 mg combined with garlic powder 900-1200 mg/day has been used to lower total cholesterol, LDL, triglycerides, and the ratios of total cholesterol to HDL, and LDL to HDL.

- For salicylate intolerance: Fish oil 10 grams daily.

Other names

Aceite de Pescado, Acides Gras Oméga-3, Acides Gras Oméga 3, Acides Gras Oméga 3 Sous Forme Ester Éthylique, Acides Gras N-3, Acides Gras Polyinsaturés N-3, Acides Gras W3, ACPI, Cod Liver Oil, EPA/DHA Ethyl Ester, Ester Éthylique de l'AEP/ADH, Fish Body Oil, Herring Oil, Huile de Foie de Morue, Huile de Hareng, Huile de Menhaden, Huile de Poisson, Huile de Saumon, Huile de Thon, Huile Lipidique Marine, Huile Marine, Huiles Marines, Lipides Marins, Marine Lipid Concentrate, Marine Fish Oil, Marine Lipid Oil, Marine Lipids, Marine Oil, Marine Oils, Marine Triglyceride, Menhaden Oil, N-3 Fatty Acids, N3-polyunsaturated Fatty Acids, Omega 3, Oméga 3, Omega-3, Oméga-3, Omega-3 Fatty Acid Ethyl Ester, Omega-3 Fatty Acids, Omega 3 Fatty Acids, Omega-3 Marine Triglycerides, PUFA, Salmon Oil, Triglycérides Marins, Tuna Fish Oil, Tuna Oil, W-3 Fatty Acids.

Methodology

To learn more about how this article was written, please see the *Natural Medicines Comprehensive Database* methodology.
Last reviewed - 09/04/2013

ω3-LC- PUFA

SECTION EIGHT

ADDITIONAL OMEGA-3 FISH OIL REFERENCES LISTED CHRONOLOGICALLY: META-ANALYSES; REVIEWS; AND RANDOMIZED, DOUBLE-BLIND CONTROLLED TRIALS

I have included these reviews, RCTs and meta-analyses for those who wish to further research this interesting subject. Combined with the references to this book, which follow, they make for a comprehensive listing of the best studies on the subject currently available today.

(Bittiner et al, 1988) (Bittiner SB, Tucker WF, Cartwright I, Bleehen SS. A double-blind randomised placebo-controlled trial of fish oil in psoriasis. Lancet 1988;1:378-80)

(DiGiacomo et al, 1989) (DiGiacomo RA, Kremer JM, Shah DM. Fish-oil dietary supplementation in patients with Raynaud's phenomenon: a double-blind, controlled, prospective study. Am J Med 1989;86:158-64)

(Astorga et al, 1991) (Astorga G, Cubillos A, Masson L, Silva JJ. Active rheumatoid arthritis: effect of dietary supplementation with omega-3 oils. A controlled double-blind trial. Rev Med Chil 1991;119:267-72)

(Grimminger et al, 1993) (Grimminger F, Mayser P, Papavassilis C, et al. A double-blind, randomized, placebo-controlled trial of n-3 fatty acid based lipid infusion in acute, extended guttate psoriasis. Rapid improvement of clinical manifestations and changes in neutrophil leukotriene profile. Clin Invest 1993;71:634-43)

(Lau et al, 1993) (Lau CS, Morley KD, Belch JJ. Effects of fish oil supplementation on non-steroidal anti-inflammatory drug requirement in patients with mild rheumatoid arthritis- a double-blind, placebo-controlled study. Br J Rheumatol 1993;32:982-9

(Onwude et al, 1995) (Onwude JL, Lilford RJ, Hjartardottir H, et al. A randomised double blind placebo controlled trial of fish oil in high risk pregnancy. Br J Obstet Gynaecol 1995;102:95-100)

(Toft et al, 1995) (Toft I, Bonaa KH, Ingebretsen OC, et al. Effects of n-3 polyunsaturated fatty acids on glucose homeostasis and blood pressure in essential hypertension. A randomized, controlled trial. Ann Intern Med 1995;123:911-8)

(Lorenz-Meyer et al, 1996) (Lorenz-Meyer H, Bauer P, Nicolay C, et al. Omega-3 fatty acids and low carbohydrate diet for maintenance of remission in Crohn's disease. A randomized controlled multicenter trial. Study Group Members (German Crohn's Disease Study Group) (abstract). Scand J Gastroenterol 1996;31:778-85)

(Mayser et al, 1998) (Mayser P, Mrowietz U, Arenberger P, et al. Omega-3 fatty acid-based lipid infusion in patients with chronic plaque psoriasis: results of a double-blind, randomized, placebo-controlled, multicenter trial. J Am Acad Dermatol 1998;38:539-47)

(von Schacky et al, 1999) (von Schacky C, Angerer P, Kothny W, et al. The effect of dietary omega-3 fatty acids on coronary atherosclerosis. A randomized, double-blind, placebo-controlled trial. Ann Intern Med 1999;130:554-62)

(Norrish et al, 1999) (Norrish AE, Skeaff CM, Arribas GL, et al. Prostate cancer risk and consumption of fish oils: a dietary biomarker-based, case-control study. Br J Cancer 1999;81:1238-42)

(Ogilvie et al, 2000) (Ogilvie GK, Fettman MJ, Mallinckrodt CH, et al. Effect of fish oil, arginine, and doxorubicin chemotherapy on remission and survival time for dogs with lymphoma: a double-blind, randomized, placebo-controlled study. Cancer 2000;88:1916-28)

(Olsen et al, 2000) (Olsen SF, Secher NJ, Tabor A, et al. Randomised clinical trials of fish oil supplementation in high risk pregnancies. Fish Oil Trials In Pregnancy (FOTIP) Team. BJOG 2000;107:382-95)

(Pradalier et al, 2001) (Pradalier A, Baudesson G, Delage A, et al. Failure of omega-3 polyunsaturated fatty acids in prevention of migraine: a double-blind study versus placebo. Cephalalgia 2001;21:818-22)

(Terry et al, 2002) (Terry P, Wolk A, Vainio H, Weiderpass E. Fatty fish consumption lowers the risk of endometrial cancer: a nationwide case-control study in Sweden. Cancer Epidemiol Biomarkers Prev 2002;11:143-5)

(Schmitz et al, 2002) (Schmitz PG, McCloud LK, Reikes ST, et al. Prophylaxis of hemodialysis graft thrombosis with fish oil: double-blind, randomized, prospective trial. J Am Soc Nephrol 2002;13:184-90)

(Maresta et al, 2002) (Maresta A, Balduccelli M, Varani E, et al. Prevention of postcoronary angioplasty restenosis by omega-3 fatty acids: main results of the Esapent for Prevention of Restenosis Italian Study (ESPRIT). Am Heart J, 2002, 143:E5)

(Woods et al, 2002) (Woods RK, Thien FC, Abramson MJ. Dietary marine fatty acids (fish oil) for asthma in adults and children. Cochrane Database Syst Rev 2002;:CD001283)

(Bruera et al, 2003) (Bruera E, Strasser F, Palmer JL, et al. Effect of fish oil on appetite and other symptoms in patients with advanced cancer and anorexia/cachexia: a double-blind, placebo-controlled study. J Clin Oncol 2003;21:129-34)

(van Gool et al, 2004) (van Gool CJ, Zeegers MP, Thijs C. Oral essential fatty acid supplementation in atopic dermatitis-a meta-analysis of placebo-controlled trials. Br J Dermatol 2004;150:728-40

(Yzebe, Lievre, 2004) (Yzebe D, Lievre M. Fish oils in the care of coronary heart disease patients: a meta-analysis of randomized controlled trials. Fundam Clin Pharmacol 2004;18:581-92)

(Fewtrell et al, 2004) (Fewtrell MS, Abbott RA, Kennedy K, et al. Randomized, double-blind trial of long-chain polyunsaturated fatty acid supplementation with fish oil and borage oil in preterm infants. J Pediatr 2004;144:471-9)

(Folsom, Demissie, 2004) (Folsom AR, Demissie Z. Fish intake, marine omega-3 fatty acids, and mortality in a cohort of postmenopausal women. Am J Epidemiol 2004;160:1005-10)

(Kojima et al, 2005) (Kojima M, Wakai K, Tokudome S, et al. Serum levels of polyunsaturated fatty acids and risk of colorectal cancer: a prospective study. Am J Epidemiol 2005;161:462-71)

(Melanson et al, 2005) (Melanson SF, Lewandrowski EL, Flood JG, Lewandrowski KB. Measurement of organochlorines in commercial over-the-counter fish oil preparations: implications for dietary and therapeutic recommendations for omega-3 fatty acids and a review of the literature. Arch Pathol Lab Med 2005;129:74-7)

(Richardson, Montgomery, 2005) (Richardson AJ, Montgomery P. The Oxford-Durham study: a randomized, controlled trial of dietary supplementation with fatty acids in children with developmental coordination disorder. Pediatrics 2005;115:1360-6)

(Mozaffarian et al, 2005) (Mozaffarian D, Geelen A, Brouwer IA, et al. Effect of fish oil on heart rate in humans: a meta-analysis of randomized controlled trials. Circulation 2005;112:1945-52)

(Seidner et al, 2005) (Seidner DL, Lashner BA, Brzezinski A, et al. An oral supplement enriched with fish oil, soluble fiber, and antioxidants for corticosteroid sparing in ulcerative colitis: a randomized, controlled trial. Clin Gastroenterol Hepatol 2005;3:358-69)

(Brouwer et al, 2006) (Brouwer IA, Zock PL, Camm AJ, et al; SOFA Study Group. Effect of fish oil on ventricular tachyarrhythmia and death in patients with implantable cardioverter defibrillators: the Study on Omega-3 Fatty Acids and Ventricular Arrhythmia (SOFA) randomized trial. JAMA 2006;295:2613-9)

(MacLean et al, 2006) (MacLean CH, Newberry SJ, Mojica WJ, et al. Effects of omega-3 fatty acids on cancer risk: a systematic review. JAMA 2006;295:403-15)

(van Gelder et al, 2007) (van Gelder BM, Tijhuis M, Kalmijn S, Kromhout D. Fish consumption, n-3 fatty acids, and subsequent 5-y cognitive decline in elderly men: the Zutphen Elderly Study. Am J Clin Nutr 2007;85:1142-7)

(Chavarro et al, 2007) (Chavarro JE, Stampfer MJ, Li H, et al. A prospective study of polyunsaturated fatty acid levels in blood and prostate cancer risk. Cancer Epidemiol Biomarkers Prev 2007;16:1364-70)

(Tavazzi et al, GISSI, 2008) (Gissi-HF Investigators; Tavazzi L, Maggioni AP, Marchioli R, et al. Effect of n-3 polyunsaturated fatty acids in patients with chronic heart failure (the GISSI-HF trial): a randomised, double-blind, placebo-controlled trial. Lancet 2008;372:1223-30)

(Amminger et al, 2010) (Amminger GP, Schafer MR, Papageorgiou K, et al. Long-chain omega-3 fatty acids for indicated prevention of psychotic disorders: a randomized, placebo-controlled trial. Arch Gen Psychiatry 2010;67:146-54)

(Wojtwicz et al, 2010) (Wojtowicz JC, Butovich I, Uchiyama E, et al. Pilot, prospective, randomized, double-masked, placebo-controlled clinical trial of an omega-3 supplement for dry eye. Cornea 2010 Oct 28. [Epub ahead of print])

(Khawaja, Djousse, 2012) (Khawaja O, Gaziano JM, Djoussé L. A meta-analysis of omega-3 fatty acids and incidence of atrial fibrillation. J Am Coll Nutr 2012;31:4-13)

(Djousse et al, 2012) (Djoussé L, Akinkuolie AO, Wu JH, et al. Fish consumption, omega-3 fatty acids and risk of heart failure: A meta-analysis. Clin Nutr 2012 Jun 6. [Epub ahead of print])

SECTION NINE

REFERENCES TO FISH OIL (OMEGA-3): FACTS, FANTASIES & FAILURES

(Aben, Danckaerts, 2010) (Aben A, Danckaerts M. Omega-3 and omega-6 fatty acids in the treatment of children and adolescents with ADHD. *Tijdschr Psychiatr.* 2010; 52(2):89-97)

(AHA 41st conf, 2001) (Fatty fish consumption and ischemic heart disease mortality in older adults: The cardiovascular heart study. Presented at the American Heart Association's 41st annual conference on cardiovascular disease epidemiology and prevention. AHA. 2001)

(Ali et al, 2014) (Quercetin and Omega 3 Ameliorate Oxidative Stress Induced by Aluminium Chloride in the Brain. Ali HA, Afifi M, Abdelazim AM, Mosleh YY. J Mol Neurosci. 2014 Feb 1)

(Andreeva et al, 2012) (B vitamin and/or ω-3 fatty acid supplementation and cancer: ancillary findings from the supplementation with folate, vitamins B6 and B12, and/or omega-3 fatty acids (SU.FOL.OM3) randomized trial. Andreeva VA, Touvier M, Kesse-Guyot E, Julia C, Galan P, Hercberg S. Arch Intern Med. 2012 Apr 9;172(7):540-7)

(Angerer, von Schacky, 2000) (Angerer P, von Schacky C. n-3 polyunsaturated fatty acids and the cardiovascular system. *Curr Opin Lipidol.* 2000;11(1):57-63)

(Ammann et al, 2012) (Ammann EM, Pottala JV, Harris WS, et al. Omega-3 fatty acids and domain-specific cognitive aging. *Neurology*. 2012)

(Ammann et al, 2013) (Ammann EM, Pottala JV, Harris WS, et al. Omega-3 fatty acids and domain-specific cognitive aging. Neurology. Published online September 25 2013)

(Anandan et al, 2009) (Anandan C, Nurmatov U, Sheikh A. Omega 3 and 6 oils for primary prevention of allergic disease: systematic review and meta-analysis. *Allergy.* 2009;64(6):840–848)

(Appleton et al, 2006) (Effects of n–3 long-chain polyunsaturated fatty acids on depressed mood: systematic review of published trials. Katherine M Appleton, Robert C Hayward, David Gunnell, Tim J Peters, Peter J Rogers, David Kessler, and Andrew R Ness. Am J Clin Nutr December 2006 vol. 84 no. 6 1308-1316)

(Appleton et al, 2010) (Appleton KM, Rogers PJ, Ness AR. Updated systematic review and meta-analysis of the effects of n-3 long-chain polyunsaturated fatty acids on depressed mood. *American Journal of Clinical Nutrition.* 2010;91(3):757–770)

(ARC, 2006) (ARC, 2006. *Arthritis Research Campaign, Diet and Arthritis* [online]. Available from: http://www.arc.org.uk/arthinfo/patpubs/6010/6010.asp [Accessed September 3 2008])

(AREDS, JAMA, 2013) (AREDS2 Research Group. "Lutein/Zeaxanthin and Omega-3 Fatty Acids for Age-Related Macular Degeneration. The Age-Related Eye Disease Study 2 (AREDS2) Controlled Randomized Clinical Trial." JAMA, published online May 5, 2013) (AREDS, JAMA Ophth, 2013) (AREDS2 Research Group. "Lutein/Zeaxanthin for the Treatment of Age-Related Cataract." JAMA Ophthalmology, published online May 5, 2013)

(AREDS2, 2013) (Lutein + Zeaxanthin and Omega-3 Fatty Acids for Age-Related Macular Degeneration The Age-Related Eye Disease Study 2 (AREDS2) Randomized Clinical Trial. The Age-Related Eye Disease Study 2 (AREDS2) Research Group* *JAMA*. Published online May 5, 2013)

(Aronson et al, 2001) (Aronson WJ, Glaspy JA, Reddy ST, Reese D, Heber D, Bagga D. Modulation of omega-3/omega-6 polyunsaturated ratios with dietary fish oils in men with prostate cancer. *Urology.* 2001;58(2):283-288)

(Bahadori, et al, 2010) (Bahadori B, Uitz E, Thonhofer R, et al. omega-3 Fatty acids infusions as adjuvant therapy in rheumatoid arthritis. *JPEN J Parenter Enteral Nutr.* 2010; 34(2):151-5)

(Balk et al, 2006) (Balk EM, Lichtenstein AH, Chung M et al. Effects of omega-3 fatty acids on serum markers of cardiovascular disease risk: A systematic review. *Atherosclerosis.* 2006 Nov;189(1):19-30)

(Ballanytyne et al, ANCHOR, 2012) (Ballanytyne CM, Bays He, Kastelein JJ, Stein E, Isaacsohn JL, Braeckman RA. Efficacy and safety of eicosapentaenoic adic dethyl ester (AMR101) therapy in statin-streated patients with persistent high triglycerides (from the ANCHOR study). Am J Carkiol. 2012;110:984-992**)**

(Barbosa et al, 2003) (Decreased oxidative stress in patients with ulcerative colitis supplemented with fish oil omega-3 fatty acids. Barbosa DS, Cecchini R, El Kadri MZ, Rodríguez MA, Burini RC, Dichi I. Nutrition. 2003 Oct;19(10):837-42)

(Baumgartner et al, 2012) (Effects of iron and n-3 fatty acid supplementation, alone and in combination, on cognition in school children: a randomized, double-blind, placebo-controlled intervention in South Africa. Baumgartner et al, The American Journal of Clinical Nutrition. December 2012 ajcn.041004)

(Bays, 2007) (Bays HE. Safety considerations with omega-3 Fatty Acid therapy. *Am J Cardiol.* 2007;99(6A):S35-43)

(Bays et al, MARINE, 2012) (Bays HE, Breackman RA, Ballantyne CM, Kastelein JJ, Otvos JD, Stirtan WG. Isosapent ethyl, a pure EPA omega-3 fatty acid: effects on lipoprotein particle concentration and size in patients with very high triglyceride levels (the MARINE study). J Clin Lipidol. 2012;6:565-572)

(Belluzzi et al, 2000) (Belluzzi A, Boschi S, Brignola C, Munarini A, Cariani C, Miglio F. Polyunsaturated fatty acids and inflammatory bowel disease. *Am J Clin Nutr.* 2000;71(suppl):339S-342S)

(Bent et al, 2009) (Bent S, Bertoglio K, Hendren RL. Omega-3 fatty acids for autistic spectrum disorder: a systematic review. *Journal of Autism and Developmental Disorders.* 2009;39(8):1145–1154)

(Berbert et al, 2005) (Berbert AA, Kondo CR, Almendra CL et al. Supplementation of fish oil and olive oil in patients with rheumatoid arthritis. *Nutrition.* 2005;21:131-6)

(Berquin et al, 2007) (Modulation of prostate cancer genetic risk by omega-3 and omega-6 fatty acids. Isabelle M. Berquin, Younong Min, Yong Q. Chen. *J Clin Invest.* 2007;117:1866-1875)

(Berson et al, 2004) (Berson EL, Rosner B, Sandberg MA, et al. Clinical trial of docosahexaenoic acid in patients with retinitis pigmentosa receiving vitamin A treatment. *Arch Ophthalmol.* 2004;122(9):1297-1305)

(Bjalakovic et al, JAMA, 2007) (Bjalakovic G, Nikolova D, Gludd LL, Smonetti RG, Gludd C. Mortality in randomized trials of antioxidant supplements for primary and secondary prevention: systematic review and meta-analysis. JAMA. 2007;297:842–857)

(Bloch, Hannestad, 2012) (Bloch MH, Hannestad J. Omega-3 fatty acids for the treatment of depression: systematic review and meta-analysis. Mol Psychiatry. 2012 Dec;17(12):1272-82. doi: 10.1038/mp.2011.100. Epub 2011 Sep 20)

(Blomhoff, 2005) (Blomhoff R. Dietary antioxidants and cardiovascular disease. Curr Opin Lipidol. 2005;16:47–54)

(Boden et al, AIM-HIGH, 2011) (AIM-HIGH Investigators, Boden WE, Probstfield JL, Anderson T, et al. Niacin inpatients with low HDL cholesterol levels receiving intensive statin therapy N Engl J Med. 2011;365:225-2267)

(Boelsma et al, 2001) (Boelsma E, Hendriks HF. Roza L. Nutritional skin care: health effects of micronutrients and fatty acids. *Am J Clin Nutr.* 2001;73(5):853-864)

(Bondi et al, 2013) (Adolescent behavior and dopamine availability are uniquely sensitive to dietary omega-3 fatty acid deficiency." Corina O. Bondi, Ameer Y. Taha, Jody L. Tock, Nelson K.B. Totah, Yewon Cheon, Gonzalo E. Torres, Stanley I. Rapoport, Bita Moghaddam, Biological Psychiatry published online 29 July 2013, doi:10.1016/j.biopsych.2013.06.007)

(Bosch et al, 2012) (Bosch J., Gerstein H.C., Dagenais G.R., Díaz R., Dyal L., Jung H., Maggiono A.P., Probstfield J., Ramachandran A., Riddle M.C. *N*-3 fatty acids and cardiovascular outcomes in patients with dysglycemia. N. Engl. J. Med. 2012;367:309–318)

(Boskou, 2000) (Boskou, D. Olive oil. *World Rev Nutr Diet.* 2000;87:56-77)

(Bradbury et al, 2004) (Bradbury J, Myers SP, Oliver C et al. An adaptogenic role for omega-3 fatty acids in stress; a randomised placebo controlled double blind intervention study (pilot)ISRCTN22569553. *Nutr J.* 2004 Nov 28;3:20)

(Bradberry, Hilleman, 2013) (Overview of omega-3 fatty acid therapies. Bradberry C, Hilleman DE, P.T. Nov 2013; 38(11): 681-687)

(Brasky et al, 2010) (Specialty supplements and breast cancer risk in the VITamins And Lifestyle (VITAL) Cohort. Brasky TM, Lampe JW, Potter JD, Patterson RE, White E. Cancer Epidemiol Biomarkers Prev. 2010 Jul;19(7):1696-708)

(Brasky et al, 2011) (Brasky TM, Till C, White E, et al. Serum phospholipid fatty acids and prostate cancer risk: results from the Prostate Cancer Prevention Trial. *Am J Epidemiol*. 2011;173(12):1429–1439)

(Brasky, 2013) (*"Plasma Phospholipid Fatty Acids and Prostate Cancer Risk in the SELECT Trial"* Theodore M. Brasky, Amy K. Darke, Xiaoling Song, Catherine M. Tangen, Phyllis J. Goodman, Ian M. Thompson, Frank L. Meyskens Jr, Gary E. Goodman, Lori M. Minasian, Howard L. Parnes, Eric A. Klein and Alan R. Kristal

Journal of the National Cancer Institute) July 11, 2013, *Journal of the National Cancer Institute*, online)

(Bucher et al, 2002) (Bucher H.C., Hengstler P., Schindler C., Meier G. *N*-3 polyunsaturated fatty acids in coronary heart disease: A meta-analysis of randomized controlled trials. Am. J. Med.2002;112:298–304)

(Buckley et al, 2004) (Buckley MS, Goff AD, Knapp WE, et al. Fish oil interaction with warfarin. *Ann Pharmacother*. 2004;38:50-2)

(Buckley, Howe, 2009) (Buckley JD, Howe PR. Anti-obesity effects of long-chain omega-3 polyunsaturated fatty acids. *Obesity Reviews*. 2009;10(6):648–659)

(Burgess et al, 2000) (Burgess J, Stevens L, Zhang W, Peck L. Long-chain polyunsaturated fatty acids in children with attention-deficit hyperactivity disorder. *Am J Clin Nutr*. 2000; 71(suppl):327S-330S)

(Burr and Burr, 1929) (Burr, G.O. and Burr, M.M., 1929. A new deficiency disease produced by rigid exclusion of fat from the diet. *Journal of Biological Chemistry*. 82, 345-367)

(Burr *et al.*, 1989) (Burr, M.L., Fehily, A.M., Rogers, S., Welsby, E., King, S. and Sandham, S., 1989. *Diet and reinfarction trial (DART): design, recruitment, and compliance. European Heart Journal*. 10 (6) 558-567)

(Burr *et al*, 2003) (Burr, M.L., Ashfield-Watt, P.A., Dunstan, F.D., Fehily, A.M., Breay, P., Ashton, T., Zotos, P.C., Haboubi, N.A. and Elwood, P.C.,

2003. Lack of benefit of dietary advice to men with angina: results of a controlled trial. *European Journal of Clinical Nutrition*. 57 (2) 193-200)

(Burr et al, 2006) (Burr ML, Dunstan FD, George CH et al. Is fish oil good or bad for heart disease? Two trials with apparently conflicting results. *J Membr Biol*. 2006;206:155-63)

(Butler, 2009) (The Fish Report - Why Public Health Policy Should Promote Plant Omega-3 in Preference to Fish Oils. Dr Justine Butler, 2009. Published by: Viva! Health, Top Suite, 8 York Court, Wilder Street, Bristol BS2 8QH T: 0117 970 5190 E: info@vegetarian.org.uk W: www.vegetarian.org.uk)

(Calder, Yaqoob, 2009) (Calder PC, Yaqoob P. Omega-3 polyunsaturated fatty acids and human health outcomes. *Biofactors*. 2009;35(3):266–272)

(Calo et al, 2005) (Calo L, Bianconi L, Colivicchi F et al. N-3 Fatty acids for the prevention of atrial fibrillation after coronary artery bypass surgery: a randomized, controlled trial. *J Am Coll Cardiol*. 2005;45:1723-8)

(Caron, White, et al, 2001) (Caron MF, White CM. Evaluation of the antihyperlipidemic properties of dietary supplements. *Pharmacotherapy*. 2001;21(4):481-487)

(Chan, Cho, 2009) (Chan EJ, Cho L. What can we expect from omega-3 fatty acids? *Cleve Clin J Med*. 2009 Apr;76(4):245-51. Review)

(Chattipakorn et al, 2009) (Chattipakorn N, Settakorn J, Petsophonsakul P, et al. Cardiac mortality is associated with low levels of omega-3 and omega-6 fatty acids in the heart of cadavers with a history of coronary heart disease. *Nutr Res*. 2009; 29(10);696-704)

(Chew et al, 2013) (Chew et al. "Long-Term Effects of Vitamins C, E, Beta-Carotene and Zinc on Age-Related Macular Degeneration." Ophthalmology, published online April 11, 2013)

(Cho et al, 2001) (Cho E, Hung S, Willet WC, Spiegelman D, Rimm EB, Seddon JM, et al. Prospective study of dietary fat and the risk of age-related macular degeneration. *Am J Clin Nutr*. 2001;73(2):209-218)

(Chong et al, 2008) (Chong EW-T, Kreis AJ, Wong TY, et al. Dietary omega-3 fatty acid and fish intake in the primary prevention of age-related macular degeneration. A systematic review and meta-analysis. *Archives of Ophthalmology*. 2008;126(6):826–833)

(Chowdhury et al, 2012) (Chowdhury R., Stevens S., Gorman D., Pan A., Warnakula S., Chowdhury S., Ward H., Johnson L., Crowe F., Hu F.B., et al. Association between fish consumption, long chain omega 3 fatty acids, and risk of cerebrovascular disease: Systematic review and meta-analysis. BMJ. 2012;345:e6698)

(Chowdhury, Van Horn, AHA, 2014) (Rajiv Chowdhury, M.D., cardiovascular epidemiologist, University of Cambridge, England; Linda Van Horn, M.D., professor of preventive medicine, Northwestern University Feinberg School of Medicine, Chicago, and member, nutrition committee, American Heart Association; Council for Responsible Nutrition, , statement, March 17, 2014; March 17, 2014, *JAMA Internal Medicine*; March 18, 2014, *Annals of Internal Medicine*)

(Christensen et al, 2001) (Christensen JH, Skou HA, Fog L, Hansen V, Vesterlund T, Dyerberg J, Toft E, Schmidt EB. Marine n-3 fatty acids, wine intake, and heart rate variability in patients referred for coronary angiography. *Circulation*. 2001;103:623-625)

(Cleland, James, Proudman, 2006) (Cleland, Leslieg; James, Michaelj; Proudman, Susannam (2006). "Fish oil: What the prescriber needs to know". Arthritis Research & Therapy 8 (1): 679–81)

(Cole, 2009) (Cole GM. Omega-3 fatty acids and dementia. *Prostaglandins Leukot Essent Fatty Acids*. 2009; 81(2-3):213-21)

(Compl., 2010) (Complementary and Alternative Medicine for the Treatment of Depressive Disorders in Women. *Psychiatric Clinics of North America*. 2010;33(2)

(Consumers' Association, 2002) (Consumers' Association, 2002. *Fish – what's the catch?* Which Magazine, October 2002 p7-9)

(Covington, 2004) (Covington MB. Omega-3 fatty acids. *American Family Physician*. 2004;70(1):133–140)

(Dangour et al, 2010) (Dangour AD, Allen E, Elbourne D, et al. Effect of 2-y n23 long-chain polyunsaturated fatty acid supplementation on cognitive function in older people: a randomized, double-blind, controlled trial. *Am J Clin Nutr*. 2010;91:1725-1732)

(Daniel et al, 2009) (Daniel CR, McCullough ML, Patel RC, Jacobs EJ, Flanders WD, Thun MJ, Calle EE. Dietary intake of omega-6 and omega-3 fatty acids and risk of colorectal cancer in a prospective cohort of U.S. men and women. *Cancer Epidemiol Biomarkers Prev.* 2009 Feb;18(2):516-25)

(De Ley et al, 2007) (De Ley M, de Vos R, Hommes DW, et al. Fish oil for induction of remission in ulcerative colitis. *Cochrane Database of Systematic Reviews.* 2007;(4):CD005986 [edited 2008]. Accessed at www.thecochranelibrary.com on November 2, 2012)

(Dewailly et al, 2001) (Dewailly E, Blanchet C, Lemieux S, et al. n-3 fatty acids and cardiovascular disease risk factors among the Inuit of Nunavik. *Am J Clin Nutr.* 2001;74(4):464-473)

(Dichi et al, 2000) (Dichi I, Frenhane P, Dichi JB, Correa CR, Angeleli AY, Bicudo MH, et al. Comparison of omega-3 fatty acids and sulfasalazine in ulcerative colitis. *Nutrition.* 2000;16:87-90)

(Dijkstra et al, 2009, the Rotterdam Study) (Dijkstra SC, Brouwer IA, van Rooij FJA, Hofman A, Witteman JCM, Geleijnse JM. Intake of very long chain n-3 fatty acids from fish and the incidence of heart failure: the Rotterdam Study. *Eur J Heart Fail.* 2009;11:922-928)

(Dopheide, Pliszka, 2009) (Dopheide JA, Pliszka SR. Attention-deficit-hyperactivity disorder: an update. *Pharmacotherapy.* 2009 Jun;29(6):656-79) (Epub ahead of print)

(EPA, 2007) (EPA (2007-01-31). "Fish Consumption Advisories". Retrieved 2007-02-08)

(Erkkilä *et al.*, 2003) (Erkkilä, A.T., Lehto, S., Pyörälä, K. and Uusitupa, M.I.J., 2003. n-3 Fatty acids and 5-y risks of death and cardiovascular disease events in patients with coronary artery disease. *American Journal of Clinical Nutrition.* 3 (78) 65–71)

(Farinotte et al, 2007) (Farinotti M, Simi S, Di Pietrantonj C, et al. Dietary interventions for multiple sclerosis. *Cochrane Database of Systematic Reviews.* 2007;(1):CD004192 [edited 2009]. Accessed at www.thecochranelibrary.com on November 2, 2012)

(Fassett et a, 2010) (Fassett RG, Gobe GC, Peake JM, et al. Omega-3 polyunsaturated fatty acids in the treatment of kidney disease. *American Journal of Kidney Diseases.* 2010;56(4):728–742)

(Fenton et al, 2001) (Fenton WS, Dicerson F, Boronow J, et al. A placebo controlled trial of omega-3 fatty acid (ethyl eicosapentaenoic acid) supplementation for residual symptoms and cognitive impairment in schizophrenia. *Am J Psychiatry*. 2001;158(12):2071-2074)

(Filaire et al, 2011) (Effects of 6 weeks of n-3 fatty acids and antioxidant mixture on lipid peroxidation at rest and postexercise. Filaire E, Massart A, Rouveix M, Portier H, Rosado F, Durand D. Eur J Appl Physiol. 2011 Aug;111(8):1829-39)

(Filion et al, 2010) (Filion KB, El Khoury F, Bielinski M, et al. Omega-3 fatty acids in high-risk cardiovascular patients: a meta-analysis of randomized controlled trials. *BMC Cardiovascular Disorders*. 2010;10:24)

(Finendegen, 2002) (Finendegen LE. Reactive oxygen species in cell responses to toxic agents. Hum Exp Toxicol. 2002;21:85–90)

(Firestein, 2008) (Firestein. *Kelley's Textbook of Rheumatology*. 8th ed. St. Louis, MO: W. B. Saunders Company; 2008)

(Flaire et al, 2010) (Flaire E. et al, Effect of 6 Weeks of n-3 Fatty-Acid Supplementation on Oxidative Stress in Judo Athletes. Int J Sport Nutr Exerc Metab. 2010 Dec;20(6):496-506)

(Fodor et al, 2014) ("'Fishing' for the origins of the 'Eskimos and heart disease' story. Facts or wishful thinking?" by George Fodor, MD, PhD, FRCPC, FAHA; Eftyhia Helis, MSc; Narges Yazdekhasti MSc; Branislav Vohnout, MD; Canadian Journal of Cardiology, DOI: 10.1016/j.cjca.2014.04.007 published by Elsevier - See more at: http://www.elsevier.com/about/press-releases/research-and-journals/investigators-find-something-fishy-with-the-classical-evidence-for-dietary-fish-recommendations#sthash.n5THIV7N.dpuf)

(Fotuhi et al, 2009) (Fotuhi M, Mohassel P, Yaffe K. Fish consumption, long-chain omega-3 fatty acids and risk of cognitive decline or Alzheimer disease: a complex association. *Nat Clin Pract Neurol*. 2009 Mar;5(3):140-52) Review.

(14th Congress, 2013) (The 14th Congress of the European Society for Biomedical Research on Alcoholism. Abstract 01.2, presented September 8, 2013_http://www.medscape.com/features/slideshow/antibrain-food?src=wnl_edit_specol&uac=67380HZ#8)

(Frangou et al, 2006) (Frangou S, Lewis M, McCrone P et al. Efficacy of ethyl-eicosapentaenoic acid in bipolar depression: randomised double-blind placebo-controlled study. *Br J Psychiatry*. 2006;188:46-50)

(Freeman et al, 2000) (Freeman VL, Meydani M, Yong S, Pyle J, Flanigan RC, Waters WB, Wojcik EM. Prostatic levels of fatty acids and the histopathology of localized prostate cancer. *J Urol.* 2000;164(6):2168-2172)

(Freund-Levi, Meydani et al, 2006) (Freund-Levi YF, Eriksdotter-Jonhagen M, Cederholm T, et al. Omega-3 fatty acid treatment in 174 patients with mild to moderate Alzheimer disease: OmegAD Study. *Arch Neurol.* 2006;63:1402-8)

(Freund-Leve, Hjorth et al, 2009) (Freund-Levi Y, Hjorth E, Lindberg C, Cederholm T, Faxen-Irving G, Vedin I, Palmblad J, Wahlund LO, Schultzberg M, Basun H, Eriksdotter Jönhagen M. Effects of omega-3 fatty acids on inflammatory markers in cerebrospinal fluid and plasma in Alzheimer's disease: the OmegAD study. *Dement Geriatr Cogn Disord.* 2009;27(5):481-90)

(FSA, 2006) (FSA, 2006. *Seven Seas Ltd withdraws a number of batches of its own brand food supplements due to the presence of dioxins* [online]. Available from:www.food.gov.uk/enforcement/alerts/2006/mar/sevenseasupdate1 [Accessed August 11 2008]).

(FSA, 2006a) (FSA, 2006a. *The Boots Company plc withdraws two batches of its own brand Super Strength Fish Oil Capsules due to the presence of dioxins.* [online]. Available from: www.food.gov.uk/enforcement/alerts/2006/apr/bootsfishoil [Accessed August 11 2008])

(FSA, 2008) (FSA, 2008. Pyne, V. (Vicki.Pyne@foodstandards.gsi.gov.uk), 14 August 2008. RE: Refs for omega 3 and cognitive function. e-Mail to J. Butler (justine@vegetarian.org.uk)

(FSA, 2009) (FSA, 2009. Fish and shellfish [online]. Available from: http://www.eatwell.gov.uk/healthydiet/nutritionessentials/fishandshellfish/?lang=en [Accessed March 26 2009])

(Fux et al, 2004) (Fux M, Benjamin J, Nemets B. A placebo-controlled cross-over trial of adjunctive EPA in OCD. J Psychiatr Res. 2004;38:323–5)

(Galan et al, 2010) (Galan P., Kesse-Guyot E., Czernichow S., Briancon S., Blacher J., Hercberg S. Effects of B Vitamins and omega 3 fatty acids on cardiovascular diseases: A randomized placebo controlled trial. BMJ. 2010;341:c6273)

(Galli, Rise, 2009) (Galli C, Risé P. Fish consumption, omega 3 fatty acids and cardiovascular disease. The science and the clinical trials. *Nutr Health.* 2009;20(1):11-20) Review

(Geelen et al, 2005) (Geelen A, Brouwer IA, Schouten EG et al. Effects of n-3 fatty acids from fish on premature ventricular complexes and heart rate in humans. *Am J Clin Nutr*. 2005;81:416-20)

(Geerling et al, 2000) (Geerling BJ, Badart-Smook A, van Deursen C, et al. Nutritional supplementation with N-3 fatty acids and antioxidants in patients iwth Crohn's disease in remission: effects on antioxidant status and fatty acid profile. *Inflamm Bowel Dis*. 2000;6(2):77-84)

(Gerstein et al, ACCORD, 2011) (ACCORD Study Group, Gerstein HC, Miller ME, Genuth S, et al. Long-term effects of intensive glucose lowering of cardiovascular outcomes. NEJM. 2011;364:818-828)

(Giuseppe et al, 2013) (Giuseppe, D., et al., "Long-term intake of dietary long-chain n-3 polyunsaturated fatty acids and risk of rheumatoid arthritis: a prospective cohort study of women," Annals of the Rheumatic Diseases, August 12, 2013)

(Goldberg, Katz et al, 2007) (Goldberg RJ, Katz J. A meta-analysis of the analgesic effects of omega-3 polyunsaturated fatty acid supplementation for inflammatory joint pain. *Pain*. 2007 Feb 28; [Epub ahead of print].)

(Gulshan et al, 2005) (Gulshan K, Rovinsky SA, Coleman ST, Moye-Rowley WS. Oxidant specific folding of Yap 1-p regulates both transcriptional activation and nuclear localization. J Biol Chem. 2005;280:40524–40533)

(Green, Hermesh, et al, 2006) (Green, Pnina; Hermesh, Haggai; Monselise, Assaf; Marom, Sofi; Presburger, Gadi; Weizman, Abraham (2006). "Red cell membrane omega-3 fatty acids are decreased in nondepressed patients with social anxiety disorder". European Neuropsychopharmacology 16 (2): 107–13)

(Gronbaek, 1999) (Grønbaek M. Fish consumption and coronary heart disease mortality. A systematic review of prospective cohort studies. Eur. J. Clin. Nutr. 1999;53:585–590)

(Grosso et al, 2014) (Role of omega-3 Fatty acids in the treatment of depressive disorders: a comprehensive meta-analysis of randomized clinical trials. Grosso G, Pajak A, Marventano S, Castellano S, Galvano F, Bucolo C, Drago F, Caraci F. PLoS One. 2014 May 7;9(5):e96905)

(Gruger, Nelson, et al, 1964) (Gruger, E. H.; Nelson, R. W.; Stansby, M. E. (1 October 1964). "Fatty acid composition of oils from 21 species of marine fish, freshwater fish and shellfish". Journal of the American Oil Chemists Society 41 (10): 662–667)

(Hagen et al, 2009) (Hagen KB, Byfuglien MG, Falzon L, Olsen SU, Smedslund G. Dietary interventions for rheumatoid arthritis. *Cochrane Database Syst Rev.* 2009 Jan 21;(1):CD006400) Review

(Halim, Newby, 2912) (Efficacy of omega-3 fatty acid supplements (eicosapentaenoic acid and docosahexaenoic acid) in the secondary prevention of cardiovascular disease: a meta-analysis of randomized, double-blind, placebo-controlled trials. Halim SA, Newby LK.Arch Intern Med. 2012)

(Hall et al, 2007) (Hall MN, Campos H, Li H, Sesso HD, Stampfer MJ, Willett WC, Ma J. Blood levels of long-chain polyunsaturated fatty acids, aspirin, and the risk of colorectal cancer. *Cancer Epidemiol Biomarkers Prev.* 2007;16(2):314-21)

(Hartweg et al, 2009) (Hartweg J, Farmer AJ, Holman RR, Neil A. Potential impact of omega-3 treatment on cardiovascular disease in type 2 diabetes. *Curr Opin Lipidol.* 2009 Feb;20(1):30-8)

(Hendriks et al, 2003) (Hendriks H.F., Brink E.J., Meijer G.W., Princen H.M., Ntanios F.Y. Safety of long-term consumption of plant sterol esters-enriched spread. Eur. J. Clin. Nutr. 2003;5:681–692)

(Hooper *et al.*, 2004) (Hooper, L., Thompson, R.L., Harrison, R.A., Summerbell, C.D., Moore, H., Worthington, H.V., Durrington, P.N., Ness, A.R., Capps, N.E., Davey Smith, G., Riemersma, R.A. and Ebrahim, S.B., 2004. *Cochrane Database of Systemic Reviews* (online). (4) CD003177)

(Hooper *et al.*, 2006) (Hooper, L., Thompson, R.L., Harrison, R.A., Summerbell, C.D., Ness, A.R., Moore, H.J., Worthington, H.V., Durrington, P.N., Higgins, J.P., Capps, N.E., Riemersma, R.A., Ebrahim, S.B. and Davey Smith, G., 2006. Risks and benefits of omega 3 fats for mortality, cardiovascular disease, and cancer: systematic review. *British Medical Journal.* 332 (7544) 752-60)

(Hosseinzadeh et al, 2012) (The effects of omega-3 on blood pressure and the relationship between serum visfatin level and blood pressure in patients with type II diabetes. Hosseinzadeh Atar MJ, Hajianfar H, Bahonar A. ARYA Atheroscler. 2012 Spring;8(1):27-31)

(HPS2-THRIVE, 2013) (HPS2-THRIVE Collaborative Group. HPS2-THRIVE randomized placebo-controlled trial in 25,673 high-risk patients of ER niacin/laropiprant: trial design, pre-specified muscle and liver outcomes, and reasons for stopping study treatment. Eur Heart J. 2013;34:1279-1291)

(Hu, Manson, 2012) (Hu FB, Manson JE. Omega-3 fatty acids and secondary prevention of cardiovascular disease—is it just a fish tale? *Archives of Internal Medicine*. 2012;172(9):694–696)

(Huang, 2010) (Huang TL. Omega-3 fatty acids, cognitive decline, and Alzheimer's disease: a critical review and evaluation of the literature. *Journal of Alzheimer's Disease*. 2010;21(3):673–690)

(Innis, Rioux, et al. 1995) (Innis, SM; Rioux, FM; Auestad, N; Ackman, RG (1995 Sep). "Marine and freshwater fish oil varying in arachidonic, eicosapentaenoic and docosahexaenoic acids differ in their effects on organ lipids and fatty acids in growing rats.". The Journal of nutrition 125 (9): 2286–93)

(Iqbal, 2014) (Trans fatty acids - A risk factor for cardiovascular disease. Iqbal MP. Pak J Med Sci. 2014 Jan;30(1):194-197)

(Irving et al, 2012) (Irving CB, Mumby-Croft R, Joy LA. Polyunsaturated fatty acid supplementation for schizophrenia. *Cochrane Database of Systematic Reviews*. 2006;(3):CD001257 [edited 2010]. Accessed at www.thecochranelibrary.com on November 2, 2012)

(Iso et al, 2001) (Iso H, Rexrode KM, Stampfer MJ, Manson JE, Colditz GA, Speizer FE et al. Intake of fish and omega-3 fatty acids and risk of stroke in women. *JAMA*. 2001;285(3):304-312)

(Itakura et al, JELIS, 2012) (Itakura H, Yokoyama M, Matsuzake NM, et al; JELIS The change in low-density lipoprotein cholesterol concentration is positively related to plasma docosahexananoic acid but not eicosapentaenoic acid. J Atheroscler Thromb. 2012;19:673-679. Epub 2012 May 26)

(Itomura et al, 2005) (Itomura M, Hamazaki K, Sawazaki S et al. The effect of fish oil on physical aggression in schoolchildren - a randomized, double-blind, placebo-controlled trial. *J Nutr Biochem*. 2005;16:163-71)

(Jacobson, 2006) (Jacobson TA. Secondary prevention of coronary artery disease with omega-3 fatty acids. Am J Cardiol. 2006;98:61i-70i. Epub 2006 May 30)

(Jacobson, 2007) (Jacobson TA. Beyond lipids: the role of omega-3 fatty acids from fish oil in the prevention of coronary heart disease. Curr Atheroscler Rep. 2007;9:145-153)

(Jans et al, 2010) (The efficacy of n-3 fatty acids DHA and EPA (fish oil) for perinatal depression. Jans LA, Giltay EJ, Van der Does AJ. Br J Nutr. 2010 Dec;104(11):1577-85)

(Jeschke et al, 2001) (Jeschke MG, Herndon DN, Ebener C, Barrow RE, Jauch KW. Nutritional intervention high in vitamins, protein, amino acids, and omega-3 fatty acids improves protein metabolism during the hypermetabolic state after thermal injury. *Arch Surg*. 2001;136:1301-1306)

(Johansen et al, 2005) (Johansen JS, Harris AK, Rychly DJ, Ergul A. Oxidative stress and the use of antioxidants in diabetes: linking basic science to clinical practice. Cardiovasc Diabetol. 2005;4:1–11)

(Joy et al, 2006) (Joy CB, Mumby-Croft R, Joy LA. Polyunsaturated fatty acid supplementation for schizophrenia. *Cochrane Database Syst Rev*. 2006 Jul 19;3:CD001257) Review

(Kang et al, 2012) (Oligomerized lychee fruit extract (OLFE) and a mixture of vitamin C and vitamin E for endurance capacity in a double blind randomized controlled trial. Kang SW, Hahn S, Kim JK, Yang SM, Park BJ, Chul Lee S. J Clin Biochem Nutr. 2012 Mar;50(2):106-13)

(Kaushik et al, 2009) (Kaushik M, Mozaffarian D, Spiegelman D, Manson JE, Willett WC, Hu FB. Long-chain omega-3 fatty acids, fish intake, and the risk of type 2 diabetes mellitus. Am J Clin Nutr. 2009;90:613-620)

(Keech et al, 2005) (Keech A, Simes RJ, Barter P, et al; FIELD study investigators. Lancet. 2005;366:1849-1861)

(Kelley et al, 2009) (Kelley DS, Siegel D, Fedor DM, Adkins Y, Mackey BE. DHA supplementation decreases serum C-reactive protein and other markers of inflammation in hypertriglyceridemic men. *J Nutr*. 2009 Mar;139(3):495-501)

(Koch *et al.*, 2008) (Koch, C., Dölle, S., Metzger, M., Rasche, C., Jungclas, H., Rühl, R., Renz, H. and Worm, M., 2008. Docosahexaenoic acid (DHA) supplementation in atopic eczema: a randomized, double-blind, controlled trial. *British Journal Dermatology*. 158 (4) 786-792)

(Kooshki et al, 2011) (Effects of marine omega-3 fatty acids on serum systemic and vascular inflammation markers and oxidative stress in hemodialysis patients. Kooshki A, Taleban FA, Tabibi H, Hedayati M. Ann Nutr Metab. 2011;58(3):197-202)

(Kotwal et al, 2012) (Kotwal S, Jun M, Sullivan D, Perkovic V, Neal B. Omega 3 fatty acids and cardiovascular outcomes: systematic review and meta-analysis. Circ Cardiovasc Qual Outcomes. 2012;5:808-818)

(Kramer et al, 1982) (Kramer, JKG and others. Reduction of Myocardial Necrosis in Male Albino Rats by Manipulation of Dietary Fatty Acid Levels. Lipids 17, 372-382, 1982)

(Krauss et al, 2000) (Krauss RM, Eckel RH, Howard B, et al. AHA Scientific Statement: AHA Dietary guidelines Revision 2000: A statement for healthcare professionals from the nutrition committee of the American Heart Association. *Circulation*. 2000;102(18):2284-2299)

(Kremer, 2000) (Kremer JM. N-3 fatty acid supplements in rheumatoid arthritis. *Am J Clin Nutr*. 2000;(suppl 1):349S-351S)

(Kris-Etherton et al, 2001) (Kris-Etherton P, Eckel RH, Howard BV, St. Jeor S, Bazzare TL. AHA Science Advisory: Lyon Diet Heart Study. Benefits of a Mediterranean-style, National Cholesterol Education Program/ American Heart Association Step I Dietary Pattern on Cardiovascular Disease. *Circulation*. 2001;103:1823)

(Kris-Etherton *et al.*, 2002) (Kris-Etherton, P.M., Harris, W.S. and Appel, L.J., 2002. Fish consumption, fish oil, omega-3 fatty acids, and cardiovascular disease. American Heart Association. Nutrition Committee. *Circulation*. 106 (21) 2747-2757)

(Krombout et al, 2010) (Kromhout D, Giltay FJ, Geleijnse JM. n-3 fatty acids and cardiovascular events after myocardial infarction. *N Engl J Med*. 2010;363:2015-2026)

(Kromhout et al, 2012) (Kromhout D., Yasuda S., Geleijnse J.M., Shimokawa H. Fish oil and omega-3 fatty acids in cardiovascular disease: Do they really work? Eur. Heart J. 2012;33:436–443)

(Kupper, Carpenter, McFiggans, 2008) (Küpper FC, Carpenter LJ, McFiggans GB, et al. (2008). "Iodide accumulation provides kelp with an inorganic antioxidant impacting atmospheric chemistry". Proceedings of the National Academy of Sciences of the United States of America 105 (19): 6954–8)

(Kwak et al, 2012) (Kwak S.M., Myung S.K., Lee Y.J., Seo H.G., Korean Meta-analysis Study Group Efficacy of Omega-3 fatty acid supplements (Eicosapentaenoic Acid and Docosahexaenoic Acid) in the secondary prevention of cardiovascular disease: A meta-analysis of randomized, double-blind, placebo-controlled trials.Arch. Intern. Med. 2012;172:686–694. doi: 10.1001/archinternmed.2012.262)

(Lau, 2006) (Lau J. Effects of omega-3 fatty acids on serum markers of cardiovascular disease risk: A systematic review. Atherosclerosis. 2006;189:19–30)

(Lee et al, 2009) (Lee JH, O'Keefe JH, Lavie CJ; Harris WS. Omega-3 fatty acids: cardiovascular benefits, sources and sustainability. *Nat Rev Cardiol.* 2009; 6(12):753-8)

(Lichtenstein, 2005) (Lichtenstein AH. Nutrient and cardiovascular disease no easy answers. Curr Opin Lipidol. 2005;16:1–3)

(Liu et al, 2011) (Liu T., Korantzopoulos P., Shehata M., Li G., Wang X., Kaul S. Prevention of atrial fibrillation with omega-3 fatty acids: A meta-analysis of randomised clinical trials. Heart.2011;97:1034–1040)

(MacLean et al, 2005) (MacLean CH, Newberry SJ, Mojica WA, et al. Effects of omega-3 fatty acids on cancer risk: a systematic review. *JAMA.* 2005;295:403-415)

(Makrides et al, 2010) (Makrides M, Gibson RA, McPhee AJ, et al. Effect of DHA Supplementation During Pregnancy on Maternal Depression and Neurodevelopment of Young Children. *JAMA.* 2010;304:1675-1683)

(Manson et al, 2012) (Manson JE, Bassuk SS, Lee IM, et al. The VITamin D and OmegA-3 TriaL (VITAL): rationale and design of a large randomized controlled trial of vitamin D and marine omega-3 fatty acid supplements for the primary prevention of cancer and cardiovascular disease. Contemp Clin Trials. 2012;33:159-171)

(Manson, 3013) (Omega-3: Fishing Out the Recent Evidence. *Medscape.* Jun 04, 2013)

(Marangell et al, 2003) (Marangell LB, Martinez JM, Zboyan HA, et al. A double-blind, placebo-controlled study of the omega-3 fatty acid docosahexaenoic acid in the treatment of major depression. Am J Psychiatry. 2003;160:996–8)

(Marik et al, 2009) (Omega-3 dietary supplements and the risk of cardiovascular events: a systematic review. Marik PE, Varon J. Clin Cardiol. 2009 Jul;32(7):365-72)

(Martins, 2009) (EPA but not DHA appears to be responsible for the efficacy of omega-3 long chain polyunsaturated fatty acid supplementation in depression: evidence from a meta-analysis of randomized controlled trials. Martins JG. J Am Coll Nutr. 2009 Oct;28(5):525-42)

(Mattar, Obeid, 2009) (Mattar M, Obeid O. Fish oil and the management of hypertriglyceridemia. *Nutr Health*. 2009;20(1):41-9) Review

(McAnulty et al, 2010) (Effect of n-3 fatty acids and antioxidants on oxidative stress after exercise. McAnulty SR, Nieman DC, Fox-Rabinovich M, Duran V, McAnulty LS, Henson DA, Jin F, Landram MJ. Med Sci Sports Exerc. 2010 Sep;42(9):1704-11)

(McAnulty et al, 2011) (Effect of n-3 fatty acids and antioxidants on oxidative stress after exercise. McAnulty SR, Nieman DC, Fox-Rabinovich M, Duran V, McAnulty LS, Henson DA, Jin F, Landram MJ. Int J Sport Nutr Exerc Metab. 2011 Aug;21(4):328-37)

(McAnulty, AOX, 2011) (Effect of mixed flavonoids, n-3 fatty acids, and vitamin C on oxidative stress and antioxidant capacity before and after intense cycling. McAnulty SR, Nieman DC, McAnulty LS, Lynch WS, Jin F, Henson DA. Int J Sport Nutr Exerc Metab. 2011 Aug;21(4):328-37)

(Medical News Today, 2013) (Oregon State University. "Potential risk in consuming excess omega-3 fatty acids." *Medical NewsToday*. MediLexicon, Intl., 30 Oct. 2013. Web. 6 Nov. 2013. <http://www.medicalnewstoday.com/releases/268054)

(Miles, Calder, 2012) (Miles EA, Calder PC. Influence of marine n-3 polyunsaturated fatty acids on immune function and a systematic review of their effects on clinical outcomes in rheumatoid arthritis. *British Journal of Nutrition*. 2012;107(Suppl 2):S171–S184)

(Miller et al, 2005) (Miller ER, Pastor –Barriuso R, Dalal D, Riemersma RA, Appel LJ, Guallar E. Meta-analysis: high dosage vitamin E supplementation may increase all cause mortality.Ann Intern Med. 2005;142:37–46)

(Mitchell et al, 1987) (Mitchell EA, Aman MG, Turbott SH, Manku M. Clinical characteristics and serum essential fatty acid levels in hyperactive children. *Clin Pediatr* (Phila). 1987;26:406-411)

(Moghadasian, 2008) (Moghadasian, Mohammed H. (2008). "Advances in Dietary Enrichment with N-3 Fatty Acids". Critical Reviews in Food Science and Nutrition 48 (5): 402–10)

(Moghaddam, 2013) ("Diets lacking omega-3s lead to anxiety, hyper-activity in teens." *Medical News Today*. MediLexicon, Intl., 31 Jul. 2013. Web.
8 Aug. 2013)

(Montori et al, 2000) (Montori V, Farmer A, Wollan PC, Dinneen SF. Fish oil supplementation in type 2 diabetes: a quantitative systematic review. *Diabetes Care*. 2000;23:1407-1415)

(Moreau et al, 2002) (Moreau R.A., Whitaker B.D., Hicks K.B. Phytosterols, phytostanols, and their conjugates in foods: Structural diversity, quantitative analysis, and health-promoting uses. Prog. Lipid Res. 2002;41:457–500)

(Mori, 2010) (Mori TA. Omega-3 fatty acids and blood pressure. *Cell Mol Biol (Nosiy-le-grand)*. 2010; 56(1):83-92)

(Moxaffarian et al, 2005) (Mozaffarian D, Geelen A, Brouwer IA et al. Effect of Fish Oil on Heart Rate in Humans. A Meta-Analysis of Randomized Controlled Trials. *Circulation*. 2005;112(13):1945-52)

(Mozaffarian, Wu, 2011) (Mozaffarian D, Wu JH. Omega-3 fatty acids and cardiovascular disease effects on risk factors, molecular pathways and clinical events. J Am Coll Cardiol. 2011;58:2047-2067)

(Mozaffarian et al, CHS, 2013) (Plasma phospholipid log-chain omega-3 fatty acids and total and cause-specific mortality in older adults: the Cardiovascular Health Study. Mozaffarian et al. Ann Int Med. Apr 2, 2013; 158(7): 515-525)

(Mozurkewich et al, 2013) (The Mothers, Omega-3, and Mental Health Study: a double-blind, randomized controlled trial. Mozurkewich EL, Clinton CM, Chilimigras JL, Hamilton SE, Allbaugh LJ, Berman DR, Marcus SM, Romero VC, Treadwell MC, Keeton KL, Vahratian AM, Schrader RM, Ren J, Djuric Z. Am J Obstet Gynecol. 2013 Apr;208(4):313)

(Murray et al, 2006) (Murray RK, Bender DA, Bothan KM, Kennelly PJ, Rodwell VW, Weid PA. Harper's illustrated biochemistry 28 in Ed. McGraw Hill. Lange. N.Y.P. 2006. p. 468–469)

(Naliwaiko,Araujo, et al. 2004) (Naliwaiko, K.;Araújo, R.L.F.; Da Fonseca, R.V.; Castilho, J.C.;Andreatini, R.; Bellissimo, M.I.; Oliveira, B.H.; Martins, E.F. et al. (2004). "Effects of Fish Oil on the Central Nervous System: A New Potential Antidepressant?". Nutritional Neuroscience 7 (2): 91–9)

(Nagakura et al, 2000) (Nagakura T, Matsuda S, Shichijyo K, Sugimoto H, Hata K. Dietary supplementation with fish oil rich in omega-3 polyunsaturated fatty acids in children with bronchial asthma. *Eur Resp J.* 2000;16(5):861-865)

(Nathan, 2003) (Nathan C. Specificity of a third kind: reactive oxygen and nitrogen intermediates in cell signaling. J Clin Invest. 2003;111:769–778)

(Nemets, Stahl, et al. 2002) (Nemets, B.; Stahl, Z; Belmaker, RH (2002). "Addition of Omega-3 Fatty Acid to Maintenance Medication Treatment for Recurrent Unipolar Depressive Disorder". American Journal of Psychiatry 159 (3): 477–9)

(Ness *et al.*, 2002) (Ness, A.R., Hughes, J., Elwood, P.C., Whitley, E., Smith, G.D. and Burr, M.L., 2002. The long-term effect of dietary advice in men with coronary heart disease: follow-up of the Diet and Reinfarction Trial (DART). *European Journal of Clinical Nutrition.* 56 (6) 512–518)

(Neubronner et al, 2011) (Neubronner J.P., Schuchardt G., Kressel G., Merkel M., von Schacky C., Hahn A.L. Enhanced increase of omega-3 index in response to long-term *n*-3 fatty acid supplementation from triacylglycerides versus ethyl esters. Eur. J. Clin. Nutr.2011;65:247–254)

(Newcomer et al, 2001) (Newcomer LM, King IB, Wicklund KG, Stanford JL. The association of fatty acids with prostate cancer risk. *Prostate.* 2001;47(4):262-268)

(Nieman et al, 2009) (n-3 polyunsaturated fatty acids do not alter immune and inflammation measures in endurance athletes. Nieman DC, Henson DA, McAnulty SR, Jin F, Maxwell KR. Int J Sport Nutr Exerc Metab. 2009 Oct;19(5):536-46)

(NIH, 2006) (NIH Medline Plus. "MedlinePlus Herbs and Supplements: Omega-3 fatty acids, fish oil, alpha-linolenic acid". Retrieved 2006-02-14)

(Nordqvist, 2013) (Joseph Nordqvist. "Omega 3 Fish Oils Linked To Increased Prostate Cancer Risk." *Medical News Today*. MediLexicon, Intl., 11 Jul. 2013. Web.

11 Jul. 2013. <http://www.medicalnewstoday.com/articles/263179.php)

(Oh, 2005) (Oh R. Practical applications of fish oil (omega-3 fatty acids) in primary care. *Journal of the American Board of Family Practice.* 2005;18(1):28–36)

(Okamoto et al, 2000) (Okamoto M, Misunobu F, Ashida K, et al. Effects of dietary supplementation with n-3 fatty acids compared with n-6 fatty acids on bronchial asthma. *Int Med.* 2000;39(2):107-111)

(Oliver et al, 2007) (Oliver C, Everard M, N'Diaye T. Omega-3 fatty acids (from fish oils) for cystic fibrosis. *Cochrane Database of Systematic Reviews.* 2007;(4):CD002201 [edited 2010]. Accessed at www.thecochranelibrary.com on November 2, 2012)

(Olsen, Secher, 2002) (Olsen SF, Secher NJ. Low consumption of seafood in early pregnancy as a risk factor for preterm delivery: prospective cohort study. *BMJ.* 2002;324(7335): 447-451)

(Otaegui-Arrazola et al, 2013) (Otaegui-Arrazola A, Amiano P, Elbusto A, et al. Diet, cognition, and Alzheimer's disease: food for thought. *European Journal of Nutrition.* 2013)

(Paulsen et al, 2014) (Vitamin C and E supplementation hampers cellular adaptation to endurance training in humans: a double-blind, randomised, controlled trial. Paulsen G, Cumming KT, Holden G, Hallén J, Rønnestad BR, Sveen O, Skaug A, Paur I, Bastani NE, Ostgaard HN, Buer C, Midttun M, Freuchen F, Wiig H, Ulseth ET, Garthe I, Blomhoff R, Benestad HB, Raastad T. J Physiol. 2014 Apr 15;592(Pt 8):1887-901)

(Pazdro, Burges, 2010) (Pazdro R, Burgess JR. The role of vitamin E and oxidative stress in diabetes complications. Mech. Ageing Dev. 2010;131:276–86)

(Philibert, Vanier, et al, 2006) (Philibert, A; Vanier, C; Abdelouahab, N; Chan, HM; Mergler, D (2006 Dec). "Fish intake and serum fatty acid profiles from freshwater fish.". The American journal of clinical nutrition 84 (6): 1299–307)

(Pocobelli et al, 2009) (Pocobelli G, Peters U, Peters U, Kristal AR, White E. Use of supplements of multivitamins, vitamin C and vitamin E in relation to mortality. Am J Epidemiol. 2009;170:472–483)

(Proudman et al, 2013) (Proudman SM, James MJ, Spargo LD, et al. Fish oil in recent onset rheumatoid arthritis: a randomised, double-blind controlled trial within algorithm-based drug use. Ann Rheum Dis. 2013 Sept 30) a randomised, double-blind controlled trial.

(Quinn et al, 2010) (Quinn JF, Rama R, Thomas RG, et al. Docosahexaenoic acid supplementation and cognitive decline in Alzheimer disease. *JAMA*. 2010;304:1903-191)

(Raitt *et al.*, 2005) (Raitt, M.H., Connor, W.E., Morris, C., Kron, J., Halperin, B., Chugh, S.S., McClelland, J., Cook, J., MacMurdy, K., Swenson, R., Connor, S.L., Gerhard, G., Kraemer, D.F., Oseran, D., Marchant, C., Calhoun, D., Shnider, R. and McAnulty, J., 2005. Fish oil supplementation and risk of ventricular tachycardia and ventricular fibrillation in patients with implantable defibrillators: a randomized controlled trial. *Journal of the American Medical Association*. 293 (23) 2884-2891)

(Rakel, 2007) (Rakel D. *Integrative Medicine*. 2nd ed. Philadelphia, PA: Saunders, An Imprint of Elsevier; 2007)

(Ratnayake et al, 2000) (WMN Ratnayake and others. Influence of Sources of Dietary Oils on the Life Span of Stroke-Prone Spontaneously Hypertensive Rats. Lipids, 2000;35(4):409-420)

(Rauch et al, 2010) (Rauch B., Schiele R., Schneider S., Diller F., Victor N., Gohlke H., Gottwik M., Steinbeck G., del Castillo U., Sack R., et al. OMEGA, a randomized, placebo-controlled trial to test the effect of highly purified Omega-3 Fatty Acids on top of modern guideline-adjusted therapy after myocardial infarction. Circulation. 2010;122:2152–2159)

(Raz, Gabis, 2009) (Raz R, Gabis L. Essential fatty acids and attention-deficit-hyperactivity disorder: a systematic review. *Developmental Medicine and Child Neurology*. 2009;51(8):580–592)

(Rice et al, 2011) (Enteral omega-3 fatty acid, gamma-linolenic acid, and antioxidant supplementation in acute lung injury. Rice TW, Wheeler AP, Thompson BT, deBoisblanc BP, Steingrub J, Rock P; NIH NHLBI Acute

Respiratory Distress Syndrome Network of Investigators. JAMA. 2011 Oct 12;306(14):1574-81)

(Richard et al, 2008) (Polyunsaturated fatty acids as antioxidants. Richard D, Kefi K, Barbe U, Bausero P, Visioli F. Pharmacol Res. 2008 Jun;57(6):451-5)

(Richardson and Montgomery, 2005) (Richardson, A.J. and Montgomery, P., 2005. The Oxford-Durham study: a randomized, controlled trial of dietary supplementation with fatty acids in children with developmental coordination disorder. *Pediatrics*. 115 (5) 1360-1366)

(Richardson, Puri, 2000) (Richardson AJ, Puri BK. The potential role of fatty acids in attention-deficit/hyperactivity disorder. *Prostaglandins Leukot Essent Fatty Acids*. 2000;63(1/2):79-87)

(Riediger et al, 2009) (Riediger ND, Othman RA, Suh M, Moghadasian MH. A systemic review of the roles of n-3 fatty acids in health and disease. *J Am Diet Assoc*. 2009 Apr;109(4):668-79) Review

(Rizos et al, 2012) (Association between omega-3 fatty acid supplementation and risk of major cardiovascular disease events: a systematic review and meta-analysis. Rizos EC, Ntzani EE, Bika E, Kostapanos MS, Elisaf MS. JAMA. 2012 Sep 12;308(10):1024-33)

(Rocha et al, 2010) (Rocha Araujo DM, Vilarim MM, Nardi AE. What is the effectiveness of the use of polyunsaturated fatty acid omega-3 in the treatment of depression? *Expert Rev Neurother*. 2010; 10(7):1117-29)

(Romano et al, 2006) (Romano C, Cucchiara S, Barabino A et al. Usefulness of omega-3 fatty acid supplementation in addition to mesalazine in maintaining remission in pediatric Crohn's disease: A double-blind, randomized, placebo-controlled study. *World J Gastroenterol*. 2006;11:7118-21)

(Roncaglioni, Tombesi et al, 2013) (Roncaglioni MC, Tombesi M, et al. Risk and Prevention Study Collaborative Group, n-3 fatty acids in patients with multiple cardiovascular risk factors. N Engl J Med. 2013;368:1800-1808)

(SACN, 2004) (SACN, 2004. *Advice on fish consumption: benefits and risks*. The Stationery Office, London. [online]. Available from http://cot.food.gov.uk/pdfs/fishreport2004full.pdf[Accessed December 8 2008])

(Sadovsky et al, 2008) (Sadovsky R, et al. Patient use of dietary supplements: a clinician's perspective. Curr Med Res Opin. 2008 Apr;24(4):1209-16)

(Salari et al, 2008) (Salari P, Rezaie A, Larijani B, et al. A systematic review of the impact of n-3 fatty acids in bone health and osteoporosis. *Medical Science Monitor.* 2008;14(3):RA37–44)

(Sarris et al, 2009) (Sarris J, Schoendorfer N, Kavanagh DJ. Major depressive disorder and nutritional medicine: a review of monotherapies and adjuvant treatments. *Nutr Rev.* 2009 Mar;67(3):125-31) Review

(Sauer et al, 1997) (Sauer, FD and others. Additional vitamin E required in milk replacer diets that contain canola oil. Nutrition Research 17(2), 259-269, 1997)

(Saravanan et al, 2010) (Saravanan P, Davidson NC, Schmidt EB, et al. Cardiovascular effects of marine omega-3 fatty acids. *Lancet.* 2010;376 (9740):540–550)

(Seddon et al, 2001) (Seddon JM, Rosner B, Sperduto RD, Yannuzzi L, Haller JA, Blair NP, Willett W. Dietary fat and risk for advanced age-related macular degeneration. *Arch Opthalmol.* 2001;119(8):1191-1199)

(Sigal Eilat-Adar, et al, 2013) (Nutritional Recommendations for Cardiovascular Disease Prevention. Sigal Eilat-Adar, Tali Sinai, Chaim Yosefy, and Yaakov Henkin. Nutrients. 2013 September; 5(9): 3646–3683) Published online 2013 September 17. doi: 10.3390/nu5093646. PMCID: PMC3798927)

(Silvers et al, 2005) (Silvers KM, Woolley CC, Hamilton FC et al. Randomised double-blind placebo-controlled trial of fish oil in the treatment of depression. *Prostaglandins Leukot Essent Fatty Acids.* 2005;72:211-8)

(Singh et al, 2010) (P. P. Singh, Anu Chandra, Farzana Mahdi, Ajanta Roy, and Praveen Sharma. Reconvene and Reconnect the Antioxidant Hypothesis in Human Health and Disease. Indian J Clin Biochem. 2010 July; 25(3): 225–243)

(Singh et al, J Physiol. 2009) (Singh S, Farzana M, Singh PP. Insinuating role of free radicals and placating behaviour of antioxidant in diabetes mellitus. J Physiol. 2009;3:5–8)

(Smith et al, 2000) (Smith W, Mitchell P, Leeder SR. Dietary fat and fish intake and age-related maculopathy. *Arch Opthamol.* 2000;118(3):401-404)

(Smith, 2012) (Association between omega-3 fatty acid supplementation and risk of major cardiovascular disease events: a systematic review and meta-analysis. Smith DA. Ann Intern Med. 2012 Aug 21;157(4):JC2-3)

(Sokol, 1984) (Sokol RJ. Vitamin E toxicity. Pediatrics. 1984;74:564–565)

(Spencer et al, 2013) (Omega-3 Fatty Acids Reduce Adipose Tissue Macrophages in Human Subjects With Insulin Resistance. Michael Spencer, Brian S. Finlin, Resat Unal, Beibei Zhu, Andrew J. Morris, Lindsey R. Shipp, Jonah Lee, R. Grace Walton, Akosua Adu, Rod Erfani, Marilyn Campbell, Robert E. McGehee Jr, Charlotte A. Peterson, Philip A. Kern. Diabetes. 2013;62(5):1709-1717)

(Stark et al, 2000) (Stark KD, Park EJ, Maines VA, et al. Effect of fish-oil concentrate on serum lipids in postmenopausal women receiving and not receiving hormone replacement therapy in a placebo-controlled, double blind trial. *Am J Clin Nutr.* 2000;72:389-394)

(Stoll et al, 1999) (Stoll AL, Severus WE, Freeman MP. Omega 3 fatty acids in bipolar disorder: a preliminary double-blind, placebo-controlled trial. Arch Gen Psychiatry. 1999;56:407–12)

(Strobel et al, 2011) (Antioxidant supplementation reduces skeletal muscle mitochondrial biogenesis. Strobel NA, Peake JM, Matsumoto A, Marsh SA, Coombes JS, Wadley GD. Med Sci Sports Exerc. 2011 Jun;43(6):1017-24)

(Studer et al, 2005) (Studer M., Briel M., Leimenstoll B., Glass T.R., Bucher H.C. Effect of different antilipidemic agents and diets on mortality: A systematic review. Arch. Intern. Med.2005;165:725–730. doi: 10.1001/archinte.165.7.725)

(Su, Huang, et al. 2003) (Su, Kuan-Pin; Huang, Shih-Yi; Chiu, Chih-Chiang; Shen, Winston W. (2003). "Omega-3 fatty acids in major depressive disorder". European Neuropsychopharmacology 13 (4): 267–71)

(Sundstrom et al, 2006) (Sundstrom B, Stalnacke K, Hagfors L et al. Supplementation of omega-3 fatty acids in patients with ankylosing spondylitis. *Scand J Rheumatol.* 2006;35:359-62)

(Szymanski et al, Am J Clin Nut. 2010) (Szymanski KM, Wheeler DC, Mucci LA. Fish consumption and prostate cancer risk: a review and meta-analysis. *American Journal of Clinical Nutrition.* 2010;92(5):1223–1233)

(Szymanski et al, 2011) (Fish consumption and prostate cancer risk: a review and meta-analysis. Konrad M Szymanski, David C Wheeler, and Lorelei A Mucci. *Am J Epidemiol.* 2011;173:1429-1439)

(Terry et al, 2001) (Terry P, Lichtenstein P, Feychting M, Ahlbom A, Wolk A. Fatty fish consumption and risk of prostate cancer. *Lancet.* 2001;357(9270):1764-1766)

(Trenholm et al, 1979) (HL Trenholm and others. An Evaluation of the Relationship of Dietary Fatty Acids to Incidence of Myocardial Lesions in Male Rats. Canadian Institute of Food Science Technology Journal, October 1979;12(4):189-193)

(Turner et al, 2009) (Turner D, Zlotkin SH, Shah PS, et al. Omega 3 fatty acids (fish oil) for maintenance of remission in Crohn's disease. *Cochrane Database of Systematic Reviews.* 2009;(1):CD006320. Accessed at www.thecochranelibrary.com on November 2, 2012)

(Venturi, Donati, et al. 2000) (Venturi S, Donati FM, Venturi A, Venturi M. 2000. "Environmental iodine deficiency: A challenge to the evolution of terrestrial life?". Thyroid 10 (8): 727–9)

(Venturi, Venturi, 2007) (Venturi S, Venturi M (2007). "Evolution of Dietary Antioxidant Defences". European Epi-Marker 11 (3): 1–12)

(Villane et al, 2013) (Fish oil administration in older adults: is there potential for adverse events? A systematic review of the literature. Villani AM, Crotty M, Cleland LG, James MJ, Fraser RJ, Cobiac L, Miller MD. BMC Geriatr. 2013 May 1;13(1):41)

(Vles et al, 1978) (R.O. Vles and others. Nutritional Evaluation of Low-Erucic-Acid Rapeseed Oils. Toxicological Aspects of Food Safety, Archives of Toxicology, Supplement 1, 1978:23-32)

(Wallsundera et al, 2000) (MN Wallsundera and others. Vegetable Oils High in Phytosterols Make Erythrocytes Less Deformable and Shorten the Life Span of Stroke-Prone Spontaneously Hypertensive Rats. Journal of the American Society for Nutritional Sciences, May, 2000;130(5):1166-78)

(Wang et al, 2006) (Wang C, Harris WS, Chung M, Lichtenstein AH, Balk EM, Kupelnick B, Jordan HS, Lau J. Tufts-New England Medical Center

Evidence-based Practice Center, Institute for Clinical Research and Health Policy Studies, Tufts-New England Medical Center, Boston, MA, USA. Am J Clin Nutr. 2006 Jul;84(1):5-17)

(Weingartner et al, 2009) (Weingärtner O., Böhm M., Laufs U. Controversial role of plant sterol esters in the management of hypercholesterolaemia. Eur. Heart J. 2009;30:404–409)

(Weinstock-Guttman, 2005) (Weinstock-Guttman B, Baier M, Park Y et al. Low fat dietary intervention with omega-3 fatty acid supplementation in multiple sclerosis patients. *Prostaglandins Leukot Essent Fatty Acids.* 2005;73:397-404)

(Weitz et al, 2010) (Weitz D, Weintraub H, Fisher E, et al. Fish oil for the treatment of cardiovascular disease. *Cardiology in Review.* 2010;18(5):258–263)

(Whiteman, 2013) (Honor Whlteman. (2013, September 11). "Fish oil could prevent alcohol-related dementia." *Medical News Today*. Retrieved from

http://www.medicalnewstoday.com/articles/265852.php)

(WHO/FAO, 2003) (WHO/FAO, 2003. Joint WHO/FAO expert consultation. *Diet, Nutrition and the Prevention of Chronic Diseases*. Geneva: World Health Organization. Pages 55-56. ISBN 92-4-120916-X. Available from: http://www.who.int/hpr/NPH/docs/who_fao_expert_report.pdf [Accessed July 23 2008])

(Weitz et al, 2010) (Weitz D, Weintraub H, Fisher E, Schwartzbard AZ. Fish oil for the treatment of cardiovascular disease. Cardiol rev. 2010;18:258-263)

(Williams, Fisher, 2005) (Williams KJ, Fisher EA. Oxidation, lipoproteins and atherosclerosis: which is wrong, the antioxidants or theory? Curr Opin Clin Nutr Care. 2005;8:139–146)

(Winther *et al.*, 2005) (Winther, K., Apel, K. and Thamsborg, G., 2005. A powder made from seeds and shells of a rose-hip subspecies (*Rosa canina*) reduces symptoms of knee and hip osteoarthritis: a randomized, double-blind, placebo-controlled clinical trial. *Scandinavian Journal of Rheumatology*. 34 (4) 302-308)

(Yashodhara, 2009) (Yashodhara BM. Omega-3 fatty acids: a comprehensive review of their role in health and disease. *Postgrad Med J.* 2009; 85(1000):84-90)

(Yehuda, Rabinovitz, 2005) (Yehuda, Shlomo; Rabinovitz, Sharon; Mostofsky, David I. (2005). "Mixture of essential fatty acids lowers test anxiety". Nutritional Neuroscience 8 (4): 265–7)

(Yokoyama et al, JELIS, 2007) (Yokoyama M, Origasa H, Matsuzake M, et al; Japa EPA lipid intervention study (JELIS) Investigators. Effects of eicosapentaenoic acid on major coronary events in hypercholesterolaemic patients (JELIS): a randomized open-label blinded endpoint analysis. Lancet. 2007;389:1090-1098)

(Yuen et al, 2005) (Yuen AW, Sander JW, Fluegel D et al. Omega-3 fatty acid supplementation in patients with chronic epilepsy: A randomized trial. *Epilepsy Behav.* 2005;7(2):253-8)

SECTION TEN

ADDENDUM

As a bonus for my readers, I have attached two of my prior papers on redox biochemistry emphasizing the crucial pathogen protective roles of hydrogen peroxide and EMODs in the killing of cancer.

Howes RM. Hydrogen Peroxide: A review of a scientifically verifiable omnipresent ubiquitous essentiality of obligate, aerobic, carbon-based life forms. *The Internet Journal of Plastic Surgery*. 2010;7(1).

HYDROGEN PEROXIDE:

A review of a scientifically verifiable omnipresent ubiquitous essentiality of obligate, aerobic, carbon-based life forms

Prof. Hon. Randolph M. Howes, M.D., Ph.D.

Abstract

Electronically modified oxygen derivatives (EMODs), such as superoxide anion and hydrogen peroxide, carry out highly sophisticated intra, inter and extra cellular signaling roles that are essential for normal biochemical functioning. Hydrogen peroxide is freely diffusible through cell membranes, can not be excluded from cells and is required for normal operation of many enzymes that maintain and promote health. Hydrogen peroxide can act as an enzymatic substrate or activate or inhibit redox sensitive enzymes. Large health related organizations, such as the American Cancer Society, continue to disregard and deride the potential beneficial involvement and contribution of EMODs, especially hydrogen peroxide, in the treatment of any disease condition, inclusive of cancer. Their position of disdain is not supported by an exhaustive review of the medical and scientific literature. Although hydrogen peroxide has on occasion been a proposed mutagen, oncogenic transformation primarily leads to an increase of cellular EMODs that renders these same cells selectively vulnerable to additional EMOD production via EMOD induced apoptosis or necrosis. Legitimate medical health agencies are obliged to embrace the widespread scientific supportive findings regarding prooxidant hydrogen peroxide existent in the literature and encourage in depth scientific investigation into prooxidant EMOD disease protection and prevention. Scientific fact must supplant unsupported skepticism or flawed conclusions based on outdated data. While emphasizing hydrogen peroxide, this review is aimed at presenting the scientific facts regarding prooxidant EMOD health applications and cancer therapy. Based on the scientific literature currently available, EMOD use has significant potential benefits in the treatment of a wide range of human pathophysiologies. To deny the crucial role of hydrogen peroxide and prooxidant EMODs in normal metabolic processes and disease protection is to deny scientific truth.

Introduction

It is perhaps amongst the greatest biochemical wonders of evolution that the most crucial and widespread small molecular weight EMODs, which are purportedly the alleged "enemies within," are ever present and essential occupants of the most sensitive biochemical control systems within obligate aerobic cells. They carry on continual cross talk with their chemical kin. The naïve notion (promulgated by the free radical theory), that EMODs are inherently toxic, is counterintuitive to very basis of the evolutionary concept itself. After all, following oxygen's arrival, they evolved with the cell, by the cell and for the cell. Logic and biochemical principles dictate that careful EMOD modulation could serve as a safe means of advancing disease protection or reversal and health promotion.

However, even with hydrogen peroxide, which is an abundant permeating cellular mediator, nonspecific inhibition or augmentation of its activities may lead to homeostatic derangements by exogenous or endogenous over- or under-production.

Refute the Old Unproven Allegation: Free Radicals are Bad, Antioxidants are Good

In discussing the history of oxidants, such as hydrogen peroxide, respected free radical research pioneer, Barry Halliwell, said that, "In the beginning, it was simple: we said free radicals are bad, antioxidants are good." However, much has changed and over half a century later, these unfounded charges remain unproven. Further, the free radial theory, upon which this was based, has failed to be verified by the scientific method because of its lack of predictability. In fact, recent findings from randomized controlled trials (RCTs) have repeatedly failed to support the free radical theory and some trial results have even shown harmful effects and increased risk of mortality from antioxidant use.

Following the 1992 US National Cancer Institute research for testing of beta carotene, Halliwell, from the National University of Singapore, said, "It was a shock. It (beta carotene) not only did no good but had the potential to do harm." Subsequently, an expert panel convened by the National Institutes of Health has concluded that there is no evidence to recommend beta carotene supplements for the general population, and strong evidence to recommend that smokers avoid it.

The story was the same with vitamin E, in which recent studies have been almost universally "disappointing." Further, in 2005, Dr. Edgar Miller of the Johns Hopkins Medical Institutions, published a meta-analysis review of 19 studies in Annals of Internal Medicine showing that vitamin E increased overall mortality.[1] Even though vitamin E appeared to be a good antioxidant in vitro, there is now serious scepticism that it acts in the same manner in vivo.[2]

Following a large RCT on vitamin C, Halliwell said, "Vitamin C is another disappointment. People are still trying to defend it, but you don't get an effect on free radical damage unless you start with people with a vitamin C deficiency. I think it is a lost cause."

Yet, the prevailing prejudice against EMODs is manifestly illustrated in the November 2003 issue of Readers Digest. In quoting Dr. Bruce Ames, a biochemist at the University of California at Berkley, he stated, "free radical oxidation doesn't just rise with aging--it causes it. The more that mitochondria 'leak' free radicals (i.e., oxygen radicals, EMODs), the more those radicals end up damaging the mitochondria, which in turn leak even more free radicals." In bold print, the article states, "The ultimate irony: The thing we need most to live--oxygen--is what's killing us." Statements such as this, which appear in both the lay press and in scientific publications, point out the currently accepted dogma which states that oxygen and its radicals are highly toxic, even lethal. To the contrary, the overall data shows that these conclusions are, at best, dubious.

History of the Flawed Free Radical Theory

In *Science* in 1954, Rebeca Gerschman and her colleagues first introduced the notion that free radicals are toxic agents. Gerschman published a paper entitled, "Oxygen poisoning and X-irradiation: a mechanism in common." This paper led to the supposed link between oxygen free radicals and cellular damage, which was later used as the basis for the free radical theory of aging and oxidative stress. In 1956, over 53 years ago, Dr. Denham Harman proposed the free radical theory of aging. The free radical theory of aging simply argues that aging results from the accumulated damage generated over time by EMODs (oxygen free radicals).[3]

Harman's theory stated that the aging process resulted from the "stochastic" or random accumulated damage caused by EMODs (reactive oxygen species, ROS), many of which are products of normal cellular metabolism.[4-7]

The mitochondrial electron transport chain (ETC) is an integral player because up to 10% of the reducing equivalents from NADH so-called "leak" to form superoxide anions and H_2O_2, although this is admittedly one of the highest "guestimates" of superoxide production by the ETC.[8] The commonly quoted range for EMOD ETC production is between 1-5%. The negative opinions regarding EMODs have changed from seeing reactive oxygen species (ROS) and redox states as only sources of damage, to viewing them as integral components in signal transduction.[9]

EMODs and the redox state act as messengers in the intricate regulation of gene expression in development, growth, and apoptosis and there is widespread scientific support for the emerging perspective that EMODs are signaling molecules crucial in numerous cellular functions that are under precise control.

EMODs and Cancer Therapy

Cancer treatments using hydrogen peroxide have been around for decades and have been referred to as some of the following: hyperoxygenation, oxymedicine, oxidative therapy, bio-oxidative therapy and oxydology. The older literature based the use of hydrogen peroxide therapy on the work of Otto Warburg, M.D. (two time Nobel Prize in Medicine recipient), who believed that cancer cells grew best and primarily in an environment with hypoxic conditions. A simplistic view of Warburg's advocates was that the administration of hydrogen peroxide, which is an oxygen-rich solution, would restore the proper oxygen balance and selectively attack and kill cancer cells. The website for the University of California, San Diego Medical Center (Moores Cancer Center) states, "According the American Cancer Society (ACS), there is no scientific evidence that hydrogen peroxide is a safe, effective or useful cancer treatment." (Accessed 9-4-09).

A review of the scientific literature is essential to evaluate the accuracy or veracity of the ACS assessment, regarding the use of hydrogen peroxide for therapeutic purposes. Such a review rebuts their assertion.

Even though there has been "the poisoning of the oxidative watering hole" by the free radical theory for over a half century, world orthodoxy is now acknowledging that EMODs, inclusive of hydrogen peroxide, are of crucial benefit and play a central role in pathogen and neoplasia protection and cellular signaling. [10]

Hydrogen Peroxide (H_2O_2)

How could the magnanimous wisdom of evolution produce a ubiquitous, omnipresent, allegedly highly damaging, powerful, toxic agent such as the accused hydrogen peroxide molecule, which, by design, is freely mobile and highly permeable through biological membranes, enabling its diffusion out of and within the cell from any intracellular production site? Such a case would defy scientific and evolutionary logic.

Hydrogen peroxide (H_2O_2) is a well-documented and essential component of aerobic living cells. It plays crucial roles in host defense and oxidative biosynthetic reactions. In addition there is growing evidence that at low levels, H_2O_2 also functions as a signaling agent, particularly in higher organisms. All aerobic organisms studied to date, from prokaryotes to humans, appear to tightly regulate their intracellular H_2O_2 concentrations at levels favorable to healthy homeostasis, i.e., 10^{-9} to 10^{-7}M. [11]

Well defined biochemical pathways involved in the response to exogenous H_2O_2 have been described in both prokaryotes and yeast. In animals and plants, many regulated enzymatic systems generate H_2O_2. In addition oxidation-dependent steps in signal transduction pathways are being uncovered, and evidence is accumulating regarding the nature of the EMOD type(s) involved in each of these pathways. Application of physiologic levels of H_2O_2 to mammalian cells has been shown to stimulate biological responses and to activate specific biochemical pathways in these cells. [12]

Oxidation serves as our first line of defense and occurs with the respiratory burst, which should more properly be referred to as a "peroxide spike," secondary to spontaneous or enzymatic dismutation of the superoxide anion. [13] Ergo, our lives are sustained, at least in part, by an innate "prooxidant-cure" and during times of need, to fight invaders or tumors, we rely on this "peroxide-spike" or "Vis medicatrix naturae" (The Healing Power of Nature). Thus, hydrogen peroxide is a formidable and influential orthomolecular agent.

Disruption of the delicate balance between prooxidants and antioxidants has been implicated in the pathophysiology of many chronic diseases, such as atherosclerosis, cancer, diabetes, strokes, arthritis and cataract formation [14] Unfortunately, far too frequently, we have been "radically misled," regarding the overstated toxicity of EMODs. (see "The Howes Selective World Library of Oxygen Metabolism," available at www.thepundit.com). [15, 16]

Prooxidants are fundamental for life and the concentrations of electronically modified oxygen derivatives (EMODs) are important signaling agents, possibly extending to virtually all cellular processes. Oxygen is an important signal in all major aspects of stem cell biology including proliferation and tumorigenesis, cell death and differentiation, self-renewal, and migration. [17] "Redox signaling" is achieved by discrete, localized redox circuitry rather than by so-called "oxidative stress." [18]

This realization represents a significant departure from traditional views that prooxidant EMODs are simply harmful by-products of normal oxidative metabolism or only a tool through which phagocytes accomplish antimicrobial action. With this paradigm shift comes the challenge of understanding how EMOD production is regulated and localized within cells in both normal and pathological circumstances. Current evidence supports a sustaining role for EMODs and a generalized "injury" and protective response in tissues and organs.

Hydrogen Peroxide Overview

The literature illustrates the wide variety of cells and the distribution of EMOD production in the living/breathing cell. This alone demonstrates their low toxicity and the important role of EMODs in aerobic cells and their wide distribution is a counter argument to their supposed pernicious activity. Noted biochemist, Barry Halliwell, said that, "Over a year, a human body makes 1.7 kilograms or 3.74# of EMODs, which is a conservative estimate." This begs the question, "Thus, how toxic are EMODs?"

$O_2^{\cdot-}$ and H_2O_2 are cellular signaling molecules and they change the behavior of proteins as diverse as transcription factors and membrane receptors by virtue of their ability to undergo redox reactions with the proteins with which they interact, converting -SH groups to disulfide bonds and changing the oxidation states of enzyme-associated transition metals.

Prevalent EMOD Presence

EMOD activity has been detected in a wide variety of different cells including mesangial cells, oocytes, Leydig cells, thyroid cells, adipocytes, tumor cells, red blood cells and platelets. $O_2^{\cdot-}$ and H_2O_2 are manufactured by many cell types, encompassing fibroblasts, endothelial and vascular smooth muscle cells, neurons, ova, spermatozoa and cells of the carotid body. Superoxide anions and hydrogen peroxide also participate in the induction of hyperactivated motility and the acrosome reaction. [19]

The carotid body is an organ located at the bifurcation of the common carotid artery that measures the oxygen tension of the blood and it produces hydrogen peroxide on a continual basis. [20]

Halliwell claims that the gastrointestinal tract, especially the stomach, with its highly acidic environment, is constantly generating reactive oxygen species from food. "Every time you drink a cup of coffee it's a dilute bowl of hydrogen peroxide," says Halliwell. The hydrogen peroxide is there because of the presence of the antioxidants – "antioxidants" is really just another way of saying reducing agent, which can react with oxygen in the water to produce hydrogen peroxide. [21]

There is a surprising number of proteins whose operation depends upon the redox state of the cell and includes the general transcription factors NF-kappa B and AP-1 (jun/fos), as well as several transcription factors that induce the synthesis of proteins that protect against so-called oxidative stress (e.g., soxR, soxS, oxyR).

Yet, some have come to view oxygen as a dangerous gift: indispensable for energy production but the alleged cause of damage that accumulates slowly over a lifetime. [22]

Peroxide, the Terrible

Some say that under normal healthy conditions, 90% of H_2O_2 is generated as a toxic by-product of the mitochondrial electron transport chain (ETC) respiratory activity.[23,24]

In the past, some believed that H_2O_2, which is long lived and highly biomembrane permeable, must be immediately neutralized at the site of production to prevent diffusion throughout the cell or to the extracellular space.[25] Specific enzyme systems exist expressly for this purpose. These H_2O_2 neutralizing anti-oxidant enzymes are catalase (E.C. 1.11.1.6) and glutathione peroxidase (GPx, E.C. 1.11.1.9) with GPx responsible for 91% of H_2O_2 consumption.[26]

Even more alarming, some believe that, if allowed to accumulate, H_2O_2 will diffuse from its site of production and generate hydroxyl radical (·OH), which is the most damaging and chemically reactive radical formed by cellular metabolism. They believe that the hydroxyl radical will indiscriminately destroy everything it encounters.[27-29]

The hydroxyl radical is believed to be principally responsible for the cytotoxic effects of oxygen in animals.[29]

Hydrogen Peroxide's Crucial Role in Normal Cellular Function

Oxygen is the ultimate electron acceptor and reacts with all elements in the periodic table except the noble gases, which have no known biological function. The mitochondrial ETC is not perfect and up to 5% of electrons fail to combine with oxygen to produce water.[27] These so-called "leaked" electrons combine directly with molecular oxygen in the immediate vicinity, instead of the next carrier in the chain, to form the superoxide (O_2- ·) radical.[30]

Likely, complex I and III, of the ETC, are the source of so-called electron leakage leading to the eventual intracellular generation of hydrogen peroxide.[31,32] This ETC "leakage" or metabolic reduction of triplet O_2 during cellular respiration produces superoxide anion ($O_2^{·-}$), which is spontaneously or enzymatically dismutated to the prooxidant, H_2O_2, within mitochondria by the enzyme superoxide dismutase (SOD).[27]

H_2O_2 has a pervasive presence in cells and is continuously being produced by the plasma membrane, cytosol and different subcellular organelles including mitochondria, peroxisomes, endoplasmic reticulum, nucleus and by almost 100 enzyme systems.[23,25]

Studies have determined that H_2O_2 is a small, diffusible, and ubiquitous molecule that can be synthesized, modified and/or destroyed rapidly in response to external stimuli, it meets all of the important criteria for an intracellular messenger, and H_2O_2 is now firmly established as a ubiquitous intracellular messenger under subtoxic conditions. [33-36]

As previously mentioned, metabolic reduction of triplet O_2 during cellular respiration produces superoxide anion radical ($O_2^{\cdot -}$), which is spontaneously or enzymatically dismutated to the prooxidant, non-radical, H_2O_2. Varying cell types produce low levels of $O_2^{\cdot -}$ and H_2O_2 in response to a variety of extracellular stimuli, including cytokines (TGF-β1, TNF-α, and IL), peptide growth factors (PDGF; EGF, VEGF, bFGF, and insulin), the agonists of heterotrimeric G protein–coupled receptors (GPCR; angiotensin II, thrombin, lysophosphatidic acid, sphingosine 1-phosphate, histamine, and bradykinin), and shear stress. Research continues to uncover additional important sources of hydrogen peroxide in aerobic cells.

Hydrogen peroxide (H_2O_2) is present in exhaled breath and condensate and is produced by airway epithelia. Additionally, H_2O_2 is a vital substrate for the airway lactoperoxidase (LPO) anti-infection system. Duox is the major NADPH oxidase expressed in airway epithelia and therefore a contributor of H_2O_2 production in the airway lumen. [37]

Although specific levels of ubiquitous H_2O_2 have been debatable, animals and humans have between 5.0 and 41 microM for aqueous humor and 115 and 187 microM for urine. [38, 39]

Again, this begs the question, "Just how toxic are EMODs?"

It was believed that oxidative stress was the hallmark of asthma and increased levels of oxidants, such as H_2O_2 were considered a marker of the inflammatory process. In contrast to this notion, current studies suggest that hydrogen peroxide serves a role in suppressing both mucus production and airway hyper-responsiveness. [40]

Hydrogen peroxide production has also been found in the nucleus of epithelial cells and it could convey redox signals altering gene expression. [41, 42] H_2O_2 is a natural orthomolecular substance and has been detected in serum and in intact liver. [43]

In mouse pancreatic beta cells, H_2O_2 hyperpolarizes the cell membrane coupled with an increase of cell membrane conductance. [44]

Moreover, it has recently been shown that H_2O_2:

increases intracellular Ca^{2+}

decreases the ATP/ADP ratio

and inhibits glucose-stimulated insulin secretion from isolated mouse islets.[45]

H_2O_2 as an Insulin Mimetic

Long ago, it was demonstrated that polyamines are able to exert insulin-like effects in fat cells through the production of hydrogen peroxide.[46]

Hydrogen peroxide is now known to cause the reversible inhibition of protein tyrosine phosphatases (PTP) in cells, thereby strengthening insulin signaling. It has also been shown that production of hydrogen peroxide chemically in cells acts as an insulin mimetic. H_2O_2 improves glucose utilization in diabetics. Membrane receptors and transporters, including the insulin receptor and receptors for certain neurotransmitters, are regulated by the redox state of the cell.

Pancreatic β-cells are extremely sensitive to oxidative stress because of the low expression and activity of antioxidant enzymes. The GSH/GSSG (reduced/oxidized glutathione) ratio in islets is low compared with other tissues.[47]

A 10-6-09 article by Tony Tiganis in the journal Cell Metabolism shows that "mice that lacked the antioxidant enzyme Gpx1 were less likely to develop insulin resistance -- an early sign of diabetes -- than normal mice. But when they treated the enzyme-deficient mice with an antioxidant, they lost this advantage and become more diabetic." Tiganis said, "Our work suggests that antioxidants may contribute to early development of insulin resistance, a key pathological hallmark of type 2 diabetes."

Other Roles for Peroxide

Hydrogen peroxide is only one of the many components that help regulate the amount of oxygen getting to cells. Its presence is vital for many other functions as well. It is required for the production of thyroid hormone and sexual hormones. Even the synthesis of thyroxin depends on the requirements of a H_2O_2 substrate for thyroid peroxidase and

it stimulates the production of interferon.

A role for EMODs in controlling oxygen-sensitive channel function in excitable cells has been demonstrated previously. Hydrogen peroxide is capable of activating potassium transport pathways in excitable cells and in alveolar epithelial cells. These data suggest that EMODs and the hydroxyl radicals, formed from O_2 in close vicinity to the cell membrane, play an important role in the oxygen-dependent activation of the K^+-Cl^- co-transporter. [48]

H_2O_2 is produced by the autooxidation of ascorbic acid (vitamin C) and catecholamines, such as dopamine, norepinephrine and serotonin. [49]

Amazingly, H_2O_2 is generated at a rate of 1.36 +/- 0.2 microM/h (3.9 +/- 0.6 nmol.h-1.g Hb-1), and a steady-state red blood cell concentration of H_2O_2 which is approximately 2 x 10(-10) M. Kinetic comparisons of H_2O_2 production and oxyhemoglobin autooxidation (which generates $O_2^{\cdot-}$ that dismutases to H_2O_2) suggests that the latter is the main source of H_2O_2 in red blood cells. [50]

Apparently, many articles and agencies are unaware of peroxide's prime importance because studies have shown that the addition of exogenous H_2O_2, or its intracellular production in response to receptor stimulation, affects the function of various proteins, including protein kinases, protein phosphatases, transcription factors, phospholipases, ion channels, and G proteins.

EMODs can induce cellular senescence and apoptosis and can therefore function as anti-tumorigenic species. [51]

Another 100+ articles related to hydrogen peroxide's varied roles, including apoptosis, can be found at: http://www.caspases.org/showcitationlist.php?keyword=hydrogen%20peroxide%20h2o2, Copyright © 2004-2007 ICMG Ltd. Medical literature citations obtained from the National Center for Biotechnology Information. Protein database information obtained from the European Bioinformatics Institute. Accessed 10-7-09.

H_2O_2 can Dilate Arteries

H_2O_2 can dilate blood vessels in the heart and brain. Mechano-sensitive mechanisms that are sensitive to deformation, pressure, stretch, and wall shear stress elicit release of NO and H_2O_2, resulting in reactive dilation of isolated coronary arterioles. [52]

On June 23, 2009, the Medical College of Wisconsin received a four year, $1.5 million grant from the National Institutes of Health's National Heart, Lung and Blood Institute to study the role of naturally produced hydrogen peroxide in controlling human blood flow. Dr. David

Gutterman's lab has observed a unique relationship between dilation in heart blood vessels from patients with coronary artery disease and the endothelial production of hydrogen peroxide and thus far, the association of vessel dilation with mitochondrial hydrogen peroxide has only been reported in human hearts.

EMOD Induced Apoptotic Cancer Cell Death

Cancer accounts for nearly 25% of all human deaths and no definitive cure is available as yet. [53] The most common treatment modalities promising a cure appear to be a combination of radiotherapy and chemotherapy and these methods, in part, utilize the reactivities of prooxidant EMODs, including hydrogen peroxide. Radiation exposure leads to the hydrolysis of water, thereby generating EMODs, which initiate chemical peroxidative processes that destroy biomolecules. [54]

The postulated mechanism of action for many forms of chemotherapy, radiation therapy, photodynamic therapy, ozone therapy, hyperbaric oxygen therapy, intravenous mega-dose of vitamin C, the Howes singlet oxygen cancer therapy system and hydrogen peroxide therapy is the generation of electronically modified oxygen derivatives (EMODs). The production of EMODs leads to the stimulation of various signaling pathways, and in particular, stress-responsive signal transduction pathways are strictly regulated by the intracellular redox state. [55, 56]

High level acute H_2O_2 treatment of various cells in vitro leads to apoptosis. [57]

However, some investigators believe that hydrogen peroxide can cause apoptosis via a non-apoptotic pathway. Recent studies in a variety of cell types have suggested that cancer chemotherapy drugs induce tumor cell apoptosis in part by inducing formation of reactive oxygen species (EMODs). Investigators demonstrated that, at least in B lymphoma cells, chemotherapy-induced apoptosis occur using a mechanism that does not involve oxidants. Hydrogen peroxide, which reportedly kills cells by a non-apoptotic pathway, caused increases in both protein and lipid oxidation. [58]

Hydrogen Peroxide and Hydroxyl Radical Antineoplastic Cytotoxicity

The cytotoxicity of the antineoplastic quinones doxorubicin, mitomycin C, and diaziridinylbenzoquinone for the Ehrlich ascites carcinoma can be significantly reduced or abolished by the antioxidant enzymes catalase and superoxide dismutase, the hydroxyl radical scavengers dimethyl sulfoxide, diethylurea, and thiourea, and the iron chelators deferoxamine, 2,2-bipyridine, and diethylenetriaminepentaacetic acid. Furthermore, treatment of intact tumor cells with doxorubicin, mitomycin C, and diaziridinylbenzoquinone required hydrogen peroxide, iron, and intact tumor cells. These results suggest that drug-induced hydrogen peroxide and hydroxyl radical production has a role in the antineoplastic action of redox active anticancer quinones.[59]

Photodynamic Therapy (PDT) and Singlet Oxygen

Photodynamic therapy (PDT) is a novel approach for destruction of malignant cells and involves the administration of nontoxic dyes known as photosensitisers (PS) either systemically or topically, followed by illumination of the lesion with visible light (usually red).[60] The PS absorbs the light, and in the presence of oxygen, transfers the energy, thereby producing cytotoxic oxygen species (either singlet oxygen or oxygen radicals, i.e., EMODs).[61,62]

This reportedly leads to a rapid tumoricidal response mediated by both direct tumor cell toxicity and photodamage to the involved microvasculature and cellular structure.[63]

Investigations have demonstrated that apoptotic and necrotic pathways are both involved in PDT-mediated cell death.[60,64]

A wide distribution of early response genes, genes associated with signal transduction pathways and cytokine expression, as well as stress response genes, are activated by PDT and primarily singlet oxygen.[65-71]

EMODs can Have Complex Interactions

Interestingly, EMODs can react and interact to produce a family of products. For example, superoxide can react with itself to produce hydrogen peroxide or it can undergo univalent reduction to form hydrogen peroxide. Superoxide can react with the hydroxyl radical to produce singlet oxygen. Superoxide can also react with nitric oxide ($NO^{\cdot}$) (also a radical) to produce peroxynitrate ($OONO^{-}$). Singlet oxygen can react with superoxide to produce hydrogen peroxide. Hydrogen peroxide can react with hypohalous acid to produce singlet oxygen. Hydrogen peroxide, in the presence of metal ions, can react to form a hydroxyl radical ($HO^{\cdot}$) and the hydroxide ion (HO^{-}). Ozone can react with water to form hydrogen peroxide. Methylene blue and superoxide dismutase produce H_2O_2. Ascorbate can react with singlet oxygen and produce hydrogen peroxide.

Examples of the cross reactivity of EMODs illustrate the generation of a family of EMODs from the more basic EMOD agents (superoxide, hydrogen peroxide and singlet oxygen).

A Role for Hydrogen Peroxide in the Pro-apoptotic Effects of Photodynamic Therapy

Although the first EMOD formed during irradiation of photosensitized cells is almost invariably singlet molecular oxygen, $^1O_2^*$, other EMODs have been implicated in the phototoxic effects of photodynamic therapy. Among these are superoxide anion radical ($O_2^{\cdot-}$), hydrogen peroxide (H_2O_2) and hydroxyl radical (OH.). Investigators studied the role of H_2O_2 in the pro-apoptotic response to PDT in murine leukemia P388 cells. A primary route for detoxification of cellular H_2O_2 involves the peroxisomal enzyme catalase. Inhibition of catalase activity by 3-amino-1,2,4-triazole led to an increased apoptotic response. PDT-induced apoptosis was impaired by addition of an exogenous recombinant catalase analog (CAT-skl) that was specifically designed to enter cells and more efficiently localize in peroxisomes. A similar effect was observed upon addition of 2,2'-bipyridine, a reagent that can chelate Fe(+2), a co-factor in the Fenton reaction that results in the conversion of H_2O_2 to the hydroxyl radical (OH). These results provide evidence that formation of H_2O_2 during irradiation of photosensitized cells contributes to PDT efficacy.[72]

H_2O_2, $O_2^{\cdot-}$ and OH. are Involved in Phototoxic Tumoricidal Action

Researchers estimated the participation of EMODs, other than singlet oxygen ($^1O_2^*$), in the antitumor effect of PDT with hematoporphyrin derivative (HPD) as well as determined the ability of photoexcited HPD to the formation of protein peroxides that are regarded as a new form of EMOD. Experiments indicated that H_2O_2 and oxygen radicals could mediate the tumoricidal action of HPD-PDT; they found that photosensitization of EAC cells with HPD leads to the formation of significant amounts of H_2O_2, superoxide ($O_2^{\cdot-}$) and hydroxyl (OH.) radicals, which along with $^1O_2^*$ were involved in photoinactivation of the cells in vitro. Their data showed that in EAC cells subjected to HPD-PDT, the generation H_2O_2, $O_2^{\cdot-}$ and OH. could be largely mediated by: (i) an increase in the activity of xanthine oxidase (XOD), due most probably to the conversion of xanthine dehydrogenase (XDH) to XOD via a Ca2+-dependent proteolytic process as well as oxidation of SH groups in XDH; and (ii) photooxidation of some cellular constituents (proteins). Another interesting finding of their studies was that in tumor cells subjected to HPD-PDT the Fenton-like reactions could play an important role in the generation of OH., and that cell-bound Cu/Zn-superoxide dismutase as well as catalase can protect tumor cells against the phototoxic action of HPD. They clearly demonstrated the ability of photoexcited HPD to the generation of protein peroxides in tumor cells. Studies suggest that $^1O_2^*$ is the main agent responsible for the generation of protein peroxides in EAC cells treated with HPD-PDT, although other EMODs (H_2O_2, $O_2^{\cdot-}$ and OH.) were also implicated in this process.[73]

Photofrin® is a purified form of hematoporphyrin derivative; it is a photosensitizer used in the treatment of cancer. Upon exposure to light it produces singlet oxygen, a highly electrophilic species that initiates oxidations that lead to cell death.[74,75]

Interestingly, singlet oxygen reacts readily with ascorbate, producing hydrogen peroxide.[76,77]

Ubiquitous and Omnipresent H_2O_2

The biochemistry of H_2O_2 is also, to a considerable extent, the biochemistry of the superoxide anion. Superoxide anion ($O_2^{\cdot-}$) converts rapidly to H_2O_2 either spontaneously or with the help of one of the superoxide dismutase enzymes (i.e., CuZnSOD, EcSOD, MnSOD, etc.). Since many of the EMODs are rapidly converted and/or transformed into other EMOD types, it also serves as a source of a large family of EMOD agents.

The two primary metabolic EMODs are $O_2^{\cdot-}$ and H_2O_2. $O_2^{\cdot-}$ is the primary stoichiometric precursor of H_2O_2 but considerable H_2O_2 can be produced directly and not via the superoxide anion.

Chance, et al. reviewed the metabolism of H_2O_2 in mammalian systems.[11]

Though controversial, many papers still state that the mitochondria are the major cellular source of hydrogen peroxide. The amount of H_2O_2 produced by brain mitochondria is up to 5% of the amount of O_2 consumed. H_2O_2 may be produced directly as a product of biological oxidations, or it may be produced by the dismutation of superoxide. The relative estimates of subcellular sources of H_2O_2 are as follows:

Endoplasmic reticulum (mixed function oxidations)	45%
Peroxisomes (metal-catalyzed oxidations)	35%
Mitochondria (oxidative phosphorylation)	15%
Cytosol (xanthine oxidation)	5%

These EMOD agents are formed continuously in all aerobic cells, either via oxygen energy metabolism, through reactions with drugs or toxins or via metabolism of fatty acids.

In 1999, Juan and Buettner calculated the steady state (ss) levels to be as follows:

$[H_2O_2]$ss in red cells is 10^{-10} M

$[H_2O_2]$ss in mitochondrial membrane is 10^{-8} M

$[H_2O_2]$ss in liver cells is 10^{-8} M

$[O_2]$ss is 10^{-5} M, much higher than $[H_2O_2]$

$[O_2^{\cdot-}]$ss in cells is 10^{-10} M

An additional source of $O_2^{\cdot-}$ and H_2O_2 is the NADPH oxidase families (NOX and DuOX), which are found on various cellular membranes. Once thought to be restricted only to phagocytes, stimulated H_2O_2 production is now known to occur in almost all cells through NOX and/or DuOX activities. Thus, H_2O_2 has been accused of contributing to pathology through its reaction with transition metals that produce hydroxyl radicals via the Fenton reaction. Yet, even though it is not discussed, two hydroxyl radicals can combine to form hydrogen peroxide. This could well represent another salutary pathway for peroxide formation and pathogen and neoplasia defense.

H_2O_2 is involved in the generation of hypohalous acids through catalysis by myeloperoxidases and lactoperoxidase. These oxidizing acids are capable of killing microorganisms and allegedly causing tissue damage during inflammation. Ubiquitous H_2O_2 acts as a secondary messenger in signal transduction through its reaction with key proteins containing critical cysteine residues. [78, 79]

Yet, the antioxidant, cysteine, itself can undergo autoxidation and form H_2O_2. This is somewhat analogous to the prooxidant EMOD activity of ascorbic acid.

The most common prooxidant in vivo is H_2O_2 and under inflammatory conditions, it is abundantly formed by dismutation of $O_2^{\cdot-}$ released from activated phagocytes and other enzymatic systems, [80] but physiologically also by intracellular NADPH oxidases. [81]

Although some H_2O_2 appears to be produced constitutively, receptor-mediated H_2O_2 formation appears to be more common. Typical examples are TNFα-induced mitochondrial $O_2^{\cdot -}$ formation, [82] or cytoplasmic increase of H_2O_2 upon growth factor receptor stimulation. [83] Nonetheless, H_2O_2 is argued to be the most common prooxidant in vivo.

In a study on synergism between tumor necrosis factor-alpha and H_2O_2, levels of cellular toxicity were found. With PC12 tumor cells, TNF alpha toxicity was seen at >50 ng/ml, and that of H_2O_2 at > 150 microM. However, when together, sub-lethal levels (25 ng/ml TNF alpha and 30 microM H_2O_2) induced toxicity. [84]

Please remember that the chemistry of superoxide is also the chemistry of hydrogen peroxide. Once activated, phagocytes produce large quantities of superoxide, on the order of 10 nmol·min-1·10^6 neuutrophils^{-1} during the oxidative burst. [80]

The rate of superoxide production in vascular cells is thought to be ~1-10% of that in leukocytes. [85, 86] Basically, all cells continuously form $O_2^{\cdot -}$ and submitochondrial particles generate $O_2^{\cdot -}$ at a rate of 4-7 nmol/ min^{-1}/mg protein^{-1}. [11]

Superoxide anion can be viewed as an innate pathway for hydrogen peroxide production. Thus, EMODs are intentionally being generated to serve as salutary cellular products intended to help regulate critical metabolic and reproductive mechanisms. [87] These prooxidant EMODs stimulate numerous transcription factors as well as signaling cascades via activation of kinases and inhibition of tyrosine phosphatases.

Under physiological conditions, the intracellular production of EMODs does not alter the redox state of cells which have large reserves of reducing agents, notably reduced glutathione, as well as extremely effective antioxidant defense mechanisms, such as SOD, catalase, and peroxidases. This allows agonist-induced increases in EMODs to function as second messengers by limiting their effecting time and space in a manner similar to other well-known intracellular signals, such as cyclic AMP or nitric oxide. [88]

Differing from $O_2^{\cdot -}$ that is charged, hardly permeable, and extremely short-lived, H_2O_2 is uncharged, relatively longer-lived, and freely diffusible. This property makes H_2O_2 an ideal signaling molecule. Clearly, this illustrates the great importance of H_2O_2, in combination with other EMODs, in the regulation of cellular homeostasis and redox status.

Under basal conditions, human cells produce about 2×10^9 (2 billion) O_2.- and H_2O_2 molecules per cell per day.[89]

EMODs are recognized as controlling key steps in cellular signal transduction cascades.[90, 91] EMODs can reversibly control gene expression and regulation at non-cytotoxic doses.[92] More specifically, there is evidence that hydrogen peroxide, H_2O_2, can modulate cellular functions through altering signal transduction in many cell types, including endothelial cells (ECs), vascular smooth muscle cells (VSMC), and T cells.[93-97]

In fact, H_2O_2 is now widely recognized as a ubiquitous intracellular messenger, under subtoxic conditions.[23, 34, 35, 36, 98-100] As of 2000, at least 127 genes and signal transducing proteins had been reported to be sensitive to reductive and oxidative (redox) states in the cell.[92] That number, as of 2009, now exceeds 200.

EMODs Kill Cancer

Otto Warburg was the primary scientist to implicate oxygen in cancer.[101] Anaerobic metabolism is favorable to many pathogenic organisms and hypoxia is the predominant condition within neoplastic cells. Hypoxia has been closely associated with pathological processes.[102] Requiring adequate oxygen levels, many anticancer drugs and radiation kill cancer cells by inducing prooxidant EMOD apoptosis.[103]

High level acute H_2O_2 treatment of various cells in vitro leads to apoptosis, with the involvement of NADPH oxidase isoforms and Src family kinases.[104]

The chemotherapeutic agents doxorubicin, mitomycin C, etoposide and cisplatin are superoxide generating agents and consequently hydrogen peroxide producers.[105]

Bleomycin and doxorubicin are agents shown to produce prooxidant oxygen agents.[106]

In reactions involving Fe(II) and oxygen, a so-called "activated" bleomycin species is generated that damages DNA through free radical intermediates.[107]

Superoxide and hydrogen peroxide can also react with Fe(II) or Fe(III) bleomycin, respectively, to produce the activated form of the drug. DNA damage from bleomycin and ionizing radiation is similar in both induction and repair.[108] Several other anti-cancer drugs are known to bring about their tumoricidal actions by an EMOD dependent mechanism. A majority of the studies reported that adriamycin, mitocmycin C, etc., augment EMOD production (superoxide anion and hydrogen peroxide) and lipid peroxidation in vitro and in vivo. [109]

The anti-estrogen tamoxifen, increasingly used alongside other breast cancer therapies, has also been shown to induce oxidative stress (EMOD production) within carcinoma cells *in vitro.* [110]

Oxygen levels are important since radiotherapy and photodynamic therapy generate oxygen radicals within the carcinoma cell. Thus, tumor hypoxia is a therapeutic concern since it can reduce the effectiveness of radiotherapy, some O_2-dependent cytotoxic agents, and photodynamic therapy. [111]

H_2O_2 Increases Doxorubicin Kill of Bladder Tumor Cells

Investigators determined whether the cytotoxicity of doxorubicin hydrochloride would be enhanced by adding hydrogen peroxide as a source of oxygen free radicals. Mouse bladder tumor cells (MBT-2) were grown in RPMI 1640 medium and treated with various concentrations of doxorubicin hydrochloride for 2 hours. They observed a dose dependent inhibition of MBT-2 cell growth after exposure to doxorubicin hydrochloride. Exposure to doxorubicin and hydrogen peroxide resulted in greater cell growth inhibition than exposure to either agent alone. The effects of hydrogen peroxide on cell proliferation were reversed by pre-incubation with alpha-tocopherol. As a source of oxygen free radicals, hydrogen peroxide enhances the anti-proliferative effect of doxorubicin hydrochloride on a mouse bladder tumor cell line. [112]

H_2O_2 Increases Sulindac Kill of Squamous Cell Carcinoma

A skin squamous cell carcinoma (SCC-25) cell line was utilized and treated with sulindac prior to exposure to tert-butyl hydroperoxide (TBHP) or hydrogen peroxide for 2 hours. The combination of sulindac and TBHP enhanced the killing of the skin cancer cells. Sulindac combined with TBHP leads to markedly increased levels of intracellular EMODs in SCC cells.

A small group of patients with actinic keratoses (AKs), were treated with the combination of sulindac and hydrogen peroxide gels. The results revealed that 60% of the treated AKs responded to therapy by exhibiting a decrease in size or becoming not visible to the naked eye. In addition, 50% of the treated AKs showed no residual AK on histopathology specimens after skin biopsy at the end of the study. Researchers concluded that the combination of sulindac and TBHP or H_2O_2 significantly enhances the killing of SCC cells. [113]

The Baylor Group Peroxide Experience

In the 1960s, a group of investigators at Baylor Medical School (the Baylor group) conducted ground breaking studies with hydrogen peroxide in the treatment of a wide range of disease conditions. Various investigators have studied the value of H_2O_2 and shrinking the size of tumors, [114] and have studied treatment advantages and increased tumor cytotoxicity by the use of regional H_2O_2 infusion. [115]

Earlier work indicated that hydrogen peroxide, a secretory product of mononuclear phagocytes, [116] accounts for a considerable portion of their nonphagocytic lysis of tumor cells in at least three circumstances: when certain secretagogues were added, when antitumor antibody was present, or when the tumor cells were coated with eosinophil peroxidase. [117]

Many clinical and experimental applications of hydrogen peroxide have been demonstrated by the Baylor group. In over 300 patients regional intra-arterial hydrogen peroxide has potentiated the effect of radiation therapy in situations of malignancy involving the head, neck, pelvis and retro-peritoneum. [118]

Increased localization of radioactive isotopes in malignant tumors has been achieved by regional and intra-arterial infusion of hydrogen peroxide. [119, 120]

Granulocytes also secrete H_2O_2, which may participate in their cytotoxic effects in a variety of conditions. Preformed or enzymatically generated H_2O_2, with or without a peroxidase, lyses tumor cells, which was shown by Nathan's group and others. [121-127]

Reports have suggested that hydrogen peroxide released by mononuclear phagocytes and neutrophils may extend the antimicrobial, antitumor, and oxidant-injury activities of these cells to adjacent tissues. [128, 129]

Nathan devised a nontoxic way to deliver hydrogen peroxide to sites of malignancy in vivo and to test its antitumor efficacy. Glucose oxidase was chosen for this purpose because its substrates, glucose and oxygen, are abundant in the body fluids and because its sole products are H_2O_2 and gluconic acid. [130] Glucose oxidase was coupled covalently to polystyrene microspheres (GOL) produced H_2O_2. Injection i.p. prolonged the survival of mice by 27% after injection of 106 P388 lymphoma cells in the same site, consistent with destruction of 97.6% of the tumor cells. Placing mice for several hours in 100% O~, the probable rate-limiting substrate for GOL, afforded a 42% prolongation of survival from P388 lymphoma, consistent with destruction of 99.6% of the tumor cells. A single injection of preformed H_2O_2 readily killed P388 cells in the peritoneal cavity, but only at doses nearly lethal to the mice. In contrast, GOL had very little toxicity. Thus, an H_2O_2-generating system confined to the tumor bed exerted clear-cut antitumor effects with little toxicity to the host.

Studies demonstrated that a combination of sub-lytic concentrations of chemically generated NO and H_2O_2 leads to death of murine lymphoma cells, in part, via induction of apoptosis. [131] In vitro studies have suggested that a reaction of nitric oxide (NO) gas and H_2O_2 produces singlet oxygen (which is the primary cytotoxic agent in PDT) or hydroxyl radicals. [132, 133] Nevertheless, this has not yet been demonstrated in cell cultures.

Others Argue That EMODs May Inhibit Apoptosis

In the past, the main focus of the importance of EMODs in oncology was that these agents were capable of inducing DNA damage, which could theoretically lead to cellular proliferation and a predisposition to cancer.

Even though an overwhelming accumulation of intracellular EMODs can create an oxidatively stressed environment leading to necrosis, a slight increase is a stimulus for cellular proliferation. [134, 135] Burdon et al interpreted this to mean that sublethal oxidative stress promotes cell proliferation *in vitro*, with both superoxide and hydrogen peroxide stimulating growth. Proliferation in response to hydrogen peroxide may be due to the activation of mitogen-activated protein kinases (MAPKs). HeLa cells treated with hydrogen peroxide undergo a sustained activation of all three MAPK pathways: extracellular signal related protein kinase; c-Jun amino-terminal kinase/stress-activated protein kinase; and p38.

However, Howes believes that a more logical explanation may be that an EMOD insufficiency "allows" for cell proliferation. [15]

Theoretically, the carcinogenic process in animal models involves initiation and promotion. Allegedly, the production of EMODs and hydrogen peroxide occurs with several known tumor promoters, including 12-*O*-tetradecanoylphorbol-13-acetate (TPA), okadaic acid (OA), thapsigargin, 2,3,7,8-tetrachlorodibenzo-*p*-dioxin (TCDD) and H_2O_2, as well as peroxisome proliferators, steroidal estrogens, phenobarbital, chlordane and aroclor. However, their specific mechanism of action is evasive and speculative. [136]

Severe oxidative stress leads to apoptosis. Conversely, persistent oxidative stress at sublethal levels may cause resistance to apoptosis. The induction of programmed cell death by EMODs is dependent on p53 in both mouse and human cell lines. [137] Current studies indicating a possible mechanism whereby H_2O_2 could promote tumor formation is sparse. [138] Further, many of these studies were carried out using non-physiological levels of H_2O_2, which can have cytotoxic activity.

However, this is in contrast to the work of others, who state that $O_2^{\cdot -}$ and H_2O_2 do not react with DNA bases at all. [139] Yet, the hydroxyl radical ($OH^{\cdot}$) generates a variety of products from all four DNA bases and this pattern is used as a diagnostic "fingerprint" of $OH^{\cdot}$ attack. [140]

Singlet oxygen selectively attacks guanine to produce the 8-hydroxyguanine (8-OHG), which is also used as an index of oxidative damage to DNA and it can be measured as the nucleoside, 8-hydroxydeoxyguanosine (8-OHdG).

Some investigators believe that H_2O_2 may act as a "genotoxicant" or "epigenetic" agent and act as a promoting agent. However, even if hydrogen peroxide could cause DNA damage, peroxide is at best a very weak mutagen in mammalian cells. [136]

Some endogenous DNA damage arises from intermediates of oxygen reduction that either attack the bases or the deoxyribosyl backbone of DNA. Yet, the study of oxidative DNA damage and its role in carcinogenesis is still controversial. [141]

The International Agency for Research on Cancer (IARC) has determined that hydrogen peroxide is not classifiable as to its carcinogenicity to humans. Even though accusations against H_2O_2 have been wide spread, there is no verified data, in man, that H_2O_2 in any way causes or promotes cancer in vivo. The WHO-IARC said, "There is inadequate evidence in humans for the carcinogenicity of hydrogen peroxide."

Hyperoxia

Under conditions of hyperoxia, mitochondrial EMOD generation increases as a linear function of the oxygen tension. [142] Oxygen is critical to aerobic metabolism, but excessive oxygen (hyperoxia) can cause cell injury and death. An oxygen-tolerant strain of HeLa cells, which proliferates even under 80% O_2, termed "HeLa-80," was derived from wild-type HeLa cells ("HeLa-20") by selection for resistance to stepwise increases of oxygen partial pressure. Unpredictably, antioxidant defenses and susceptibility to oxidant-mediated killing do not differ between these two strains of HeLa cells. However, under both 20 and 80% O_2, intracellular reactive oxygen species (EMODs) production is significantly (~2-fold) less in HeLa-80 cells. In both cell lines the source of EMODs is evidently mitochondrial. Although HeLa-80 cells consume oxygen at the same rate as HeLa-20 cells, they consume less glucose and produce less lactic acid. Most importantly, the oxygen-tolerant HeLa-80 cells have significantly higher cytochrome *c* oxidase activity (~2-fold), which may act to deplete upstream electron-rich intermediates responsible for EMOD generation. Indeed, preferential inhibition of cytochrome *c* oxidase by treatment with *n*-methyl protoporphyrin (which selectively diminishes synthesis of heme a in cytochrome *c* oxidase) enhances EMOD production and abrogates the oxygen tolerance of the HeLa-80 cells. Thus, it appears that the remarkable oxygen tolerance of these cells derives from tighter coupling of the electron transport chain and reduced EMOD production. [143]

Vitamin C

The ultimate agent to treat cancer would be cytotoxic only to tumor cells and non-toxic to normal cells. Vitamin C has been theorized to meet these requirements but has been criticized by conventional medicine in favor of more powerful and toxic chemotherapeutic agents. [144] Riordan found that at a dose of 7.04 mg/dl, vitamin C is completely toxic to cancer cells while being completely non-toxic to normal cells. Only at eight times the dose needed to kill cancer cells does vitamin C become toxic to normal cells. This reveals its considerable clinical potential. [145]

Metabolically, vitamin C produces dehydroascorbate (DHA), an oxidant. Normal cells take in DHA, which is then converted to ascorbate and H_2O_2, by an oxidation/reduction (redox) electron transfer. Benade et al at the National Cancer Institute found that, in Ehrlich ascites carcinoma cell cultures, vitamin C selectively destroyed cancer cells by generating excess intracellular H_2O_2. [146]

It has been observed for a long time that ascorbic acid and ascorbic acid salts are preferentially toxic to tumor cells, which were thought to be related to intracellular generation of hydrogen peroxide. [147-149] It is theorized that cancer cells are less able than normal cells to neutralize

H_2O_2 because they are deficient in catalase. Dr.Agus et al reported that cancer cells have extra glucose channels that rapidly bring in glucose and excess DHA. [150]

Cancer cells are defective in that they cannot fully distinguish between glucose and DHA. This may explain why vitamin C is safe in large doses for normal cells but toxic to cancer cells. The good results of Cameron and Hoffer with humans confirm the National Cancer Institute lab tests.

Mark Levine's group published a study on line for PNAS on September 12, 2005, with results showing that, "Pharmacologic ascorbic acid concentrations selectively kill cancer cells: Action as a pro-drug to deliver hydrogen peroxide to tissues." Human lymphoma cells were studied because of their sensitivity to ascorbate (EC50 of 0.5 mM) and suitability for evaluating mechanisms. Extracellular, but not intracellular, ascorbate resulted in cell death, which occurred by apoptosis and pyknosis/necrosis. Cell death was independent of metal chelators and absolutely dependent on H_2O_2 formation. [151]

Investigators stated that it was not known why it killed cancer cells but not normal cells. They felt that it was possible the hydrogen peroxide caused damage that was repaired in normal cells but not in sensitive cancer cells. The main mechanism thought to be responsible for this is the lack or relative deficiency of catalase in tumor cells. [152]

Therefore, it takes a smaller amount of H_2O_2 to reach or "trigger" apoptosis. This is the point of selectivity for toxicity to cancer cells, wherein there is no harm to normal cells. Interestingly, there is a reported 10- to 100-fold greater content of catalase in normal cells than in tumor cells. [146]

Humans lack gulonolactone oxidase, which is necessary to synthesize vitamin C and H_2O_2 is produced as a by-product in the process. It is incredibly ironic, that in the synthesis of one of the most touted of all of the antioxidants, ascorbate, that "dreaded H_2O_2" is generated stochiometrically on a molecule per molecule basis. This illustrates the fact that H_2O_2 is very important in maintaining homeostasis within the cell and as a secondary messenger and that antioxidants and prooxidants may be considered to be flip sides of the same redox coin.

H_2O_2 Induced Apoptosis in Human Gastric Cancer Cells

Investigations were made into the molecular mechanism by which ascorbic acid (AA) induces apoptosis in human gastric cancer cells, AGS cells. High concentration (more than 5mM) of AA increased cellular iron uptake by increasing transferrin receptor (TfR) expression and induced AGS cell apoptosis which was inhibited by catalase. Interestingly, p38 mitogen-activated protein kinase (MAPK) inhibitor inhibited the upregulation of TfR and increased cell survival by AA. TfR-siRNA-transfected cells reduced apoptosis by AA. H_2O_2 increased TfR expression in AGS cells. Taken together, investigators concluded that high concentration of AA, through H_2O_2, induces apoptosis of AGS cells by p38-MAPK-dependent upregulation of TfR.[153]

H_2O_2 Regulation of T Cells

The immune system is vital to protect us against infectious agents (bacteria, viruses, fungi, protozoans and cancer). Patients with T Cell immunodeficiencies are prone to infections and to certain types of cancers, especially leukemias and lymphomas.

There is evidence that T cells themselves produce H_2O_2 upon stimulation of their antigen receptor.[154, 155] A potential source for the unique production of H_2O_2 is the T cell receptor itself. This proposal comes from studies with isolated antibodies, which have the ability to catalyze a light-dependent reaction between molecular oxygen and water that leads to the production of H_2O_2.[156, 157]

These events occur in all antibodies, regardless of source or antigenic specificity. The reaction is initiated by singlet oxygen that reacts with H_2O to ultimately produce H_2O_2 via intermediates such as H_2O_3 and ozone.[158]

H_2O_2 Safety

The Food & Drug Administration (FDA) in Federal Regulation Vol. 46, Number 6, Jan 9, 1981, in effect gave the food industry a green light to use hydrogen peroxide in the "Aseptic" packaging process. The FDA has further ruled that hydrogen peroxide can be used in the processing of cheese and related cheese products (part 133), eggs and egg products (part 160), and as an anti-microbial agent in whey processing. They have also ruled it to be used in cleaning and healing mouth injuries and as a mouthwash (1% to 3% food grade H_2O_2).

As previously stated, "The International Agency for Research on Cancer (IARC) has determined that hydrogen peroxide is not classifiable as to its carcinogencity to humans. Even though accusations against H_2O_2 have been wide spread, there is no verified data, in man, that H_2O_2 in any way causes or promotes cancer in vivo." The WHO-IARC said, "There is inadequate evidence in humans for the carcinogenicity of hydrogen peroxide."

Information from the Hazardous Substances Data Bank (HSDB), a database of the National Library of Medicine's TOXNET system (http://toxnet.nlm.nih.gov) indicates in general, ingestion, ocular or dermal exposure to small amounts of dilute hydrogen peroxide will cause no serious problems.

In 5 persons who accidentally drank 50 mL of a 33% H_2O_2 solution (not the readily available 3%), symptoms included stomach and chest pain, retention of breath, foaming at the mouth and loss of consciousness. Later, motor and sensory disorders, fever, microhemorrhages and moderate leukocytosis were noted. Still, *all recovered completely within 2-3 weeks.* [159] Yet, it may rarely be the cause of accidental death. [160]

A review by Howes found a total of 13 deaths due to the accidental or intentional use of H_2O_2 in the entire history of recorded medical literature available on the internet. [16]

Compare the record of safety with hydrogen peroxide with that of pharmaceutical drugs, which kill 12 per hour, every hour of the day, for 365 days a year (106,000/year). A 2000 report published in the Journal of the American Medical Association by Barbara Starfield, M.D., MPH reported that drugs kill over 106,000 annually, as a conservative estimate. [161]

Pravda has discussed the possible role of hydrogen peroxide in the induction of ulcerative colitis secondary to non-physiological concentrations of peroxide used in peroxide enemas. [162]

Caveat: Some references do not provide access to the original article or to an abstract. Most of the references available to Howes on the internet do not go beyond 1979. Thus, there may be cases of which I am unaware. Many of the articles concerning ingestion or infusion of peroxide are non-conclusive. Clinical histories are incomplete and documentation is scanty. One thing for certain is that many cases of over-zealous or accidental ingestion of concentrated hydrogen peroxide (20-40%) have had a surprisingly uneventful recovery. Actually, the ingestion or infusion of 3% H_2O_2 has resulted in very few patients who developed serious complications or severe outcomes.

A retrospective review of all exposures reported to a regional poison center over a 36 month period and found that of 95,052 exposures reported, 325 (.34%) were due to hydrogen peroxide. The pediatric population (< 18 years) accounted for 71% of hydrogen peroxide exposures and ingestion was the most common route of exposure (83%). Nausea and vomiting were the most common symptoms secondary to ingestion. Ocular and dermal exposures to dilute solutions resulted in transient symptoms without permanent sequelae. While most exposures by all routes resulted in a benign outcome (no effect or minor effect), there was a trend toward more severe outcomes in those who ingested a concentration greater than 10% ($p = 0.011$). [163] (Division of Emergency Medicine, University of Utah School of Medicine, Utah Poison Control Center, Salt Lake City).

Reports have described levels of H_2O_2 over 50 mM as being cytotoxic for a wide range of plants and animal cells in vitro, but is dependent upon many factors such as, pH, media used, cell type used, length of exposure, etc. Paradoxically, acatalasemia in humans appears to produce no significant phenotype, nor does "knockout" of glutathione peroxidase in mice except under conditions of "abnormally high oxidative stress." This is contrary to the teachings of the free radical theory and consistent with Howes' Unified Theory. [164]

Discussion

It is important to reemphasize the fact that antioxidants have repeatedly failed to prevent, control or reverse cancer and a host of so-called oxidative stress diseases. Thus, the free radical theory lacks predictability and consequently, according to the scientific method, it is unfounded. It is inexcusable that researchers continue to incriminate EMODs as only deleterious, noxious or mutagenic agents. In vitro studies may have little resemblance to the events occurring in living/breathing cells, which have considerable EMOD levels omnipresent.

Previously, investigators suggested that anything which served as an antioxidant was good and anything which oxidized something else was bad. That has repeatedly been proven to be untrue. All antioxidants can serve as prooxidants of greater or lesser reactivity. Further, H_2O_2 is now well recognized as an important and widespread second messenger for all aerobic cells. Based on scientific investigations, implying or giving the false impression that the presence of H_2O_2 is categorically bad is another example of unfounded and erroneous reporting.

Rethinking the Free Radical Theory

Any critical evaluation of EMODs must address the misconceptions propagated by the free radical theory of oxidative stress and aging. Hard data has yielded the following: [15]

- high levels of the antioxidant bilirubin cause kernicterus and permanent brain damage

- the antioxidant β-carotene increases the rate of lung cancer development in smokers

- the antioxidant CoQ, ubiquinone, when deleted from the diet of C. elegans, increases its lifespan

- SOD/catalase mimetics decrease the lifespan of house flies

- the antioxidant α-tocopherol, vitamin E, increases the rate and number of heart attacks and strokes

- high levels of the antioxidant, uric acid, cause gout and cardiovascular disease

- acatalasemic patients live basically normal lives

Many molecules are designed to accept and receive electrons as a natural part of their reactivity, especially the transitlons metals and the heme proteins. Oxygen's varlous modified derivatives, electronic configuratlons and states, are the primary agents that protect us from infections and neoplastic growths throughout our lives, from conception to death. Report after report shows that mitochondria play a crucial role in apoptosis. [165]

A growing body of evidence favors the involvement of intracellular reactive oxygen species (EMODs) at some point during apoptotic execution. [166-170] Apoptosis is carried out by a multistage chain of reactions in which EMODs act as triggers and essential mediators. [171, 172] The level of lipid peroxidation in patients with cancer was significantly reduced compare with that in healthy control subjects. [173] The lower level of lipid peroxidation in the cancer patients may be indicative of low EMOD levels, which would allow for the development of cancer.

Even death signaling by anticancer drugs generally relies on positive input from the mitochondria, as is evidenced by the resistance of tumor cells over-expressing the death-inhibitory protein Bcl-2 that is localized to the membranes of mitochondria, endoplasmic reticulum, and nucleus. [174-176] Repeatedly, the critical role of cellular redox status in the regulation of death signaling has been demonstrated. [177-180]

These findings become more important considering the critical role of the mitochondria during apoptosis and the fact that mitochondria have been implicated directly as a prime source of EMODs during drug-induced apoptosis. [181-183] As the mitochondria are a major source of intracellular EMODs, it is tempting to speculate that EMODs, such as

H_2O_2, may function both upstream and downstream of the mitochondria. Tumor cells lacking Bax (Bax–/–) are resistant to the effect of some anti-cancer drugs. [184]

Analysis of subcellular distribution of Bax (in HCT116, HL60, and CEM cells) revealed that Bax redistributed to the mitochondrial fraction from the cytosol on exposure to H_2O_2, which could be significantly blocked by the H_2O_2 scavenger, catalase.

Recruitment of Bax to the mitochondria during apoptotic signaling has been linked to the activation of upstream caspase 8 and caspase 8-mediated cleavage of the proapoptotic protein Bid. This is particularly true on ligation of death receptors, such as CD95 (Apo1/Fas). Additionally, H_2O_2 and anticancer drugs have been shown to up-regulate the expression of the CD95 receptor or its ligand (CD95L) in some systems. [185, 186]

Investigators utilized the ability of certain anticancer drugs to increase intracellular production of EMODs, specifically H_2O_2. [187] Indeed, exposure of HCT116 Bax+/– or HL60 cells to a novel anticancer compound C1 resulted in an increase in intracellular H_2O_2 and translocation of Bax to the mitochondria. This translocation of Bax was inhibited by catalase, thus establishing the critical role of intracellular H_2O_2 in mitochondrial recruitment during drug-induced apoptosis of tumor cells. These data indicate that Bax translocation triggered in tumor cells during drug (C1)-induced apoptosis was a direct result of intracellular H_2O_2 production, independent of the upstream caspase 8 or ceramide pathways. [187]

Cytosolic Acidification

Cytosolic acidification is an early event in apoptosis and provides an intracellular milieu permissive for efficient death execution. In this regard, exposure of cells to H_2O_2 or drugs that trigger intracellular increase in H_2O_2 results in a significant drop in cytosolic pH. [187]

Accordingly, signals that inhibit apoptotic acidification impede death signaling as demonstrated in a recent study. [188] Investigators results provided strong evidence that the link between H_2O_2 and Bax translocation could be the drop in cytosolic pH brought about by exposure of cells to exogenous H_2O_2 or endogenous production of H_2O_2 on drug exposure. It is possible that this indicates the pivotal role of H_2O_2 in cancer cell killing or apoptotic execution.

This shows that apoptosis is likely initiated with EMOD production, especially H_2O_2. H_2O_2 is, for the most part, essential for cancer killing and a shift to an acidic intracellular environment may also aid in its tumoricidal activity and the production of other agents within the EMOD family. Studies demonstrated the ability of commonly used chemotherapeutic drugs vincristine and daunorubicin to trigger an early increase in intracellular H_2O_2.[188]

Pro-oxidant intracellular milieu is a hallmark of many tumor cells and is believed to endow tumor cells with a survival advantage over their normal counterparts.[189, 190] It has been shown previously that maintaining a slightly elevated intracellular O_2^- promotes cellular proliferation [135] and inhibits apoptotic signaling.[191] Fortunately, this is one specific feature which provides us with an opportunity to selectively kill cancer cells by increasing EMOD levels even further.

Many investigators have demonstrated the critical role of intracellular H_2O_2 in rendering the cytosolic milieu permissive for efficient apoptotic execution.[169, 170, 192] Further, these data strongly support and underscore the critical role of H_2O_2 in creating a permissive intracellular milieu for efficient drug-induced execution of tumor cells.[193]

Dicumarol Increased EMODs Killing Human Pancreatic Cancer Cells

Dicumarol is a naturally occurring anticoagulant derived from coumarin that induces cytotoxicity and oxidative stress in human pancreatic cancer cells. Dicumarol increased intracellular levels of superoxide ($O_2^{\cdot -}$), as measured by hydroethidine staining, and inhibited cell growth.[194] Mitochondrial production of EMODs mediates the increased susceptibility of cancer cells to dicumarol-induced cytotoxicity.[195]

MnSOD Overexpression and Inhibition of H_2O_2 Removal Increases Cancer Cell Cytotoxicity

Overexpression of manganese superoxide dismutase (MnSOD) and inhibition of H_2O_2 removal, increases cancer cell cytotoxicity. Investigators hypothesized that increasing endogenous $O_2^{\cdot -}$ production in cells that were pretreated with adenoviral MnSOD (AdMnSOD) plus 1,3-bis(2-chloroethyl)-1-nitrosourea (BCNU) would lead to an increased level of intracellular H_2O_2 accumulation and increased cell killing. The cytotoxic effects of Adriamycin or radiation, agents known to produce $O_2^{\cdot -}$, were determined in MDA-MB-231 breast cancer cells pretreated with AdMnSOD plus BCNU both in vitro and in vivo. In vitro, AdMnSOD plus BCNU sensitized cells to the cytotoxicity of Adriamycin or radiation. In vivo, AdMnSOD, BCNU, and Adriamycin or ionizing radiation inhibited tumor growth and prolonged survival. Thus, agents that produce $O_2^{\cdot-}$ in combination with AdMnSOD plus BCNU may represent a powerful new antitumor regimen against breast cancer.[196]

Myeloperoxidase Involvement in H_2O_2-induced Apoptosis of HL-60 Human Leukemia Cells

Investigators examined the mechanism of H_2O_2-induced cytotoxicity and its relationship to oxidation in human leukemia cells. The HL-60 promyelocytic leukemia cell line was sensitive to H_2O_2, and at concentrations up to about 20-25 uM, the killing was mediated by apoptosis. When HL-60 cells were incubated with methimazole or 4-aminobenzoic acid hydrazide, which are inhibitors of myeloperoxidase, they no longer underwent H_2O_2-induced apoptosis.[197] This strongly supports the primary role of EMOD induced apoptosis in cancer cell cytotoxicity.

Antitumor Therapy via Enzymatic Generation of Hydrogen Peroxide

Investigators studied the antitumor activity of an H_2O_2-generating enzyme, D-amino acid oxidase (DAO), and its conjugate with polyethylene glycol (PEG; PEG-DAO). To generate cytotoxic H_2O_2 at the tumor site, PEG-DAO was first administrated i.v. to tumor-bearing mice. After an adequate lag time, the substrate of DAO, D-proline, was injected i.p. This treatment resulted in significant suppression of tumor growth.

PEG-DAO thus delivered together with D-proline produces remarkable antitumor activity via extensive generation of H_2O_2.[198]

SOD Over Expression Increases Peroxide Levels and Suppresses Human Prostate Cancer Cells

Investigators studied the role of the antioxidant enzyme manganese superoxide dismutase (MnSOD) in androgen-independent human prostate cancer (PC-3) cells' growth rate in vitro and in vivo. Production of extracellular H_2O_2 was increased in the MnSOD-overexpressing clones. Results are consistent with MnSOD being a tumor suppressor gene in human prostate cancer.[199]

This supports the assertion that prooxidant EMODs, such as H_2O_2, contribute to a continually functional oxidative protective system to curtail cancer growth. The increased SOD resulted in increased peroxide levels, which in turn suppressed tumor growth, via EMOD induced apoptosis.

Increased EMODs Increases Cancer Cell Cytotoxicity

Relative to normal cells, neoplastic cells demonstrate increased sensitivity to glucose-deprivation-induced cytotoxicity. To determine whether oxidative stress mediated by $O_2^{\cdot-}$ and hydroperoxides contributed to the differential susceptibility of human epithelial cancer cells to glucose deprivation, the oxidation of DHE (dihydroethidine; for $O_2^{\cdot-}$) and CDCFH(2) [5- (and 6-)carboxy-2',7'-dichlorodihydrofluorescein diacetate; for hydroperoxides] was measured in human colon and breast cancer cells (HT29, HCT116, SW480 and MB231) and compared with that in normal human cells [FHC cells, 33Co cells and HMECs (human mammary epithelial cells)]. HCT116 and MB231 cells were more susceptible to glucose-deprivation-induced cytotoxicity and oxidative stress, relative to 33Co cells and HMECs. HT29 cells were also more susceptible to 2DG (2-deoxyglucose)-induced cytotoxicity, relative to FHC cells. Overexpression of manganese SOD (superoxide dismutase) and mitochondrially targeted catalase significantly protected HCT116 and MB231 cells from glucose-deprivation-induced cytotoxicity and oxidative stress and also protected HT29 cells from 2DG-induced cytotoxicity. These results show that cancer cells (relative to normal cells) demonstrate increased steady-state levels of EMODs (reactive oxygen species; i.e. $O_2^{\cdot-}$ and H_2O_2) that contribute to differential susceptibility to glucose-deprivation-induced cytotoxicity and oxidative stress. These studies support the hypotheses that cancer cells increase glucose metabolism to compensate for excess metabolic production of EMODs and that inhibition of glucose and hydroperoxide metabolism may provide a biochemical target for selectively enhancing cytotoxicity and oxidative stress in human cancer cells. [200]

EMODs are Positive Signals in the Fruit Fly Immune System

The September 24, 2009 issue of the journal Nature, carried an article by Dr. Utpal Banerjee et al, UCLA's Jonsson Comprehensive Cancer Center researchers found much to their surprise, that in Drosophila, the common fruit fly, moderately elevated levels of EMODs are a good thing. Banerjee said, "These small molecules act as an internal communicator, signaling certain blood precursor cells, or blood stem cells, to differentiate into immune-bolstering cells in reaction to a threat. After the progenitor cells differentiate, the EMOD levels return to normal, ensuring the safety and survival of the mature blood cells."

Thus, he asks, "could excessive use of antioxidants deplete our immune systems?" Alleged;y, reducing levels of reactive oxygen is usually the goal, and what Banerjee found was surprising, in that when EMODs were taken away from the blood stem cells, they failed to differentiate into the immune-bolstering cells, called macrophages. On the other hand, when levels of EMODs were further increased by genetic means, the blood stem cells "differentiated like gang busters," Banerjee said, making a large number of macrophages.

The EMODs, Banerjee said, acted as a signaling mechanism that kept the blood stem cells in a certain state - when levels rose, it was a message to the cell to differentiate. Keeping their EMOD levels slightly elevated puts the cells on alert, sensitized and ready to respond to any threat quickly.

That work prompted the obvious question: If fruit fly blood stem cells and mammalian blood stem cells operate in the same way, is it a good thing for people to be taking antioxidants? Are antioxidants dulling the immune system and its ability to react to threats? It is interesting, however, that these types of blood progenitors in mammals also give rise to macrophages, Banerjee said.

Banerjee said, "If we find that those blood stem cells aren't primed to respond because the ROS levels are reduced, that would not be a good thing. Our findings raise the possibility that wanton overdose of antioxidant products may in fact inhibit formation of cells participating in innate immune response." Once again, this data emphasizes the crucial role of EMODs in aerobic cells. http://www.medicalnewstoday.com/articles/165268.php Accessed 9-25-09.

Just to Add Further Complications

Pro-senescent Effect of Hydrogen Peroxide on Cancer Cells and Tumor Suppression

Mild oxidative stress is known to induce premature senescence, termed stress-induced premature senescence (SIPS), in normal human diploid cells. Investigators determined whether mild oxidative stress would trigger SIPS in a human tumor cell line, human lung adenocarcinoma A549. The results showed that sublethal concentrations of H_2O_2 induced SIPS in A549 cells and consequently attenuated, but did not completely eliminate, the tumorigenicity of these cells. They next investigated the reasons for this incomplete impairment of tumorigenicity in A549 cells in SIPS. The results suggested that H_2O_2 treated A549 cells are composed of a heterogeneous cell population: one is sensitive to H_2O_2 and the other is resistant or undergoes reversal; the latter reverted to their original tumorigenic form. The molecular mechanisms determining the cellular fate of tumor cells in SIPS should be identified in order to make use of SIPS and oncogene-induced senescence in tumor cells as methods of tumor suppression. [201]

Indirect Evidence for EMOD Induced Apoptosis Via Antioxidant Studies

The US is experiencing epidemics of cancer, diabetes, obesity and fatigue, which may be related to increased ingestion of antioxidant vitamins and dietary supplements, which are now commonly found as supplements or fortifiers of many foods and are aggressively marketed to an ever-growing segment of the population. These agents could be interfering with or modifying our continually operational prooxidant protective system.

Despite two decades of controversy regarding the use of dietary antioxidant supplementation during conventional chemotherapy and radiation therapy, questions remain about their efficacy and safety. However, on the basis of published randomized clinical trials, the use of supplemental antioxidants during chemotherapy and radiation therapy should be discouraged because of the possibility of tumor protection and reduced patient survival. [202]

Several new reports are raising concerns about the safety and efficacy of vitamin and mineral supplements in healthy individuals and cancer patients and survivors. Some experts see a need for further studies; whereas, others say that there are sufficient negative data to stop vitamin trials altogether. [203]

Significant in vitro data exists showing that antioxidants can block EMOD-induced apoptosis for a wide variety of cancerous cell types, such as leukemia, lymphoma, retinoblastoma, myeloma, pheochromocytoma and human cancers of the breast, lung, pancreas, liver, colon, rectum and endometrium. [204] This data can not be ignored.

However, it has recently been shown that EMODs may have an alternative activity, by modulating tumor cell signaling and that tumor cell signaling mediated by EMODs are readily reversible upon treatment with antioxidants. This emerging evidence may serve as bona fide signal transduction modifiers for cancer. A re-examination is warranted. [205]

However, in the words of one investigator, "If you suppress free radicals, you suppress programmed cell death." [206]

One Final Note

Philipp Niethammer, Harvard Medical School postdoctoral researcher and biologist, accidentally discovered while analyzing the severed tail of zebrafish that the hydrogen peroxide in their wounds appeared in bursts at the wound about 17 minutes before the leukocytes that were supposed to be producing them appeared too. On 6-4-09, ScienceNow reported that hydrogen peroxide summons reinforcements from the immune system, and more specifically white blood cells, which in turn aid with the healing process. Please view the video of peroxide migration in the wound of a zebrafish http://www.youtube.com/watch?v=a7PJ8yXyPVU. "Hydrogen peroxide marshals immune system." Accessed 10-9-09. This interesting video illustrates the rapid wound response and permeability of H_2O_2.

However, due to the complex nature of the interactions of EMODs and antioxidants within the body, it is difficult to clearly and definitively interpret the results of many experiments and observations.

Conclusion

Unarguably, EMODs are intricately, inextricably and crucially involved in cancer cell killing via their prominent role in apoptosis. Statements of the ineffectiveness in the killing of cancerous cells via hydrogen peroxide or other EMOD types are baseless, inaccurate and irresponsible. The lingering inaccuracies of the free radical theory must be countered by the obvious omnipresent and ubiquitous known salutary effects of the prooxidant EMODs. Their presence in steady state quantities testifies to their essential nature in healthy homeostasis and their low toxicity. EMODs, and especially hydrogen peroxide, are produced throughout the body in steady state levels on an as needed and when needed basis and serve to support the interrelated highly complex redox systems of the body. It is inconceivable that they only exist for pernicious purposes. Because of their relatively short half lives, their localized instantaneous concentrations can remain at low levels. Yet, their synthesis and availability can be called upon at any given moment to combat impending pathogens or neoplasia.

EMODs have bactericidal, fungicidal, virucidal and anti-protozoan and anti-neoplastic roles but also have far reaching cellular signaling control functions. The peroxide spike during the respiratory burst classically serves as a protective role against infectious pathogens, as does EMOD induced apoptosis to combat neoplasia. Hydrogen peroxide is likely the most ubiquitous member of the family of EMOD agents. Its important and prominent biochemical role is ever expanding.

REFERENCES

1. Miller ER III, Pastor-Barriuso R, Dalal D, Riemersma RA, Appel LJ, Guallar E. Meta-analysis: high-dosage vitamin E supplementation may increase all-cause mortality. *Ann Intern Med.* 2005;142:37-46.

2. Howes M.D., PhD., R. (2007). Antioxidant Vitamins A, C & E; Death in Small Doses and Legal Liability? *PHILICA.COM Article number 89*. Published April 5, 2007.

3. Harman D. Aging: a theory based on free radical and radiation chemistry. J Gerontol 11: 298–300, 1956.

4. Harman, D., 1981. The aging process. Proc. Natl Acad. Sci. USA 78, 7124–7128.

5. Beckman, K.B., Ames, B.N., 1998. The free radical theory of aging matures. Physiol. Rev. 78, 547–581.

6. Finkel, T., Holbrook, N.J., 2000. Oxidants, oxidative stress and the biology of ageing. Nature 408, 239–247.

7. Balaban, R.S., Nemoto, S., Finkel, T., 2005. Mitochondria, oxidants, and aging. Cell 120, 483–495.

8. Marnett LJ, Riggins JN, West JD. Endogenous generation of reactive oxidants and electrophiles and their reactions with DNA and protein. J Clin Invest. 2003; 111: 583–593.

9. Darley-Usmar, V., Starke-Reed, P.E., 2000. Antioxidants: strategies for interventions in aging and age-related diseases, a workshop sponsored by the National Institute on aging and by the office of dietary supplements. Antioxid. Redox. Signal. 2, 375–377.

10. Howes R.M. The Free Radical Fantasy: A Panoply of Paradoxes. Ann. N.Y. Acad. Sci. 2006;1067:22-26.

11. Chance B, Sies, H, Boveris A. Hydroperoxide metabolism in mammalian organs. Physiol Rev 1979; 59: 527-605.

12. Hydrogen Peroxide: A Signaling Messenger. James R. Stone, Suping Yang. Antioxidants & Redox Signaling. March/April 2006, 8(3-4): 243-270.

13. Howes, R. M. *U.T.O.P.I.A. - Unified Theory of Oxygen Participation in Aerobiosis.* © 2004. Free Radical Publishing Co. Kentwood, LA, available at www.iwillfindthecure.org.

14. Halliwell B. Oxidants and human disease: some concepts. FASEB J. 1987;1:358–364.

15. Howes, R.M. © 2005. The Medical and Scientific Significance of Oxygen Free Radical Metabolism. Free Radical Publishing Co. Kentwood, LA. available at www.iwillfindthecure.org.

16. Howes, R.M. Hydrogen Peroxide Monograph 1: Scientific, Medical and Biochemical Overview & Monograph 2: Antioxidant Vitamins A, C, & E: Equivocal Scientific Studies, © 2006. Free Radical Publishing Co. Kentwood, LA. available at www.iwillfindthecure.org.

17. Marie Csete. Oxygen in the Cultivation of Stem Cells. Ann. N.Y. Acad. Sci. 1049: 1–8 (2005.

18. Go YM, Gipp JJ, Mulcahy RT, and Jones DP. H_2O_2-dependent activation of GCLC-ARE4 reporter occurs by mitogen-activated protein kinase pathways without oxidation of cellular glutathione or thioredoxin-1. J Biol Chem 279: 5837–5845, 2004.

19. Aitken J, Fisher H. Reactive oxygen species generation and human spermatozoa: the balance of benefit and risk. Bioessays. 1994 Apr;16(4):259-67.

20. Acker H, Bolling B, Delpiano MA, Dufau E, Gorlach A & Holtermann G (1992). The meaning of H_2O_2 generation in carotid body cells for pO_2 chemoreception. Journal of the Autonomic Nervous System, 41: 41-51.

21. Lisa Melton. The antioxidant myth: a medical fairy tale – from New Scientist. http://www.newscientist.com/article/mg19125631.500.html (5 August 2006) New Scientist. Pg. 40-43. volume 191; issue 2563.

22. B.M. Barbior. Superoxide: a two-edged sword. Braz J Med Biol Res, February 1997, Volume 30(2) 141-155.

23. Thannical VJ, Fanburg BL. Reactive oxygen species in cell signaling. Am J Physiol Lung Cell Mol Physiol 2000; 279: L1005-L1028.

24. Eaton JW, Qian M. Molecular basis of cellular iron toxicity. Free Radic Biol Med 2002; 32: 833-840.

25. Harman, D. 1957. Prolongation of the normal life span by radiation protection chemicals. J. Gerontol. 12: 257-263.

26. Boveris A, Cadenas E. Mitochondrial production of hydrogen peroxide regulation by nitric oxide and the role of ubisemiquinone. IUBMB Life 2000; 50: 245-250.

27. Eberhardt MK. Reactive Oxygen Metabolites: Chemistry and Medical Consequences. CRC Press 2001.

28. Chen S, Schopfer P. Hydroxyl radical production in physiological reactions. Eur J Biochem 1999; 260: 726-735.

29. Fridovich I. Oxygen toxicity: A radical explanation. J Exp Biol 1998; 20: 1203-1209.

30. Cadenas E, Davies KJ. Mitochondrial free radical generation, oxidative stress, and aging. Free Radic Biol Med 2000; 29:222-230.

31. Lemasters J, Nieminen A. Mitochondria in Pathogenesis. Kluwer Academic/Plenum Publishers 2001: 281-286) 90.

32. St-Pierre, J., Buckingham, J.A., Roebuck, S.J. and Brand, M.D. Topology of superoxide production from different sites in the mitochondrial electron transport chain. J Biol Chem 2002; 277:44784-44790.

33. Rhee SG, Bae YS, Lee SR, Kwon J: Hydrogen peroxide:A key messenger that modulates protein phosphorylation through cysteine oxidation. Science's stke. Available at: www.stke.sciencemag.org/cgi/content/full/OC_sigtrans; 2000/53/pe1.

34. Rhee SG: Redox signaling: Hydrogen peroxide as intracellular messenger. Exp Mol Med 31: 53–59, 1999.

35. Finkel T: Oxygen radicals and signaling. Curr Opin Cell Biol 10: 248–253, 1998.

36. Suzuki YJ, Ford GD: Redox regulation of signal transduction in cardiac and smooth muscle. J Mol Cell Cardiol 31: 345–353, 1999.

37. Radia Forteza et al. Regulated Hydrogen Peroxide Production by Duox in Human Airway Epithelial Cells. American Journal of Respiratory Cell and Molecular Biology. Vol. 32, pp. 462-469, 2005.

38. Ramachandran S, Morris SM, Devamanoharan P, Henein M, Varma SD. Radio-isotopic determination of hydrogen peroxide in aqueous humor and urine. Exp Eye Res. 1991 Oct;53(4):503-6.

39. García-Castiñeiras S. Hydrogen peroxide in the aqueous humor: 1992-1997. P R Health Sci J. 1998 Dec;17(4):335-43.

40. Niki L. Reynaert et al. Catalase Overexpression Fails to Attenuate Allergic Airways Disease in the Mouse. The Journal of Immunology, 2007, 178: 3814-3821.

41. Li JM and Shah AM. (2002) Intracellular localization and preassembly of the NADPH oxidase complex in cultured endothelial cells. J Biol Chem 277:19952–19960.

42. Grandvaux N, Grizot S, Vignais PV, Dagher MC. (1999) The Ku70 autoantigen interacts with p40phox in B lymphocytes. J Cell Sci 112:Pt 4503–513.

43. IARC, 1985). (IARC. 1985. International Agency for Research on Cancer. Hydrogen Peroxide. In: IARC Monographs on the Evaluation of Carcinogenic Risk if Chemicals to Humans: Allyl compounds, Aldehydes, Epoxides and Peroxides, Vol. 36. IARC, Lyon, pp. 285-314.

44. Krippeit-Drews, P., Lang, F., Haussinger, D. and Drews, G. Pflugers. H_2O_2 induced hyperpolarization of pancreatic β-cells. Pflügers Arch. 426: 552-554, 1994.

45. Krippeit-Drews, P., Kramer, C., Welker, S., Lang, F., Ammon, H.P. and Drews, G. Interference of H_2O_2 with stimulus-secretion coupling in mouse pancreatic □-cells. J Physiol (Lond) 1999; 514(Pt 2): 471-481.

46. Livingston J, Gurny P, Lockwood D: Insulin-like effects of polyamines in fat cells. Mediation by H_2O_2 formation. J Biol Chem 1977, 252:560-562.

47. Lenzen S, Drinkgern J, Tiedge M. Low antioxidant enzyme gene expression in pancreatic islets compared with various other mouse tissues. Free Radical Biology & Medicine. 1996;20:463–466.

48. Anna Yu Bogdanova and Mikko Nikinmaa. Reactive Oxygen Species Regulate Oxygen-sensitive Potassium Flux in Rainbow Trout Erythrocytes. The Journal of General Physiology, Volume 117, Number 2, February 1, 2001 181-190.

49. Halliwell B. Reactive oxygen species and the nervous system. 1992. J. Neurochemistry 59, 1609-1623.

50. C Giulivi, P Hochstein, KJ Davies. Hydrogen peroxide production by red blood cells. Free Radic Biol Med (1994) 16: 123-9.

51. Valko M, Leibfritz D, Moncol J, Cronin MT, Mazur M, Telser J. Free radicals and antioxidants in normal physiological functions and human disease. Int J Biochem Cell Biol. 2007;39(1):44-84.

52. Akos Koller and Zsolt Bagi. Nitric oxide and H_2O_2 contribute to reactive dilation of isolated coronary arterioles. Am J Physiol Heart Circ Physiol 287: H2461-H2467, 2004.

53. Balachandran P and Govindarajan R. Cancer—an ayurvedic perspective Pharmacol Res 2005; 51: 19–30.

54. Papa S and Shulachev VP. Reactive oxygen species, mitochondria, apoptosis and aging. Mol Cell Biochem 1997; 174: 305–19.

55. Matsuzawa A, Ichijo H. Stress-responsive protein kinases in redox-regulated apoptosis signaling. Antioxid Redox Signal. 2005;7:472–481.

56. Han H, Wang H, Long H, Nattel S, Wang Z. Oxidative preconditioning and apoptosis in L-cells. Roles of protein kinase B and mitogen-activated protein kinases. J Biol Chem. 2001;276:26357–26364.

57. Reinehr R, Becker S, Eberle A, Grether-Beck S, Haussinger D. Involvement of NADPH oxidase isoforms and Src family kinases in CD95-dependent hepatocyte apoptosis. J Biol Chem. 2005; 280(29):27179-27194.

58. Senturker, S., Tschirret-Guth, R., Morrow, J., Levine, R. and Shacter, E. Induction of apoptosis by chemotherapeutic drugs

without generation of reactive oxygen species. Arch of Biochem and Biophy 2002; 397(2): 262-272.

59. J H. Doroshow. Role of Hydrogen Peroxide and Hydroxyl Radical Formation in the Killing of Ehrlich Tumor Cells by Anticancer Quinones. PNAS June 15, 1986, vol. 83, no. 12, 4514-4518.

60. Dougherty TJ, Gomer CJ, Henderson BW, Jori G, Kessel D, Korbelik M, Moan J, Peng Q (1998) Photodynamic therapy. J Natl Cancer Inst 90: 889–905.

61. Ochsner M (1997) Photophysical and photobiological processes in the photodynamic therapy of tumours. J Photochem Photobiol *B* 39: 1–18.

62. Fisher A. M. R., Murphree A. L., Gomer C. J. Clinical, and preclinical photodynamic therapy. Lasers Surg. Med., *17:* 2-31, 1995.

63. Henderson B.W., Dougherty T. J. How does photodynamic therapy work? Photochem. Photobiol., *55:* 145-157, 1992.

64. Oleinick N. L., Evans H. E. The photobiology of photodynamic therapy: cellular targets and mechanisms. Radiat. Res., *150:* S146-S156, 1998.

65. Luna M. C., Wong S., Gomer C. J. Photodynamic therapy mediated induction of early response genes. Cancer Res., 53: 1374-1380, 1994.

66. Gollnick S. O., Liu X., Owczarczak B., Musser D., Henderson B. W. Altered expression of interleukin 6 and interleukin 10 as a result of photodynamic therapy *in vivo*. Cancer Res., *57:* 3904-3909, 1997.

67. Tao J-S., Sanghera J. S., Pelech S. L., Wong G., Levy J. G. Stimulation of stress-activated protein kinase and p38 HOG1 kinase in murine keratinocytes following photodynamic therapy with benzoporphyrin derivative. J. Biol. Chem., *271:* 27107-27115, 1996.

68. Gomer C. J., Luna M., Ferrario A., Rucker N. Increased transcription and translation of heme oxygenase in Chinese hamster fibroblasts following photodynamic stress or Photofrin II incubation. Photochem. Photobiol., *53:* 275-279, 1991.

69. Gomer C. J., Ferrario A., Rucker N., Wong S., Lee A. Glucose regulated protein induction and cellular resistance to oxidative stress mediated by porphyrin photosensitization. Cancer Res., *51:* 6574-6579, 1991.

70. Gomer C., Ryter S., Ferrario A., Rucker N., Wong S., Fisher A. Photodynamic therapy mediated oxidative stress can induce heat shock proteins. Cancer Res., *56:* 2355-2360, 1996.

71. Curry P. M., Levy J. Stress protein expression in murine tumor cells following photodynamic therapy with benzoporphyrin derivative. Photochem. Photobiol., *58:* 374-379, 1993.

72. Price M, Terlecky SR, Kessel D. A Role for Hydrogen Peroxide in the Pro-apoptotic Effects of Photodynamic Therapy. Photochem Photobiol. 2009 Jul 21.

73. Chekulayeva LV, Shevchuk IN, Chekulayev VA, Ilmarinen K. Hydrogen peroxide, superoxide, and hydroxyl radicals are involved in the phototoxic action of hematoporphyrin derivative against tumor cells. J Environ Pathol Toxicol Oncol. 2006;25(1-2):51-77.

74. Redmond RW, Gamlin JN. A compilation of singlet oxygen yields from biologically relevant molecules. Photochem. Photobiol. 1999;70:391–475.

75. Dysart JS, Patterson MS. Characterization of Photofrin photobleaching for singlet oxygen dose estimation during photodynamic therapy of MLL cells in vitro. *Phys. Med. Biol.* 2005;50:2597–2616.

76. Buettner GR, Need MJ. Hydrogen peroxide and hydroxyl free radical production by hematoporphyrin derivative, ascorbate and light. Cancer Lett. 1985;25:297–304.

77. Galina G. Kramarenko, Stephen G. Hummel, Sean M. Martin, and Garry R. Buettner. Ascorbate Reacts with Singlet Oxygen to Produce Hydrogen Peroxide. Photochem Photobiol. 2006; 82(6): 1634–1637.

78. Henry Jay Forman. Hydrogen Peroxide: The Good, The Bad, and The Ugly. Contained in: . Springer Netherlands. ISBN 978-1-4020-8398-3. 2008.

79. James R. Stone, Suping Yang. Hydrogen Peroxide: A Signaling Messenger. Antioxidants & Redox Signaling. March/April 2006, 8(3-4): 243-270.

80. Babior, B.M. NADPH oxidase: An update. Blood 1999; 93: 1464-1476.

81. Bayraktutan, U., Blayney, L. and Shah, A.M. Molecular characterization and localization of the NADPH oxidase components gp91-phox and p22-phox in endothelia cells. Arterioscler Thromb Vasc Biol 2000; 20: 1903-1911.

82. Goossens, V., Grooten, J., DeVos, K. and Fiers. W. Direct evidence for tumor necrosis factor-induced mitochondrial reactive oxygen intermediates and their involvement in cytotoxicity. Proc Natl Acad Sci USA 1995; 92: 8115-8119.

83. Finkel, T. Redox-dependent signal transduction. FEBS Lett 2000; 476: 52-54.

84. Trembovler, V., Abu-Raya, S. and Shohami, E. Synergism between tumor necrosis factor-alpha and H_2O_2 enhances cell damage in rat PC12 cells. Neurosci Lett. 2003 Dec 19; 353(2):115-118.

85. Hohler, B.; Holzapfel, B., and Kummer W. NADPH oxidase submits and superoxide production in porcine pulmonary artery endothelial cells. Histochem Cell Biol 2000; 114: 29-37.

86. Rueckschloss, U. Galle, J., Zerkowski H. R. and Morawietz, H. Induction of NAD(P)H oxidase by oxidized low-density lipoprotein in human endothelial cells: antioxidative potential of hydroxymethylglutaryl coenzyme A reductase inhibitor therapy. Circulation 2001; 104: 1767-1772.

87. Signal Transduction by reactive Oxygen and Nitrogen Species: Pathways and Chemical Principles. Edited by H.J. Forman, J. Fukuto and M. Torres, Kluwer Academic Publishers, 2003.

88. Schafer, F. Q. and Buettner, G. R. Redox environment of the cell as viewed through the redox state of the glutathione disulfide/glutathione couple. Free Radic Biol Med 2001; 30: 1191-1212.

89. Hoidal, J.R. Reactive oxygen species and cell signaling. Am J Respir Cell Mol Biol 2001; 25: 661-663.

90. Schreck, R., Rieber, P. and Baeuerle, P.A. Reactive oxygen intermediates as apparently widely needed messengers in the activation of the NK-k B transcription factor and HIV-1. Embo J 1991; 10: 2247-2258.

91. Sen, C.K. and Packer, L. Antioxidant and redox regulation of gene transcription. Faseb J 1996; 10: 709-720.

92. Allen, R.G. and Tresini, M. Oxidative stress and gene regulation. Free Rad Biol Med 2000; 28: 463-499.

93. Los, M., W. Droege, K. Stricker, P.A. Baeuerle, K. Schulze-Osthoff. 1995. Hydrogen peroxide as a potent activator of T lymphocyte functions. Eur. J. Immunol. 25:159.

94. Harlan, J. M., K. S. Callahan. 1984. Role of hydrogen peroxide in the neutrophil-mediated release of prostacyclin from cultured endothelial cells. J. Clin. Invest. 74:442.

95. Lewis, M. S., R. E. Whatley, P. Cain, T. M. McIntyre, S. M. Prescott, G.A. Zimmerman. 1988. Hydrogen peroxide stimulates the synthesis of platelet-activating factor by endothelium and induces endothelial cell-dependent neutrophil adhesion. J. Clin. Invest. 82:2045.

96. Sundaresan, M., Z-X. Yu, V. J. Ferrans, K. Irony, T. Finkel. 1995. Requirement for generation of H_2O_2 for platelet-derived growth factor signal transduction. Science 270:296.

97. Rao, G. N., B. C. Berk. 1992. Active oxygen species stimulate vascular smooth muscle cell growth and proto-oncogene expression. Circ. Res. 70:593.

98. Griendling, K.K. and Ushio-Fukai, M. Reactive oxygen species as mediators of angiotensin II signaling. Regul Pept 2000; 91: 21-27.

99. Patel, R.P., Moellering, D., Murphy-Uhrich, J., Jo., H., Beckman, S. and Darley-Usmar, V.M. Cell signaling by reactive nitrogen and oxygen species in atherosclerosis. Free Radic Biol Med 2000; 28: 1780-1794.

100. Forman, H.J. and Torres, M. Signaling by the respiratory burst in macrophages. IUBMB Life 2001; 51: 365-371.

101. Warburg, O. On the origin of cancer cells. Science 1956; 123: 309-314.

102. Einar K. Rofstad, Heidi Rasmussen, Kanthi Galappathi, Berit Mathiesen, Kristin Nilsen and Bjørn A. Graff. Hypoxia Promotes Lymph Node Metastasis in Human Melanoma Xenografts by Up-Regulating the Urokinase-Type Plasminogen Activator Receptor. Cancer Research 62, 1847-1853, March 15, 2002.

103. Hickman, J.A. Apoptosis induced by anticancer drugs. Cancer Metast Rev 1992; 11: 121-139.

104. Reinehr R, Becker S, Eberle A, Grether-Beck S, Haussinger D. Involvement of NADPH oxidase isoforms and Src family kinases in CD95-dependent hepatocyte apoptosis. J Biol Chem. 2005; 280(29):27179-27194.

105. Yokomizo A, Ono M, Nanri H, Makino Y, Ohga T, Wada M, Okamoto T,Yodoi J, Kuwano M, Kohno K. Cellular levels of thioredoxin associated with drug sensitivity to cisplatin, mitomycin C, doxorubicin, and etoposide. Cancer Res 1995;55:4293–4296.

106. Hasinoff B. B., Davey J. P.Adriamycin and its iron(III) and copper(III) complexes, glutathione-induced dissociation, cytochrome *c* oxidase inactivation and protection: binding to cardiolipin. Biochem. Pharmacol., *37:* 3663-3669, 1988.

107. Burger R. M. Cleavage of nucleic acids by bleomycin. Chem. Rev., *98:* 1153-1169, 1998.

108. Byfield J. E., Lee Y. C., Tu L., Kullhanian F. Molecular interactions of the combined effects of bleomycin and X-rays on mammalian cell survival. Cancer Res., *36:* 1138-1143, 1976.

109. Sangeetha, P., Das, U.N., Koratkar, R. and Suryaprabha, P. Increase in free radical generation and lipid peroxidation following chemotherapy in patients with cancer. Free Radic Biol Med 1990; 8(1): 15-19.

110. Ferlini C, Scambia G, Marone M, Distefano M, Gaggini C, Ferrandina G, Fattorossi A, Isola G, Benedetti Panici P, Mancuso S. Tamoxifen induces oxidative stress and apoptosis in estrogen receptor-negative human cancer cell lines. Br J Cancer 1999;79:257–263.

111. P. Vaupel and L. Harrison. Tumor Hypoxia: Causative Factors, Compensatory Mechanisms, and Cellular Response. Oncologist, November 1, 2004; 9(suppl_5): 4 – 9.

112. Loughlin KR; Manson K; Cragnale D; Wilson L; Ball RA; Bridges KR. The use of hydrogen peroxide to enhance the efficacy of doxorubicin hydrochloride in a murine bladder tumor cell line J Urol. 2001; 165(4):1300-4.

113. Lionel Resnick, Harold Rabinovitz, David Binninger, Maria Marchetti, Herbert Weissbach. Topical sulindac combined with hydrogen peroxide in the treatment of actinic keratoses. Journal of Drugs in Dermatology. January 1, 2009. Volume: 8 Issue: 1 Page: 29(4).

114. Aronoff, B.L. Regional oxygenation in neoplasms. Cancer 1965; 18: 1250.

115. Mallams, J.T., Balla, G.A. and Finney, J.W. Regional oxygenation and irradiation in the treatment of malignant tumors. Prog in Clin Cancer 1965; 1: 137.

116. Nathan, C. F., and R. K. Root. 1977. Hydrogen peroxide release from mouse peritoneal macrophages. Dependence on sequential activation and triggering.]. *Exp. Med.* 146:1648.

117. Nathan CF, Cohn ZA. Antitumor effects of hydrogen peroxide in vivo. J Exp Med. 1981 Nov 1;154(5):1539–1553.

118. Mallams, J.T., Balla, G.A. and Finney, J.W. Regional oxygenation and irradiation in the treatment of malignant tumors. Prog Clin Cancer 1965; 1: 137.

119. Finney, J.W., Collier, R.E., Balla, G.A., Tomme, J.W., Wakley, J., Race, G.J., Urschel, H.C., D'Errico, A.D. and Mallams, J.T. The preferential localization of radioisotopes in malignant tissue by regional oxygenation. Nature 1961; 202: 1172.

120. Finney, J.W., Balla, G.A., Collier, R.E., Wakely, J., Urschel, H.C. and Mallams, J.T. Differential localization of isotopes in tumors through the use of intra-arterial hydrogen peroxide: Part 1: Basic science. Amer J Roentgen 1965; 94: 783.

121. Nathan, C. F., L, H. Brukner, S. C. Silverstein, and Z. A. Cohn. 1979. Extracellular cytolysis by activated macrophages and

granulocytes. I. Pharmacologic triggering of effector cells and the release of hydrogen peroxide. J. Exp. Med. 149:84.

122. Philpott, G. W., W. T. Shearer, R. J. Bower, and C. W. Parker. 1973. Selective cytotoxicity of hapten-substituted cells with an antibody-enzyme conjugate. J. Immunol. 111:921.

123. Edelson, P. J., and Z. A. Cohn. 1973. Peroxidase-mediated mammalian cell cytotoxicity. J. Exp. Med. 138:318.

124. Clark, R. A., S. J. Klebanoff, A. B. Einstein, and A. Fefer. 1975. Peroxidase-H20-halide system: cytotoxic effect on mammalian tumor cells. Blood. 45:161.

125. Nathan, C. F. 1979. The role of oxidative metabolism in the cytotoxicity of activated macrophages after pharmacologic triggering. *In* Immunobiology and Immunotherapy of Cancer. W. D. Terry and Y. Yamamura, editors. Elsevier North-Holland, Inc., New York. 59.

126. Philpott, G. W., A. Kulczycki, Jr., E. H. Grass, and C. W. Parker. 1980. Selective binding and cytotoxicity of rat basophilic leukemia cells (RBL-1) with immunoglobulin E-biotin and avidin-glucose oxidase conjugates. J. Immunol. 125:1201.

127. Nathan, C. F., B. A. Arrick, H. W. Murray, N. M. DeSantis, and Z. A. Cohn. 1981. Tumor cell antioxidant defenses: inhibition of the glutathione redox cycle enhances macrophage mediated cytolysis. J. Exp. Med. 153:766.

128. Nathan CF, Brukner LH, Silverstein SC, Cohn ZA. Extracellular cytolysis by activated macrophages and granulocytes. I. Pharmacologic triggering of effector cells and the release of hydrogen peroxide. J Exp Med. 1979 Jan 1;149(1):84–99.

129. Nathan CF, Silverstein SC, Brukner LH, Cohn ZA. Extracellular cytolysis by activated macrophages and granulocytes. II. Hydrogen peroxide as a mediator of cytotoxicity. J Exp Med. 1979 Jan 1;149(1):100–113.

130. Keilin, D., and E. F. Hartree. 1948. Properties of glucose oxidase (notatin). Biochem. J. 42:221.

131. Filep, J.G., Lapierre, C., Lachance, S. and Chan, J.S.D. Nitric oxide cooperates with hydrogen peroxide in inducing DNA

fragmentation and cell lysis in murine lymphoma cells. Biochem J 1997; 321: 887-901.

132. Kanner, J., Harel, S. and Granit, R. Arch Biochem Biophys 1991; 289: 130-136.

133. Noronha-Dutra, A.A., Epperlein, M.M. and Woolf, N. FEBS Lett 1993; 321: 59-62.

134. Burdon R. H., Gill V., Rice-Evans C. Cell proliferation and oxidative stress. Free Radic. Res. Commun., *7:* 149-159, 1989.

135. Burdon R. H. Superoxide and hydrogen peroxide in relation to mammalian cell proliferation. Free Radic. Biol. Med., 18: 775-794, 1995.

136. Takeuchi, T., Matsugo, S. and Morimoto, K. (1997) Mutagenicity of oxidative DNA damage in Chinese hamster V79 cells. Carcinogenesis, 18, 2051–2055.

137. Yin Y, Solomon G, Deng C, Barrett JC. Differential regulation of p21 by p53 and Rb in cellular response to oxidative stress. Mol Carcinog 1999;24:15–24.

138. Huang, et al, Tumor promotion by hydrogen peroxide in rat liver epithelial cells. Carcinogenesis, Vol. 20, No. 3, pp. 485-492, 1999.

139. Dizdaroglu, M. (1993) In DNA and Free Radicals (Halliwell, B., and Aruoma, O.I. eds.), pp. 19-39, Ellis Horwood, Chichester.

140. Halliwell, B. and Aruoma, O.I. DNA damage by oxygen-derived species. (1991) FEBS Lett. 281, 9-19.

141. L.J. Marnett. Oxyradicals and DNA damage. Carcinogenesis 2000 Mar;21(3):361-70.

142. Turrens, J.F. Mitochondrial formation of reactive oxygen species. (2003) Journal of Physiology-LONDON 552(2):335-344.

143. Campian, J.L., Qian, M., Gao, X., and Eaton, J.W. Oxygen tolerance and coupling of mitochondrial electron transport. 279(45): 46580-46587, 2004.

144. Riordan N, Riordan H and Casiari J. Clinical and experimental experiences with intravenous vitamin C. Journal of Orthomolecular

Medicine, Special Issue: Proceedings from Vitamin C as Cancer Therapy Workshop, Montreal. 15(4): 201-13. 1999.

145. Riordan N et al. Intravenous ascorbate as a tumour cytotoxic chemotherapeutic agent. Medical Hypothesis. 9(2): 207-13. 1994.

146. Benade L, Howard T and Burke D. Synergistic killings of Ehrlich ascites carcinoma cells by ascorbate and 3 amino-1, 2, 4-triazole. Oncology. 1969;23:33-43.

147. Tsao C, Dungham B and Ping Y. In vivo antineoplastic activity of ascorbic acid for human mammary tumour. In vivo. 2: 147-50. 1988.

148. Bram S et al. Vitamin C preferential toxicity for malignant melanoma cells. Nature. 284: 629-31. 1980.

149. Matsuda, T., Kuroyanagi, M., Sugiyama, S., Umehara, K., Ueno, A. and Nishi, K. Role of hydrogen peroxide for cell death induction by sodium 5,6-Benzylidene-L-ascorbate. Chem Pharm Bull 1994; 6: 1216-1225.

150. Agus DB, Vera JC and Golde DW. Stromal cell oxidation: a mechanism by which tumors obtain vitamin C. Cancer Research. 1999;59:4555-4558.

151. Chen Q, Espey MG, Krishna MC, Mitchell JB, Corpe CP, Buettner GR, Shacter E, and Levine L. Pharmacologic ascorbic acid concentrations selectively kill cancer cells: Action as a pro-drug to deliver hydrogen peroxide to tissues. PNAS. September 20, 2005. Vol. 102. No. 38. pp. 13604-13609.

152. Maramag C et al. Effect of vitamin C on prostate cancer cells in vitro: effect on cell number, viability, and DNA synthesis. Prostate. 32: 188-95. 1997.

153. Ha YM, Park MK, Kim HJ, Seo HG, Lee JH, Chang KC. High concentrations of ascorbic acid induces apoptosis of human gastric cancer cell by p38-MAP kinase-dependent up-regulation of transferrin receptor. Cancer Lett. 2009 May 8;277(1):48-54.

154. Devadas S, Zaritskaya L, Rhee SG, Oberley L, Williams MS. Discrete generation of superoxide and hydrogen peroxide by T cell receptor stimulation: selective regulation of mitogen-acti-

vated protein kinase activation and Fas ligand expression. J Exp Med 195(1):59-70, 2002.

155. Williams MS, Kwon J. T cell receptor stimulation, reactive oxygen species and cell signaling. Free Rad Biol Med 37(8):1144-1151, 2004.

156. Wentworth et al., 2000) (Wentworth AD, Jones LH, Wentworth P Jr, Janda KD, Lerner RA. Antibodies have the intrinsic capacity to destroy antigens. PNAS 97(20):10930-10935, 2000).

157. Wentworth P Jr, Jones LH, Wentworth AD, Zhu X, Larsen NA, Wilson IA, Xu X, Goddard WA III, Janda KD, Eschenmoser A, Lerner RA. Antibody catalysis of the oxidation of water. Science 293 (5536):1806-1811, 2001.

158. Wentworth P Jr, Wentworth AD, Zhu X, Wislon IA, Janda KD, Eschenmoser A, Lerner RA. Evidence for the production of trioxygen species during antibody-catalyzed chemical modification of antigens. PNAS 100(4):1490-1493, 2003.

159. IARC. 1985. International Agency for Research on Cancer. Hydrogen Peroxide. In: IARC Monographs on the Evaluation of Carcinogenic Risk if Chemicals to Humans: Allyl compounds, Aldehydes, Epoxides and Peroxides, Vol. 36. IARC, Lyon, pp. 285-314.

160. Cina SJ, Downs JC, Conradi SE. Hydrogen peroxide: a source of lethal oxygen embolism. Case report and review of the literature. Am J Forensic Med Pathol. 1994 Mar;15(1):44-50.

161. Starfield, B. Is US Health Really the Best in the World? JAMA 2000 Jul 26;284[4]:483-5.

162. Jay Pravda. Radical induction theory of ulcerative colitis. J Gastroenterol April 28, 2005 April;11(16):2371-2384.

163. Dickson KF, Caravati EM. Abstract: Hydrogen peroxide exposure--325 exposures reported to a regional poison control center. J Toxicol Clin Toxicol. 1994;32(6):705-14.

164. Howes, R. M. *U.T.O.P.I.A. - Unified Theory of Oxygen Participation in Aerobiosis.* © 2004. Free Radical Publishing Co. Kentwood, LA Available at www.iwillfindthecure.org.

165. Kroemer, G., Zamzami, N. and Susin, S.A. Mitochondrial control of apoptosis. Immunol Today 1997; 18: 44-51.

166. Fleury C, Mignotte B, Vayssiere JL Mitochondrial reactive oxygen species in cell death signaling. Biochimie 2002;84:131-41.

167. Mansat-de Mas V, Bezombes C, Quillet-Mary A, et al Implication of radical oxygen species in ceramide generation, c-Jun N-terminal kinase activation and apoptosis induced by daunorubicin. Mol Pharmacol 1999;56:867-74.

168. Simizu S, Umezawa K, Takada M, Arber N, Imoto M Induction of hydrogen peroxide production and Bax expression by caspase-3(-like) proteases in tyrosine kinase inhibitor-induced apoptosis in human small cell lung carcinoma cells. Exp Cell Res 1998;238:197-203.

169. Hirpara JL, Clement MV, Pervaiz S Intracellular acidification triggered by mitochondrial-derived hydrogen peroxide is an effector mechanism for drug-induced apoptosis in tumor cells. J Biol Chem 2001;276:514-21.

170. Clement MV, Ponton A, Pervaiz S Apoptosis induced by hydrogen peroxide is mediated by decreased superoxide anion concentration and reduction of intracellular milieu. FEBS Lett 1998;440:13-18.

171. Kerr, J.F.R., Winterfold, C.M. and Harmon, B.V. Apoptosis, its significance in cancer and cancer therapy. Cancer 1994; 73: 2013-2026.

172. Blackstone, N.W. and Green, D.R. The evolution of a mechanism of cell suicide. Bio Essays 1999; 21: 84-88.

173. Khyshiktyev BS, Khyshiktueva NA, Ivanov VN, Darenskaia SD, Novikov SV. Diagnostic value of investigating exhaled air condensate in lung cancer. Vopr Onkol 1994; 40: 161-164.

174. Tsujimoto Y., Shimizu S. VDAC regulation by the Bcl-2 family of proteins. Cell Death Differ., *7:* 1174-1181, 2000.

175. Korsmeyer S. J. *BCL-2* gene family and the regulation of programmed cell death. Cancer Res., *59:* 1693-1700S, 1999.

176. Harris M. H., Thompson C. B. The role of the Bcl-2 family in the regulation of outer mitochondrial membrane permeability. Cell Death Differ, *7:* 1182-1191, 2000.

177. Clement M.V., Pervaiz S. Reactive oxygen intermediates regulate cellular response to apoptotic stimuli: an hypothesis. Free Radic. Res., *30:* 247-252, 1999.

178. Clement M.V., Pervaiz S. Intracellular superoxide and hydrogen peroxide concentrations: a critical balance that determines survival or death. Redox. Rep., *6:* 211-214, 2001.

179. Pervaiz S., Clement M.V. Hydrogen peroxide-induced apoptosis: oxidative or reductive stress?. Methods Enzymol., *352:* 150-159, 2002.

180. Pervaiz S., Clement M.V. A permissive apoptotic environment: function of a decrease in intracellular superoxide anion and cytosolic acidification. Biochem. Biophys. Res. Commun., *290:* 1145-1150, 2002.

181. Fleury C, Mignotte B, Vayssiere JL Mitochondrial reactive oxygen species in cell death signaling. Biochimie 2002;84:131-41.

182. Childs AC, Phaneuf SL, Dirks AJ, Phillips T, Leeuwenburgh C Doxorubicin treatment in vivo causes cytochrome C release and cardiomyocyte apoptosis, as well as increased mitochondrial efficiency, superoxide dismutase activity, and Bcl-2:Bax ratio. Cancer Res 2002;62:4592-8.

183. Quillet-Mary A, Jaffrezou JP, Mansat V, Bordier C, Naval J, Laurent G Implication of mitochondrial hydrogen peroxide generation in ceramide-induced apoptosis. J Biol Chem 1997;272:21388-95.

184. Zhang L, Yu J, Park BH, Kinzler KW, Vogelstein B Role of BAX in the apoptotic response to anticancer agents. Science 2000;290:989-92.

185. Hug H, Strand S, Grambihler A, et al Reactive oxygen intermediates are involved in the induction of CD95 ligand mRNA expression by cytostatic drugs in hepatoma cells. J Biol Chem 1997;272:28191-3.

186. Suhara T, Fukuo K, Sugimoto T, et al Hydrogen peroxide induces up-regulation of Fas in human endothelial cells. J Immunol 1998;160:4042-7.

187. Hirpara JL, Clement MV, Pervaiz S. Intracellular acidification triggered by mitochondrial-derived hydrogen peroxide is an effector mechanism for drug-induced apoptosis in tumor cells. J Biol Chem 2001;276:514-21.

188. Ahmad KA, Clement MV, Hanif IM, Pervaiz S. Resveratrol inhibits drug-induced apoptosis in human leukemia cells by creating an intracellular milieu nonpermissive for death execution. Cancer Res 2004;64:1452-9.

189. Cerutti P. A. Prooxidant states and tumor promotion. Science (Wash. DC), *227:* 375-381, 1985.

190. Burdon R. H., Gill V., Rice-Evans C. Oxidative stress and tumour cell proliferation. Free Radic. Res. Commun., *11:* 65-76, 1990.

191. Fadeel B., Ahlin A., Henter J. I., Orrenius S., Hampton M. B. Involvement of caspases in neutrophil apoptosis: regulation by reactive oxygen species. Blood, *92:* 4808-4818, 1998.

192. Hampton M. B., Orrenius S. Dual regulation of caspase activity by hydrogen peroxide: implications for apoptosis. FEBS Lett., *414:* 552-556, 1997.

193. Tze Wei Poh and Shazib Pervaiz. LY294002 and LY303511 Sensitize Tumor Cells to Drug-Induced Apoptosis via Intracellular Hydrogen Peroxide Production Independent of the Phosphoinositide 3-Kinase-Akt Pathway. Cancer Research 65, 6264-6274, July 15, 2005.

194. Cullen, J. J., Hinkhouse, M. M., Grady, M., Gaut, A. W., Liu, J., Zhang, Y., Weydert, C. J. D., Domann, F. E., and Oberley, L. W. (2003) *Cancer Res.* 63, 5513–5520.

195. Juan Du, David H. Daniels, Carla Asbury, Sujatha Venkataraman, Jingru Liu, Douglas R. Spitz, Larry W. Oberley, and Joseph J. Cullen. Mitochondrial Production of Reactive Oxygen Species Mediate Dicumarol-induced Cytotoxicity in Cancer Cells. The Journal of Biological Chemistry Vol. 281, No. 49, pp. 37416–37426, December 8, 2006.

196. Sun Wenqing; Kalen Amanda L; Smith Brian J; Cullen Joseph J; Oberley Larry W. Enhancing the antitumor activity of adriamycin and ionizing radiation. Cancer research 2009;69(10):4294-300.

197. Wagner B A; Buettner G R; Oberley L W; Darby C J; Burns C P. Myeloperoxidase is involved in H_2O_2-induced apoptosis of HL-60 human leukemia cells. The Journal of biological chemistry 2000;275(29):22461-9.

198. Jun Fang, Tomohiro Sawa, Takaaki Akaike and Hiroshi Maeda. Tumor-targeted Delivery of Polyethylene Glycol-conjugated D-Amino Acid Oxidase for Antitumor Therapy via Enzymatic Generation of Hydrogen Peroxide. Cancer Research 62, 3138-3143, June 1, 2002.

199. Venkataraman Sujatha; Jiang Xiaohong; Weydert Christine; Zhang Yuping; Zhang Hannah J; Goswami Prabhat C; Ritchie Justine M; Oberley Larry W; Buettner Garry R. Manganese superoxide dismutase overexpression inhibits the growth of androgen-independent prostate cancer cells.

200. Oncogene 2005;24(1):77-89.

201. Aykin-Burns Nùkhet; Ahmad Iman M; Zhu Yueming; Oberley Larry W; Spitz Douglas R. Increased levels of superoxide and H_2O_2 mediate the differential susceptibility of cancer cells versus normal cells to glucose deprivation. The Biochemical Journal 2009;418(1):29-37.

202. Yoshizaki K, et al. Pro-senescent effect of hydrogen peroxide on cancer cells and its possible application to tumor suppression. Biosci Biotechnol Biochem. 2009 Feb;73(2):311-5.

203. Brian D. Lawenda, Kara M. Kelly, Elena J. Ladas, Stephen M. Sagar, Andrew Vickers, Jeffrey B. Blumberg. Should Supplemental Antioxidant Administration Be Avoided During Chemotherapy and Radiation Therapy? JNCI Journal of the National Cancer Institute 2008 100(11):773-783.

204. Vicki Brower. An Apple a Day May Be Safer Than Vitamins. JNCI Journal of the National Cancer Institute 2008 100(11):770-772.

205. Howes M.D., PhD., R. (2009). Dangers of Antioxidants in Cancer Patients: A Review. PHILICA.COM Article number 153. Published 7th February, 2009.

206. Nima Sharifi. Commentary: Antioxidants for Cancer: New Tricks for an Old Dog? The Oncologist, Vol. 14, No. 3, 213-215, March 2009.

207. Salganik, R. I., Albright, C. D., Rodgers, J., Kim, J., Zeisel, S. H., Sivashinskiy, M. S. & Van Dyke, T. A. (2000) Dietary antioxidant depletion: enhancement of tumor apoptosis and inhibition of brain tumor growth in transgenic mice. Carcinogenesis 21: 909–914.

CANCER THERAPY:

A Review with Scientific Validation for the Role of Electronically Modified Oxygen Derivatives in Oncologic Treatment Modalities

Prof. Hon. Randolph M. Howes, M.D., Ph.D.

Adjunct Assistant Professor of Plastic Surgery, The Johns Hopkins Hospital, Baltimore, Md., U.S.A., Espaldon Professor of Plastic and Reconstructive Surgery, University of Santo Tomas, Manila, Philippines. Adjunct Professor of Biological Sciences, Southeastern Louisiana University, Hammond, La.

Address for communication: 27439 Highway 441, Kentwood, Louisiana 70444-8152, USA. Email: net

Abstract

The American Cancer Society and the British Columbia Cancer Agency state that electronically modified oxygen derivatives, such as hydrogen peroxide and other "oxidative therapies," are basically ineffective, harmful or even lethal in the treatment of cancer. A compelling body of evidence over the past few decades demands that the therapeutic role of oxygen derivatives be reevaluated. The free radical theory defined oxygen free radicals or reactive oxygen species as being destructive and as the cause of the majority of common human diseases. Yet, decades of experimentation have shown that the free radical theory lacks predictability, fails to meet the requirements of the scientific method and is therefore invalidated. This nullification requires reexamination of oxidative oncologic complementary, alternative and integrative treatment modalities.

Prooxidants, some of which are oxygen free radicals or reactive oxygen species, have been blamed for cancer causation and unscrupulous marketers have brought discredit to oxygen based therapies and disregard to oxidative centered treatments. In contrast, a review of currently effective tumoricidal methods reveals a "commonality of oxygen based, anti-neoplastic action," in that many successful cytotoxic agents, procedures or methods have been shown to proceed primarily via prooxidants. Discussions will compare chemotherapy, radiation therapy, megadose intravenous vitamin C therapy, photodynamic therapy, sonodynamic therapy, the Howes' singlet oxygen tumoricidal system, ozone therapy, hyperbaric oxygen therapy and hydrogen peroxide therapy. Various prooxidant delivery systems currently offer beneficial, unique tumoricidal properties and approach the "Holy Grail" for cancer treatments, allowing for selective killing of cancer cells while sparing normal cells.This review describes these prooxidant EMOD agents and areas of possible complementarity of oxidative therapies (prooxidant stacking) based on the available scientific literature. Decades of scientific study have shown that prooxidant antineoplastic therapeutic agents provide significant clinical advantage and offer safe, effective and economical promise in the future treatment of cancer.

Introduction

The widely held flawed notions promulgated by the free radical theory have so biased world orthodoxy, regarding the true role of oxygen in disease causation and prevention that it is best to start over with a new, well configured, open minded scientific paradigm.To this end, prior "oxidative" prejudicial terminology will be eschewed.

Unproven therapies and misrepresented products, offered over the internet and at various clinics, local and abroad, have created a generalized negative attitude towards so-called "oxygen therapies" and "oxidative medicine," because it has been used to refer to any number of worthless products or ineffective treatments, which were not based on scientific facts regarding oxygen metabolism. The therapeutic potential of prooxidant electronically modified oxygen derivatives (EMODs) have been demonstrated for decades by their use in academic oncology treatment programs. Many so-called oxidative therapies prompted the British Columbia Cancer Agency (a part of the Canadian Provincial Health Services Authority) and the American Cancer Society (ACS) to recommend against their use. These therapies go by many names including "Oxygen Therapies, Hyperoxygenation Therapy, Oxymedicine, Bio-Oxidative Therapy, Oxidative Therapy, Oxidology, Ozone therapy, Autohemotherapy, Hydrogen peroxide therapy and Germanium sesquioxide therapy." To be sure, some of these approaches are subject to fraudulent practices and lack credibility but others are based on a solid scientific principles and investigations. (ACS website accessed 12-7-09).

The BC Cancer Agency website presents the following summary: "Patients with cancer should not consider oxygen therapies as either alternative (first-line) or adjunct (complementary) therapies. Researchers now understand that cancer cells "lower-than-normal respiration" is due to the fact that tissue surrounding cancer cells receives less oxygen because it has fewer blood vessels feeding it. Oxygen therapies have not been found useful against cancer and are not used as mainstream cancer treatments." They also state that, "Oxygen therapy can destroy cells, including those of the blood-forming organs. Very high doses can seriously damage health or even cause death." (BC Cancer Agency website accessed 8-31-09).

The American Cancer Society website gives the following overview: "Available scientific evidence does not support claims that putting oxygen-releasing chemicals into a person's body is effective in treating cancer. It may even be dangerous. There have been reports of patient deaths from this method."

Contrary to disputed statements of major cancer agencies, this review clearly demonstrates that prooxidant EMODs have been scientifically confirmed as essential, effective and safe clinical agents in the battle against cancer. Undeniably, for decades, prooxidant EMOD cancer therapeutic modalities have been a mainstay for our most effective oncologic treatment programs, which utilize chemotherapy, radiation therapy and photodynamic therapy.

Simultaneously, a persuasive assemblage of scientific data shows that EMODs are crucial agents for gene regulation, maintenance of cellular oxidation/reduction (redox) homeostasis and pathogen and neoplasia protection.

At first glance, oxygen has obvious medical benefits in emergency or critical care situations but upon closer review of the available scientific literature, it becomes readily apparent that EMODs have already made significant contributions in fighting disease, maintaining healthy homeostasis and in combatting cancer. As it relates to cancer therapy, prooxidant EMOD-induced apoptosis and necrosis is currently used in a wide spectrum of modalities to successfully treat neoplasia. There appears to be "a prooxidant point of convergence" in these EMOD applications, which includes a role in chemotherapy, radiation therapy, intravenous vitamin C mega-dose therapy, photodynamic therapy, sonodynamic therapy, the Howes singlet oxygen tumoricidal system, ozone therapy, hyperbaric oxygen therapy and intravenous hydrogen peroxide therapy.

Conversely, hypoxia and so-called antioxidants can effectively modify or block cancer cell kill by interfering with electronically modified oxygen derivative (EMOD)-induced apoptosis. EMODs possess the levels of reactivity to serve as tumoricidal agents.

Ground state triplet oxygen (O_2) does not have the same level of reactivity as the prooxidants referred to in this article, such as: the superoxide anion (O_2.-), hydrogen peroxide (H_2O_2), metastable excited singlet oxygen ($^1O_2$*), the hydroxyl radical (OH.), hypochlorous acid (HOCl), nitric oxide (NO), peroxynitrite (OONO-), ozone (O_3), etc. However, ground state triplet oxygen serves as the source for the production of the entire family of EMOD agents. EMODs are formed by basic alterations of the electron structure of ground state triplet oxygen, such as addition or removal of electrons, altered electron spin configurations, altered pi electron orbital positions, combinations with nitrogen, exposure to ultraviolet light or wave specific white light, altered pressure other than atmospheric, etc.

Gathering EMOD agents into inaccurate and misleading categorizations is no longer suitable with the use of terms such as oxygen free radials or reactive oxygen species. The usage of incorrect biochemical terminology is no longer acceptable and its taint must be abandoned. Ignorance of the literature does not allow health care agencies the latitude of making scientifically unsupported statements. As Carl Nathan said in a 2003 *Journal of Clinical Investigation* article, "terms of discourse" need to be addressed.

Because of the common use of varying terms, such as reactive oxygen species (ROS), reactive oxygen intermediates (ROI), reactive oxygen metabolites (ROM), active oxygen species (AOS), oxygen species (OS), etc., confusion abounds as to precise nature of the oxygen entities being discussed in various articles. Thus, in 2005, in *The Medical and Scientific Significance of Oxygen Free Radical Metabolism*. pg. 39, I stated, " It is also time to discard ROS, RONS, OS, ROI, ROM, AOS, etc. and utilize a more meaningful and accurate term. I propose the term "electronically modified oxygen derivative(s)" (EMODs). This term does not imply charge, radicality, or reactivity. It merely indicates that an electron(s) of oxygen has (have) been altered or changed from its ground state orbit. This avoids all of the inaccuracies of terms such as reactive oxygen species, reactive oxygen metabolites, or oxygen intermediates, all of which should be discarded from usage. Thus, EMODs include superoxide anion, singlet oxygen, hydrogen peroxide, hypochlorous acid, peroxynitrite, hydroxyl radical, nitric oxide, alkyl radicals, alkoxyl radicals, etc. The term does not limit itself to oxygen covalent bonding or hydrogen abstraction and addition. Thus, oxygen-containing sulfates, nitrates, phosphates, etc. would also qualify as EMODs. Further, it includes all of the nitrative and oxidative forms of oxygen."

Further, according to Barry Halliwell, EMODs such as superoxide anion are barely "reactive" at all and are redox ambivalent at a physiological pH. EMODS, such as hydrogen peroxide, singlet oxygen, ozone and hypochlorous acid are not free radicals but are frequently erroneously placed in this chemical category.

In 1971, President Nixon launched the "War Against Cancer," which was designed to fight the escalating incidence of cancer that had assumed epidemic proportions. According to Samuel S. Epstein's book, *Cancer-GATE: How to Win the Losing Cancer War*, only incremental progress has been made in this overall crusade. The development of agents that improve or enhance the efficacy of cancer therapy is one of the most important areas of research in current medical oncology. Biological oxidation/reduction (redox) reactions are central to metabolism, cellular energy production and cancer therapy.

Many in vitro *studies have shown support of prooxidant cancer therapies and even though it should not be assumed that they will be identically effective* in vivo *in the cure of cancer, clinical studies cited in this review are increasingly showing support for this thesis.*

Discussion

Harman's free radical theory

Harman's free radical theory hypothesized that diseases, such as cancer and aging, resulted from the random or "stochastic" accumulation of oxidative damage purportedly caused by EMODs, from environmental sources and from by-products of normal cellular metabolism. [1-5] When investigators found that their results were not as predicted by the free radical theory, they either discounted their results or referred to them as a paradox. Countless examples of this are in the literature but can be best illustrated by the 1995 tome edited by Kelvin J.A. Davies and Fulvio Ursini entitled, *THE OXYGEN PARADOX*.

The alleged damaging derivatives of oxygen were defined as being inherently deleterious and harmful. However, this notion has been rebuffed by Howes. [6] Apoptosis, necrosis, and growth arrest have been shown to be regulated to a significant degree by prooxidant EMOD species. [7-10] Apoptosis, in part, controls the neoplastic process as genetically damaged or mutated cells can be eliminated by inducement of the apoptotic process. [11] Apoptosis involves caspases (cysteine proteases cleaving after particular aspartate residues), mitochondrial pathways and/or EMODs, which are usually, but not always, key components. [12] Many apoptosis-inducing agents function as prooxidants *in vitro.* [13]

Prooxidant EMOD generating agents have repeatedly been shown to kill cancer cells selectively, while sparing normal cells and this tumoricidal action can be modified or blocked by antioxidants, which may accelerate cancer growth both *in vitro* and *in vivo.* [14-17] Since therapeutic agents (radiation therapy, chemotherapy or photodynamic therapy, PDT) work, to a considerable extent, by releasing prooxidant free radicals (EMODs), it is logical that antioxidants likely interfere with their action. EMOD levels and cellular redox tone appear to be uniquely exploitable targets in cancer chemoprevention via the stimulation or induction of cytoprotection in normal cells and/or the induction of apoptosis in transformed malignant cells.

Antioxidants and apoptosis

Yet, some believe that antioxidants may play a central role in apoptosis and cancer therapy. Some investigators have made claims that antioxidants can actually kill cancer cells and argue that antioxidants are beneficial during chemotherapy. A review on the use of antioxidants during chemotherapy, published in Cancer Treatment Reviews, was a collaborative effort led by Dr. Keith Block and researchers from the University of Illinois at Chicago and M.D. Anderson Cancer Center in Houston. After reviewing articles, only 33 of 965 articles considered, including 2,446 subjects, met the inclusion criteria. Antioxidants evaluated were: glutathione, melatonin, vitamin A, an antioxidant mixture, N-acetylcysteine, vitamin E, selenium, L-carnitine, Co-Q10 and ellagic acid. Nine studies reported no difference in toxicities between the 2 groups. Only 1 study (vitamin A) reported a significant increase in toxicity in the antioxidant group. This review provides some evidence that antioxidant supplementation during chemotherapy might reduce dose-limiting toxicities but it must be kept in mind that many of these so-called antioxidants have considerable prooxidant activity to which their salutary effects could also be attributed. Larger, well-designed studies of antioxidants impact on PDT, chemotherapy and tumoricidal radiation therapy are warranted. [18]

However, until such data is available, considerations for utmost patient safety must prevail. The mechanisms of action of chemotherapeutic drugs and antioxidants are sufficiently understood to predict their resultant interactions and to suggest that considerable care should be exercised with respect to both clinical decisions and study interpretations.

[19] Additionally, antioxidants have a wide variety of biochemical actions and are capable of interfering selectively with EMOD initiation, propagation and termination. EMODs have been studied for their positive effects in the prevention or cure of many cancers, cardiovascular disease, age-related diseases, and other disorders. [20-23]

Nonetheless, there seems to be agreement that the antioxidant N-acetylcysteine (NAC), a derivative of the naturally occurring amino acid cysteine, should be avoided by cancer patients because of studies showing interference with chemotherapeutic agents, such as cisplatin and doxorubicin. [24, 25] A 2005 report concluded that cancer patients should avoid antioxidant supplements while receiving chemotherapy or radiation treatment. [26] Directed towards informing the public, a *Wall Street Journal* article argued that antioxidants could block the beneficial effects of standard cancer therapy. [27]

Those who recommend the use of antioxidants in cancer patients claim that antioxidants such as vitamin C, vitamin E, coenzyme Q10, glutathione, and selenium can reduce the toxicity of free radicals. [28-31] Thus, EMOD-induced prooxidant apoptosis and the cancer conundrum leave us with unanswered questions regarding their interactions, auto-oxidation of antioxidants and the prooxidant character of many antioxidants. [32]

A 2007 article not only defends the use of antioxidants in cancer patients, it states that, "In 15 human studies, 3,738 patients who took non-prescription antioxidants and other nutrients actually had increased survival." [33] In contrast, a 2008 article in the *Journal of the National Cancer Institute* reviewed randomized trial data, which suggested that cancer patients should avoid the routine use of antioxidant supplements because they may potentially decrease the efficacy of cancer therapy by protecting the tumor and reducing survival. They looked at clinical trials investigating the impact of antioxidants on radiation therapy and found evidence suggesting that antioxidant supplementation reduced overall survival. [34]

Hypoxia (low oxygen levels)

Threshold levels of oxygen (O_2)

Hypoxia (defined as the fraction of measured O_2 partial pressures of <5 mmHg) is a statistically significant adverse prognostic factor of disease-free survival. Considerable data indicates that low O_2 in tumor cells is an adverse prognostic sign. In general, low tumor O_2 is associated with: increased aggressiveness of primary cancerous lesions, their ability to metastasize, and an increased resistance to treatments with irradiation, chemotherapeutics and surgery.

In general, median O_2 partial pressures of less than 10 mmHg result in intracellular acidosis, ATP depletion, a drop in the energy supply and increasing levels of inorganic phosphate. Mitochondrial oxidative phosphorylation is limited at O_2 partial pressures of less than approximately 0.5 mmHg but there are exceptions to this generality.

Overall, a number of key findings have been described as follows: 1) most tumors have lower median O_2 partial pressures than their tissue of origin; 2) many solid tumors contain areas of low O_2 partial pressure than cannot be predicted by clinical size, stage, grade, histology and site; 3) tumor-to-tumor variability in oxygenation is usually greater than intra-tumoral variability in oxygenation; and 4) recurring tumors have a poorer oxygenation status than the corresponding primary tumors.

Cancer cell apoptosis or cellular suicide (apoptotic execution) is considered to be a needed means for controlling the growth or proliferation of neoplastic cells, which is highly desirable and the goal of cancer therapy.

Tumor hypoxia and *oxygen deficiency is strongly implicated in the growth of tumors and is a known adverse factor in the effectiveness of conventional radiation and chemotherapy.* [35, 36] Hypoxia can induce programmed (apoptotic) cell death in normal and neoplastic cells. The level of p53 in cells increases under hypoxic conditions, and the increased level of p53 induces apoptosis by a pathway involving Apaf-1 and caspase-9 as downstream effectors. [37] However, hypoxia also initiates p53-dependent apoptosis pathways involving hypoxia-inducible factor-1 (HIF-1), genes of the BCL-2 family, and other unidentified genes. [38]

Hypoxia stimulates the transcription of glycolytic enzymes, glucose transporters (GLUT1 and GLUT3), angiogenic molecules, survival and growth factors (e.g. vascular endothelial growth factor [VEGF], angiogenin, platelet-derived growth factor-B, transforming growth factor-B, and insulin-like growth factor-II), enzymes, proteins involved in tumor invasiveness (e.g., urokinases-type plasminogen activator), chaperones, nuclear factor kB (NFkB) and other resistance-related proteins.

Anoxia/hypoxia-induced proteome changes in neoplastic and stroma cells may lead to the arrest or impairment of neoplastic growth through molecular mechanisms, resulting in cellular quiescence, differentiation, apoptosis and necrosis. Cells exposed to hypoxia are generally arrested at the G1/S-phase boundary.[39] Under anoxia, most cells are arrested immediately, regardless of their position in the cell cycle.

Studies on tumors of the uterine cervix have demonstrated that tumor hypoxia is independent of patient and tumor characteristics such as, patient age, menopausal status, and parity, International Federation of Gynecology and Obstetrics (FIGO) stage, clinical tumor size, histopathological and grade of malignancy. In fact, tumor oxygenation was the strongest independent prognostic factor.[40]

Adequate levels of oxygen are essential to effectively generate adequate tumoricidal prooxidant EMOD levels and to kill a wide range of cancer cell types and tumor hypoxia can be a serious limiting factor in reducing the effectiveness of radiotherapy, some O_2-dependent cytotoxic agents and photodynamic therapy.[41]

Prooxidant Chemotherapeutic Agents

Cancer therapy can be aimed at the cell cycle, which consists of four phases, i.e., the G_1, S, G_2, and M phases. Based on their specificity, chemotherapy drugs can be classified as cell-specific agents (effective during certain cell cycle phases) and cell-cycle non-specific (effective during all phases of the cell cycle). Based on their specific characteristics and nature of treatment, chemotherapeutic agents can be classified as alkylating agents, anti-metabolites, anthracyclines, antitumor antibiotics, monoclonal antibodies, platinums, or plant alkaloids.

Prooxidant EMOD production by chemotherapeutic agents

Many chemotherapeutic drugs have well-defined mechanisms of actions, including traditional alkylating agents and anthracycline antitumor antibiotics, which generate EMODs. Depending upon specifics of oxidation/reduction potentials, these EMODs are uniformly subject to transformation to altered compounds by antioxidants through the simple process of electron transfer.

Doxorubicin, arsenic-induced apoptosis and 2-Methoxyestradiol induced apoptosis

Antineoplastic therapy can be based on the cell cycle and/or it can be based on the involvement of electronically modified oxygen derivatives (EMODs), formerly called oxygen free radicals or reactive oxygen species. These prooxidant EMOD reactants induce apoptosis and appear to be essential as activators for removing or killing cells that have accumulated mutations. 2-Methoxyestradiol induces apoptosis in Ewing sarcoma cells through mitochondrial hydrogen peroxide production. [42-44] Daunorubicin and doxorubicin can undergo redox cycling and produce EMODs, which can have a variety of effects, including damage to cell membranes and DNA-damage. [45]

Bleomycin and doxorubicin

Bleomycin and doxorubicin are two agents known to generate pro-oxidant oxygen species. [46] In reactions involving Fe(II) and oxygen, an "activated" bleomycin species is formed that damages DNA through free radical intermediates. [47] Superoxide and hydrogen peroxide can also react with Fe(II) or Fe(III) bleomycin, respectively, to produce the activated form of the drug. DNA damage from bleomycin and ionizing radiation is similar in both induction and repair. [48]

Tamoxifen, doxorubicin, mitomycin C, etoposide and cisplatin

Many chemotherapeutic drugs, such as tamoxifen, doxorubicin, mitomycin C, etoposide and cisplatin are superoxide (EMOD) generating agents and induce oxidative stress and apoptosis. [49,50]

Anthracyclines

Reduction in EMOD levels generated by chemotherapeutic agents has the same effect as a reduction in dose. [51] NADPH-flavin reductase, cytochrome p450 reductase and mitochondrial NADH reductase can all reduce anthracyclines to a semiquinone radical. [52] This semiquinone radical can donate its free electron to molecular oxygen to generate the superoxide radical ($O^{\bullet}_2$). [52] Like hydrogen peroxide (H_2O_2), $O^{\bullet}_2$ can generate hydroxyl radicals ($^{\bullet}OH$) upon interaction with metal ions. [52] This results in lipid peroxidation of plasma membranes, leading to a loss of mitochondrial inner membrane potential and consequent cytochrome c release and apoptosis. EMODs can also directly damage DNA through generation of strand breaks and oxidized nucleic bases such as guanine to 8-hydroxyguanine, giving rise to G-T transversions. [52]

However, as a caution, free radical generation by anthracyclines is thought to be responsible for the cardiotoxicity that puts some limits on their therapeutic use. [53,54]

Additional prooxidant EMOD apoptosis inducing agents

Ideal treatment should aim to selectively kill the cancer cells, without harming normal cells. Elegant regulation of prooxidant EMOD levels may be a means to this exalted goal.

Cancer therapy seeks to utilize the sensitivity of transformed cells towards apoptotic signals, which allows the execution of apoptotic cell death. [55, 56] Contrary to Harman's free radical theory in which EMODs are only deleterious, EMODs have been found to play a crucial beneficial role in intracellular apoptotic execution (cellular suicide). [57-61]

Glioma pathogenesis-related protein 1 (GLIPR1), a p53 target gene

Glioma pathogenesis-related protein 1 (GLIPR1), a novel p53 target gene, is down-regulated by methylation in prostate cancer and has p53-dependent and -independent proapoptotic properties in tumorous cells. Investigators reported that the expression of GLIPR1 is significantly reduced in human prostate tumor tissues compared with adjacent normal prostate tissues and in multiple human cancer cell lines and that overexpression of GLIPR1 in cancer cells leads to suppression of colony growth and induction of apoptosis. Mechanistic analysis indicated that GLIPR1 up-regulation increases EMOD production leading to apoptosis through activation of the c-Jun–NH_2 kinase (JNK) signaling cascade. These results identify GLIPR1 as a proapoptotic tumor suppressor acting through EMODs and the ROS-JNK pathway and support the therapeutic potential for this protein. [62]

Elesclomol (formerly STA-4783)

Elesclomol (formerly STA-4783) is a novel small molecule undergoing clinical evaluation in a pivotal phase III melanoma trial (SYMMETRY). In a phase II randomized, double-blinded, controlled, multi-center trial in 81 patients with stage IV metastatic melanoma, treatment with elesclomol plus paclitaxel showed a statistically significant doubling of progression-free survival time compared with treatment with paclitaxel alone. Elesclomol induces apoptosis in cancer cells through the induction of oxidative stress (EMOD generation). Treatment of cancer cells *in vitro* with elesclomol resulted in the rapid generation of EMODs and the induction of a transcriptional gene profile characteristic of an oxidative stress response. Inhibition of oxidative stress by the antioxidant *N*-acetylcysteine (NAC) blocked the induction of gene transcription by elesclomol. In addition, *N*-acetylcysteine blocked drug-induced apoptosis, indicating that EMOD generation is the primary mechanism responsible for the proapoptotic activity of elesclomol. Excessive EMOD production and elevated levels of oxidative stress is believed by some to cause critical biochemical alterations that contribute to cancer cell growth. Thus, the induction of oxidative stress by elesclomol exploits this unique characteristic of cancer cells by increasing EMOD levels beyond a threshold that triggers cell death. [63]

Imexon

The antitumor agent imexon activates oxidative stress and antioxidant gene expression, which is evidence for EMOD production. Results show that a predominant biological effect of imexon is a change in redox state that can be detected in surrogate normal tissues as increased redox-sensitive transcription factor binding, EMOD generation and increased antioxidant gene expression. [64]

Chaetocin

Investigators found that Chaetocin, a thiodioxopiperazine natural product previously unreported to have anticancer effects, was found to have potent antimyeloma activity in IL-6–dependent and –independent myeloma cell lines in freshly collected sorted and unsorted patient CD138$^+$ myeloma cells and *in vivo*. Chaetocin displays superior *ex vivo* antimyeloma activity and selectivity than does doxorubicin and dexamethasone, and dexamethasone- or doxorubicin-resistant myeloma cell lines are largely non–cross-resistant to chaetocin. Mechanistically, chaetocin is dramatically accumulated in cancer cells via a process inhibited by glutathione and requiring intact/unreduced disulfides for uptake. Its anticancer (antimyeloma) *in vitro* and *in vivo* activity appears to be mediated primarily via the imposition of oxidative stress (prooxidant EMODs) and consequent apoptosis induction. [65]

PCI-24781 (histone deacetylase [HDAC] inhib)

Investigators examined the cytotoxicity and mechanisms of cell death of the broad-spectrum histone deacetylase (HDAC) inhibitor PCI-24781, alone and combined with bortezomib in Hodgkin lymphoma and non-Hodgkin lymphoma cell lines and primary lymphoproliferative (CLL/SLL) cells. PCI-24781 resulted in increased EMODs, oxidative stress and NF-κB inhibition, leading to caspase-dependent apoptosis. They showed that bortezomib is synergistic with PCI-24781.This combination or PCI-24781 alone has potential therapeutic value in lymphoma. [66]

Zinc

Zinc is becoming increasingly important in regulating cancer cell growth and proliferation. Investigators showed that the anticancer agent motexafin gadolinium (MGd) disrupted zinc metabolism in A549 lung cancer cells, leading,in the presence of exogenous zinc, to cell death.They reported the effect of MGd and exogenous zinc on intracellular levels of free zinc, oxidative stress, proliferation, and cell death in exponential phase human B-cell lymphoma and other hematologic cell lines. They found that increased levels of oxidative stress, EMOD production and intracellular free zinc precede and correlate with cell cycle arrest and apoptosis. [67]

Quinones

Many naturally occurring quinones can be isolated from biological tissues. [68] Also, chemotherapeutic drugs (adriamycin, daunorubicin,and mitomycin), acetaminophen (Tylenol), and air pollutants (cigarette smoke and automobile exhaust) are common source of quinones. Some quinones have potential to markedly induce the generation of prooxidant EMODs and may serve as the molecular mechanism of quinone cytotoxicity. [68]

Radiation Therapy

Hypoxic cancer cells are radio-resistant, which contributes dramatically to the inability of radiotherapy to control neoplastic growth and metastasis. Methods or therapies that provide increased prooxidant oxygen to cancer cells help radiation work more effectively by enabling more EMOD or free-radical formation. Radiation kills cancer cells by concentrating massive amounts of prooxidant free radicals directly into tumors.

Ionized radiation releases reactive oxygen species, i.e., EMODs, from the water molecule. [69] Thus cancer patients who undergo radiation therapy may be exposed to significant quantities of reactive prooxidant species.This may produce overkill or generate dangerously high prooxidant levels in areas outside of the treatment target site. Radiotherapy aims to alter cellular homeostasis, modify signal transduction pathways, alter redox states and induce cellular apoptosis. Exposure to ionizing radiation produces prooxidant oxygen-derived free radicals including hydroxyl radicals (the most damaging), superoxide anion radicals, hydrogen peroxide and other oxidants. [70]

And finally, as reported on 2-04-09 in the journal Nature, Stanford researcher, Robert Cho, found that breast cancer stem cells make much higher levels of protective antioxidants than other cancer cells. Use of a drug to block the antioxidant, glutathione, caused the cancer stem cells to become far more vulnerable to radiation. Using cells from mice and human breast cancer, the antioxidant glutathione protected the cancer cells from being killed by radiation EMOD-induced apoptosis.

However, even though EMODs are effective in killing tumor cells, they may threaten the integrity and survival of surrounding normal cells, which is dependent upon inherent tissue sensitivity and repair. Yet, the bottom line is that oxygen and its prooxidant EMOD agents are usually essential for effective radiation therapy and the induction of either apoptosis and/or necrosis.

Hydrogen Peroxide Therapy

Hydrogen peroxide appears to have medical attributes but has received little support in modern medicine. Hydrogen peroxide (H_2O_2) is a moderate oxidant that induces apoptosis of tumor cells *in vitro.* [71]

Even though the Baylor group's research on cancer, heart disease, wound healing and infections in the 1960s on hydrogen peroxide was ground breaking, it has remained in obscurity. Still, it teaches the therapeutic potential of hydrogen peroxide in the treatment of cancer, wound healing, atherosclerosis, shock management and infectious diseases. Peroxide has been used widely in Europe and has had an impressive record of safety and effectiveness.

Many clinical and experimental applications of hydrogen peroxide have been demonstrated. In over 300 patients regional intra-arterial hydrogen peroxide potentiated the effect of radiation therapy for malignancy involving the head, neck, pelvis and retro-peritoneum. [72] Increased localization of radioactive isotopes in malignant tumors was achieved by regional and intra-arterial infusion of hydrogen peroxide. [73, 74] Oxygen enhanced environments were shown to be bactericidal for most clostridia species and inhibited alpha toxin release. Hyperbaric oxygen was shown to be a beneficial adjunct to therapy in Bacteroides fragilis, Fusobacterium infections and nonclostridial anaerobic soft tissue infections. [75]

Results with hyperbaric oxygen are similar to that obtained by the Baylor investigators using intra-arterial and intra-venous H_2O_2.

Hydrogen peroxide appears to have two distinct effects. It initially inhibits the caspases and delays apoptosis. Then, depending on the degree of the initial oxidative stress, the caspases are activated and the cells die by apoptosis, or they remain inactive and necrosis occurs.[76,77] Some investigators believe that AIDS and cancer can be helped with hydrogen peroxide because of its induction of interferon-gamma production and its interactions which can produce a wide variety of oxygen derivatives.[78]

In a simple but rather elegant experiment, Davies showed that cellular division or cell death is EMOD concentration dependent, when utilizing the EMOD, H_2O_2. Cellular responses go from proliferation, to arrest, to apoptosis.[77] Those opposing hydrogen peroxide use have accused it of acting as a "genotoxicant or epigenetic" agent but although H_2O_2 can cause DNA damage, it is, at best, a very weak mutagen in mammalian cells.[79]

Intravenous Vitamin C Megadoses and Hydrogen Peroxide

Vitamin C (ascorbate, ascorbic acid) has had a controversial history in the prevention of cancer. Based on the pioneering work of Dr. Hugh Riordan, there have been some significant subsequent developments. One clinical case report by Drisko et al showed that vitamin C together with other oxidants, when added adjunctively to first-line chemotherapy, prevented recurrence in two ovarian cancer patients.[80] This high dose, intravenous vitamin C therapy was believed to operate through the generation of hydrogen peroxide. Ascorbate-mediated cell death was due to protein-dependent extracellular H_2O_2 generation (i.e., pro-oxidant EMOD generation). Ascorbate, an electron-donor in such reactions, ironically initiates prooxidant chemistry and H_2O_2 formation. It was concluded that ascorbate at pharmacologic concentrations in blood is a pro-drug for H_2O_2 delivery to tissues.[81,82]

Vitamin C acts as a cosubstrate for hydroxylase and oxygenase enzymes for the biosynthesis of procollagen, carnitine, and neurotransmitters.[83] These enzymes produce EMODs and ascorbate acts as a cosubstrate for them and thus, acts as a prooxidant.[84] Chen et al showed that at pharmacologic concentrations, ascorbate acts as a prooxidant, hydrogen peroxide generating agent, which exhibits selective cytotoxicity towards a wide variety of cancer cells *in vitro* and *in vivo*.[85,86] Even though there is much to be discovered in the ascorbate and hydrogen peroxide system, this appears to be an area of great potential.[87]

Yet, in contrast, several vitamin C and iron co-supplementation studies, both in animals and humans, indicate that vitamin C inhibits rather than promotes iron-dependent oxidative damage.[88]

Photodynamic Therapy

Photodynamic therapy (PDT) holds considerable promise in treating cancer but current terminology leads to confusion.

First, we need a definition of terms:

Phototherapy - light, UV, etc., is shown on to the skin, such as treating hyperbilirubinemia in babies.

Photochemotherapy - uses a photosensitizer like, psoralin

Photodynamic therapy - uses a photosensitizer given to the patient to produce $^1O_2^*$ (excited singlet oxygen).

Photo-oxidative therapy - also referred to as photo irradiative therapy, uses UV light shown on blood which is returned to the body.

Bio-oxidative therapy - aerobic exercise.

Autohemotherapy - ozone.

Photodynamic effect - a photon is absorbed by a photosensitizer and raises it to its lowest triplet excited state, it diffuses until it collides with O_2 and raises it to its lowest singlet state.

Photodynamic therapy requires a photosensitive compound and a light source (usually a laser) capable of energizing electrons to higher orbitals (excited states). These excited molecules in turn excite triplet oxygen to one of its singlet excited states in accordance with the amount of energy transferred to oxygen's outer orbital electrons.

The unique property of photosensitizers to selectively accumulate in malignant and dysplastic tissues is exploited in the treatment of malignancies. PDT can selectively destroy tumors with this simple concept. Compared to surgery and conventional thermal Yag and argon laser treatment, there is much less damage and disruption of the underlying and adjacent normal tissue structures with photodynamic therapy, since there is essentially no thermal damage to the tissues. Superficial treatments do not require sterile theater conditions and can be delivered in an outpatient setting. There is little post-treatment discomfort and the only significant side effect is residual photosensitivity.

Availability of ground state oxygen within the tumor can dramatically influence and limit direct tumor cell kill.[89] Photodynamic therapy (PDT) is a novel therapeutic method for the treatment of malignant tumors, which utilizes prooxidant EMOD generation and in particular meta-stable singlet oxygen ($^1O_2$*). By combining PDT with hyperoxygenation, any underlying hypoxic condition is improved and the cell killing rate at various time points after PDT is dramatically enhanced.[90,91]

In 1991, investigators described an apoptotic response to PDT.[92] Prooxidant species, especially singlet oxygen, produced by photosensitization or derived from cytotoxic agents, can activate apoptotic pathways.[93] However, malignant cell types can exhibit an impaired ability to undergo apoptosis. PDT-mediated oxidative stress induces a transient increase in the downstream early response genes c-fos, c-jun, c-myc, and egr-1.[94]

The *in vivo* tumoricidal reaction after PDT is accompanied by a complex immune response. PDT is a highly effective means of generating tumor-sensitized immune cells that can be recovered from lymphoid sites distant to the treated tumor at protracted time intervals after PDT, which asserts their immune memory character.[95,96] Vascular shutdown is clearly an important aspect of PDT.[97]

Clearly, when generated under carefully controlled conditions using exogenous sensitizers and light in the visible range (400 -700 nm), $^1O_2$* can be exploited for therapeutic purposes, as in antineoplastic photodynamic therapy (PDT). In biological systems, singlet oxygen has a short lifetime of <0.04 ms and has also been shown to have a short radius of action of <0.02 mm.[98]

However, in a cell with quenchers or scavengers abounding, $^1O_2$* lifetime can be <50 nsec with a diffusion distance <10 nm from its point of origin, which is less than 0.1% of the radius of an average eukaryotic cell. This short distance of reactivity can have clinical and therapeutic benefits and limit the target area or "zone of reactivity."

Although controversial, it is important to remember that all antibodies apparently go through a singlet oxygen and ozone step. Antibodies can generate hydrogen peroxide (H_2O_2) from singlet molecular oxygen ($^1O_2$*). This process is catalytic, and investigators identified the electron source for a quasi-unlimited generation of H_2O_2. Antibodies produce up to 500 mole equivalents of H_2O_2 from $^1O_2$*, without a reduction in rate. This work shows the enormous potential for H_2O_2 production by antibodies and their prooxidant mechanism of action.[99,100]

The Howes Singlet Oxygen ($^1O_2^*$) Cancer Therapy System

Howes proposed a singlet oxygen generating system composed of physiological agents for the eradication of cancer, which did not have the limitations of conventional photodynamic therapy, radiation therapy or chemotherapeutic systems. In a pilot study at Tuft's Medical School, athymic mice, which had received human squamous cell carcinoma, experienced a 22.7% tumor disappearance rate in the "high dose group" following injection with the Howes singlet oxygen producing system. [101]

Even more encouraging results were seen, with an initial 80% disappearance rate, when basal cell skin cancers were similarly injected with this singlet oxygen delivery system. [102]

PDT generates similar products, in particular $^1O_2^*$, with similar chemical reactivity as the Howes Singlet Oxygen Delivery system.

Commonality Between PDT and the Howes Singlet Oxygen Therapy System

Pioneering work in the 1970s by Howes and Steele on microsomal lipid peroxidation [103] and aryl-hydroxylations [104] demonstrated evidence for the generation and participation of electronic excitation states, namely singlet oxygen. This was the first demonstration of a functional generation of an electronic excitation state, exclusive of vision, in mammalian systems. Their proposal, that singlet oxygen is the identity of the long sought out "active oxygen" acting on the cytochrome P 450 microsomal mixed function oxidases, has more recently been supported by the work of Yasui et al in 2002. [105]

While studying widely divergent biological electronic excitation generating systems, such as the microsomal mixed function oxidases, the neutrophil respiratory burst [106] and proline hydroxylation for collagen biosynthesis, one of the investigators (Howes) believed that these oxidative systems shared a point of convergence, expressed in the Howes Excytomer Pathway, involving superoxide anion and electronically excited singlet oxygen. [107]

Furthermore, Howes saw an additional commonality with generation of singlet oxygen produced by the steady-state physiological oxidative reagents containing an organic peroxide and the salt of hypohalous acid [108]

Subsequently, Howes reasoned that the peroxide/hypochlorite oxidative system may represent an ideal method of singlet oxygen delivery for effectively treating premalignant and malignant lesions, while simultaneously eliminating many of the drawbacks associated, not only with PDT, but with all other conventional methods of cancer therapy, including chemotherapy and irradiation. The peroxide/hypochlorite oxidative system has been shown to generate primarily singlet oxygen exclusively, as opposed to hydroperoxide/hypochlorite systems which have been shown to produce peroxyl and alkoxyl radicals. [109]

Ozone Therapy

Ozone therapy is practiced in most mainland European countries and the recently passed Alternative Therapy Legislation has made ozone therapy an option for patients in the USA in Alaska, Arizona, Colorado, Georgia, Minnesota, New York, New Jersey, North Carolina, Ohio, Oklahoma, Oregon, South Carolina, and Washington. Ozone therapy is not prohibited in Bulgaria, Cuba, Czech Republic, France, Germany, Greece, Israel, Italy, Japan, Malaysia, Mexico, Poland, Romania, Russia, Switzerland, Turkey, United Arab Emirates and Ukraine. Still, it remains on the fringe of mainstream medicine in America and the American Cancer Foundation has always strongly advised cancer patients against ozone therapy, as it does for other "Questionable methods of cancer management: hydorgen peroxide and other 'hyperoxygenation' therapies." [110]

However, scientific studies have found support for ozone therapy and investigators *at Washington University discovered ozone inhibited growth of lung, breast and uterine cancer cells in a dose dependent manner while healthy tissues were not damaged by ozone.* [111]

French studies have shown that ozone enhanced the treatment of chemo-resistant tumors and acted adjunctively with 5-fluorouracil chemotherapy in tumors derived from the colon and breast. [112]

Research has shown that ozone therapy can improve oxygenation in hypoxic tumors. [113-115] *A 2004 study at Oxford University, using a human trial of ozone therapy, involving 19 patients with incurable head and neck tumors receiving radiotherapy and tegafur, plus either chemotherapy or ozone therapy, concluded that results warrant further research of ozone as a treatment for cancer.* [116]

Cuban studies in rats [117, 118] *and Russian human trials report benefits of complimentary ozone treatment and as regards drug complications.* [119-121]

A 2008 study by Schulz et al, published in the International Journal of Cancer, found that survival of New Zealand White rabbits with head and neck squamous cell carcinoma could be enhanced by peritoneal insufflation of a medical ozone/oxygen gas mixture.

Hyperbaric Oxygen Therapy

It has been reported that hyperbaric oxygen therapy, using pressures at or less than 2.5 ATA, do not significantly increase EMODs in the presence of normal antioxidant defenses. Hyperbaric oxygen increases the oxygen in tumor tissue, as well as EMOD and prooxidant levels, and appears to enhance the efficiency of PDT. [122, 123] Hyperoxygenation appears to provide effective ways for improving PDT efficiency by oxygenating both preexisting and treatment-induced cell hypoxia. [124]

Relevant General Information

Lest we forget, oxygen and prooxidant EMODs play a central protective role against pathogens, as well as a crucial role in cancer therapy.

Polymorphonuclear cells (PMNs) require oxygen to kill organism by producing prooxidant superoxide, hydrogen peroxide, singlet oxygen and other products via the respiratory burst. [125] The PMN is protected by detoxifying free radicals with superoxide dismutase, catalase and glutathione. It has been shown in numerous studies that the degree of polymorphonuclear cell function in killing of bacteria is directly dependent on oxygen tension. [126, 127]

Scientists at The Ohio State University (OSU) have identified a way to predict very early in the treatment process the outcome of radiation and chemotherapy for cervical cancer patients and it is based on oxygen levels within the tumor. According to Jian Z. Wang, the oxygenation of a tumor is critical for the success of cancer treatment because the amount of oxygen in a cell is directly correlated with the ability of that cell to repair radiation damage. Wang stated that, "Inevitably, those well-oxygenated tumor cells die, tumors are less likely to return, and patient survival rates rise." The research was described in the talk, "When the Oxygen Level Matters Mostly During Radiation Therapy of Cervical Cancer?" presented July 31, 2008 at the 50th annual meeting of the American Association of Physicists in Medicine.

Men with a low oxygen supply to their prostate tumor have a higher chance of the prostate cancer returning, as found by increasing prostate-specific antigen (PSA) levels following treatment, according to Benjamin Movsas, M.D., senior study author and chair of the Department of Radiation Oncology at Henry Ford Hospital. Moreover, recent studies suggest the same finding also appears to apply to patients treated with surgery. Movsas stated that "A tumor's oxygen supply can significantly predict outcome following treatment, independent of tumor stage or Gleason score (a classification of the grade of prostate cancer)." [128]

In short, consideration of oxygen levels in cancer chemotherapy is crucial for successful eradication of neoplasia.

Various cancer chemopreventive agents can induce apoptosis in premalignant and malignant cells *in vivo* and/or *in vitro,* which serve as an anti-cancer mechanism. Many of these apoptogenic-inducing agents function as prooxidants *in vitro*.

Significant *in vitro* data exists showing that antioxidants can block EMOD-induced apoptosis for a wide variety of cancerous cell types, such as leukemia, lymphoma, retinoblastoma, myeloma, pheochromocytoma and human cancers of the breast, lung, pancreas, liver, colon, rectum and endometrium. This data can not be ignored when considering effective prooxidant cancer therapy. [129]

In 2001, Harvard Medical School investigators observed a dose dependent inhibition of MBT-2 cell (murine bladder cancer) growth after exposure to doxorubicin hydrochloride, which could be enhanced by hydrogen peroxide and inhibited by preincubation with alpha tocopherol. They concluded that hydrogen peroxide may be a relatively inexpensive, nontoxic method of augmenting the cytotoxicity of doxorubicin hydrochloride. [130]

To avoid the confusion with terms of the past, it is suggested that current scientific oxygen related therapies should be referred to as "prooxidant EMOD therapies."

Conclusion

The salutary role of EMODs in oncologic therapy has been scientifically substantiated by the use of prooxidant EMODs in currently available anti-cancer therapeutic methods, such as chemotherapy, radiation, photodynamic therapy, etc. Points of confluence exist within the many cancer methods available to treat cancer and many share the interaction of prooxidants. It also suggests potential courses of action clinicians may take when patients express an interest in prooxidant therapies or combinations thereof. Prooxidant EMODs have been proven to exhibit tumoricidal activity in both *in vitro* and *in vivo* studies. We must move forward and beyond the outdated and negative history surrounding so-called "oxidative therapies." Many prooxidant agents suggest selectivity in promoting the death of cancerous cells and avoidance of harm to normal cells. The prooxidant approach to cancer therapy begs for further scientific inquiry and additional validation.

Contrary to the unsupported and irresponsible statements of some major cancer agencies, this review clearly demonstrates that some pro-oxidant EMODs (a.k.a. oxidative therapies) are currently and have been for decades, integral, effective and safe theoretical and clinical agents in the battle against cancer. To deny the scientific facts supporting prooxidant EMOD therapies is to deny patients significant treatment modalities, which may be crucial to their survival. Various medically related organizations may deny the truth surrounding prooxidant cancer therapy but they can not change the truth, which is exposed to all by a review of the literature.

RMH Note: Hydrogen peroxide is fundamental to the apoptotic process and tumoricidal activity.

I believe that hydrogen peroxide is the most prevalent, and perhaps the most significant EMOD in the body, even exceeding the well recognized importance of nitric oxide. Page 32, Medical and Scientific Significance of Oxygen Metabolism. Prof. R.M. Howes MD, PhD, © 2005.

References

1. Harman D, Aging: a theory based on free radical and radiation chemistry. *J Gerontol* 11: 298–300, 1956.

2. Harman D, 1981. The aging process. Proc. Natl Acad. Sci. USA 78, 7124–7128.

3. Beckman KB, Ames, B.N., 1998. The free radical theory of aging matures. Physiol. Rev. 78, 547–581.

4. Finkel T, Holbrook NJ, 2000. Oxidants, oxidative stress and the biology of ageing. Nature 408, 239–247) (Harman D. 1961. Mutation, cancer and aging. Lancet 1: 200-201.

5. Harman D. 1961. Mutation, cancer and aging. Lancet 1: 200-201.

6. Howes RM, The Free Radical Fantasy: A Panoply of Paradoxes. Ann. N.Y. Acad. Sci. 2006; 1067:22-26.

7. Aw TY, 1999. Molecular and cellular responses to oxidative stress and changes in oxidation–reduction imbalance in the intestine. Am. J. Clin. Nutr. 70, 557–565.

8. Kwon YW, Masutani H., Nakamura H, Ishii Y, Yodoi J, 2003. Redox regulation of cell growth and cell death. Biol. Chem. 384, 991–996.

9. Duranteau J, Chandel NS, Kulisz A, Shao Z, Schumacker PT, 1998. Intracellular signaling by reactive oxygen species during hypoxia in cardiomyocytes. J. Biol. Chem. 273, 11619–11624.

10. Valko M, et al. Free radicals and antioxidants in normal physiological functions and human disease. Int J Biochem Cell Biol. 2007;39(1):44-84. Epub 2006 Aug 4.

11. White MK. and McCubrey JA. (2001) Suppression of apoptosis: role in cell growth and neoplasia. Leukemia, 15, 1011–10121.

12. Fiers W, Beyaert R, Declercq W, Vandenabeele P. More than one way to die: apoptosis, necrosis and reactive oxygen damage. Oncogene (1999) 18: 7719-30.

13. Howes M.D., PhD., R, (2007). Cancer, Apoptosis and Reactive Oxygen Species: A New Paradigm. *PHILICA.COM Article number 86*. Feb. 26th, 2007.

14. Begin ME, Ells G, Horrobin DF. Polyunsaturated fatty acid induced cytotoxicity against tumor cells and its relationship to lipid peroxidation. J Natl Cancer Inst 1988;80:188–94.

15. Begin ME. Effects of polyunsaturated fatty acids and of their oxidation products on cell survival. Chem Phys Lipids 1987;45:269–313.

16. Das UN, Begin ME, Ells G, HuangYS, Horrobin DF. Polyunsaturated fatty acids augment free radical generation in tumor cells in vitro. Biochem Biophys Res Commun 1987;145:15–24.

17. Lhuillery C, Cognault S, Germain E, Jourdan ML, Bougnoux P. Suppression of the promoter effect of polyunsaturated fatty acids by the absence of dietary vitamin E in experimental mammary carcinoma. Cancer Lett 1997;114:233–4.

18. Block KI, Koch AC, Mead MN, Tothy PK, Newman RA, Gyllenhaal C. Impact of antioxidant supplementation on chemotherapeutic toxicity: a systematic review of the evidence from randomized controlled trials. International journal of cancer. Journal international du cancer 2008;123(6):1227-39.

19. Chabner BA, Collins JM: Cancer Chemotherapy: Principles and Practice, pp 276-297, 314-333. Philadelphia, JB Lippincott, 1990.

20. Enger SM, Longnecker MP, Shikany JM, et al: Questionnaire assessment of intake of specific carotenoids. Cancer Epidemiol Biomarkers Prev 4(3):201-205, 1995.

21. Jarvinen R, Carotenoids, retinoids, tocopherols, and tocotrienols in the diet—the Finnish mobile clinic health examination survey. Int J Vitam Nutr Res 65(1):24-30, 1995.

22. Taylor PR, Wang GQ, Sanford MD, et al: Effect of nutrition intervention on intermediate end points in esophageal and gastric carcinogenesis. Am J Clin Nutr 62(suppl):1420S-1423S, 1995.

23. Frommel TO, Sohrab M, Doria M, et al: Effect of beta-carotene supplementation on indices of colonic cell proliferation. J Natl Cancer Inst 87(23):1781-1787, 1995.

24. Olson RD, Stroo WE, Boerth RC. Influence of N-acetylcysteine on the antitumor activity of doxorubicin. Semin Oncol 1983;10:S29-S34.

25. Roller A, Weller M. Antioxidants specifically inhibit cisplatin cytotoxicity of human malignant glioma cells. Anticancer Res 1998;18:4493-4497.

26. D'Andrea GM. Use of antioxidants during chemotherapy and radiotherapy should be avoided. *CA* 2005;55:319–21.

27. Parker-Pope T. Cancer and Vitamins: Patients Urged to Avoid Supplements During Treatment; *The Wall Street Journal* 2005 Sep 20 Sect. D:1.

28. Weijl NI, Cleton FJ, Osanto S. Free radicals and antioxidants in chemotherapy-induced toxicity. *Cancer Treat Rev* 1997.23:209–40.

29. Judy WV, Hall JH, Dugan W, et al. Coenzyme Q10 reduction of adriamycin cardiotoxicity. In: Folkers K, Yamamura Y, eds. *Biomedical and Clinical Aspects of Coenzyme Q*, Vol. 4, Elsevier, 1984:231–41.

30. Sieja K, Talerczyk M. Selenium as an element in the treatment of ovarian cancer in women receiving chemotherapy. *Gynecol Oncol* 2004;93:320–27.

31. Cascinu S, Cordella L, Del Ferro E, et al. Neuroprotective effect of reduced glutathione on cisplatin-based chemotherapy in advanced gastric cancer: a randomized double-blind placebo-controlled trial. *J Clin Oncol* 1995;13:26–32.

32. Seifried, HE, McDonald, SS, Anderson, DE, Greenwald, P & Milner, JA, (2003) The antioxidant conundrum in cancer. Cancer Res 63:4295-4298.

33. Simone CB 2nd, Simone NL, Simone V, Simone CB. Antioxidants and other nutrients do not interfere with radiation or chemotherapy. Altern Ther Health Med. 2007 Mar-Apr;13(2):40-7.

34. Lawenda BD, Kelly KM, Ladas EJ, Sagar SM, Vickers A, Blumberg J. 2008. Should supplemental antioxidant administration be avoided during chemotherapy and radiation therapy?. Journal of the National Cancer Institute. May 27, 2008. 100(11)773-783.

35. *Gray LH, Conger AD, Ebert M, Hornsey S, Scott OC, "The concentration of oxygen dissolved in tissues at the time of irradiation as a factor in radiotherapy". Br J Radiol. (December 1953) 26 (312): 638–48).*

36. *Dunn T, "Oxygen and cancer". N C Med J. (1997). 58 (2): 140–3.*

37. Soengas, MS, Alarcon, RM, Yoshida, H, Giaccia, AJ, Hakem, R and Mak, TW, et al. Apaf-1 and caspace-9 in p53-dependent apoptosis and tumor inhibition. Science 1999; 284: 156-159.

38. Shimizu, S, Eguchi, Y, Kosaka, H, Kamiike, W, Matsuda, H and Tsujimoto, Y, Prevention of hypoxia-induced cell death by Bel-2 and Bel-xL. Nature 1995; 374: 811-813.

39. Giaccia, AJ, Hypoxic stress proteins: Survival of the fittest. Semin Radiat Oncol 1996; 6: 45-58.

40. Howes, RM, *U.T.O.P.I.A. - Unified Theory of Oxygen Participation in Aerobiosis.* © 2004. Free Radical Publishing Co. Kentwood, LA. (available at www.thepundit.com and www.iwillfindthecure.org)

41. Vaupel P and Harrison L, Tumor Hypoxia: Causative Factors, Compensatory Mechanisms, and Cellular Response. Oncologist, November 1, 2004; 9(suppl_5): 4 – 9.

42. Tsang WP., Chau SP., Kong SK., Fung KP. and Kwok TT, (2003) Reactive oxygen species mediate doxorubicin induced p53-independent apoptosis. Life Sci., 73, 2047–2058.

43. Liu L, Trimarchi JR., Navarro P, Blasco MA. and Keefe DL. (2003) Oxidative stress contributes to arsenic-induced telomere attrition, chromosome instability and apoptosis. J. Biol. Chem., 278, 31998–32004.

44. Djavaheri-Mergny M, Wietzerbin J and Besancon F, (2003) 2-Methoxyestradiol induces apoptosis in Ewing sarcoma cells through mitochondrial hydrogen peroxide production. Oncogene, 22, 2558–2567.

45. Gewirtz DA: A critical evaluation of the mechanisms of action proposed for the antitumor effects of the anthracycline antibiotics Adriamycin and daunorubicin. Biochem Pharmacol 1999, 57:727-741.

46. Hasinoff BB, Davey JP. Adriamycin and its iron(III) and copper(III) complexes, glutathione-induced dissociation, cytochrome *c* oxidase inactivation and protection: binding to cardiolipin. Biochem. Pharmacol., *37:* 3663-3669, 1988.

47. Burger RM, Cleavage of nucleic acids by bleomycin. Chem. Rev., *98:* 1153-1169, 1998.

48. Byfield JE, Lee YC, Tu L, Kullhanian F, Molecular interactions of the combined effects of bleomycin and X-rays on mammalian cell survival. Cancer Res., *36:* 1138-1143, 1976.

49. Ferlini C, Scambia G, Marone M, Distefano M, Gaggini C, Ferrandina G, Fattorossi A, Isola G, Benedetti Panici P, Mancuso S. Tamoxifen induces oxidative stress and apoptosis in estrogen receptor-negative human cancer cell lines. Br J Cancer 1999;79:257–263.

50. Yokomizo A, Ono M, Nanri H, Makino Y, Ohga T, Wada M, Okamoto T, Yodoi J, Kuwano M, Kohno K. Cellular levels of thioredoxin associated with drug sensitivity to cisplatin, mitomycin C, doxorubicin, and etoposide. Cancer Res 1995;55:4293–4296.

51. Erhola M, Kellokumpu-Lehtinen P, Metsa-Ketela T, et al: Effect of anthracycline-based chemotherapy on total plasma antioxidant capacity in small-cell lung cancer patients. Free Radic Biol Med 21(3):383-390, 1996.

52. Halliwell B, Gutteridge JMC: *Free Radicals in Biology and Medicine.* Oxford University Press; 1989.

53. Davies KJ, Doroshow JH: Redox cycling of anthracyclines by cardiac mitochondria. I. Anthracycline radical formation by NADH dehydrogenase. J Biol Chem 1986, 261:3060-3076.

54. Doroshow JH, Davies KJ: Redox cycling of anthracyclines by cardiac mitochondria. II. Formation of superoxide anion, hydrogen peroxide, and hydroxyl radical. J Biol Chem 1986, 261:3068-3074.

55. Nicholson DW, ICE/CED3-like proteases as therapeutic targets for the control of inappropriate apoptosis. Nature Biotechnol., 1996. 14, 297–301.

56. Nicholson DW, (1996) From bench to clinic with apoptosis-based therapeutic agents. Nature, 407, 810–816.

57. Fleury C, Mignotte B, Vayssiere JL, Mitochondrial reactive oxygen species in cell death signaling. Biochimie 2002; 84:131-41.

58. Clement MV, Ponton A, Pervaiz S, Apoptosis induced by hydrogen peroxide is mediated by decreased superoxide anion concentration and reduction of intracellular milieu. FEBS Lett 1998; 440:13-18.

59. Hirpara JL, Clement MV, Pervaiz S, Intracellular acidification triggered by mitochondrial-derived hydrogen peroxide is an effector mechanism for drug-induced apoptosis in tumor cells. J Biol Chem 2001;276:514-521.

60. Simizu S, Umezawa K, Takada M, Arber N, Imoto M, Induction of hydrogen peroxide production and Bax expression by caspase-3(-like) proteases in tyrosine kinase inhibitor-induced apoptosis in human small cell lung carcinoma cells. Exp Cell Res 1998;238:197-203.

61. Mansat-de Mas V, Bezombes C, Quilletary A, et al. Implication of radical oxygen species in ceramide generation, c-Jun N-terminal kinase activation and apoptosis induced by daunorubicin. Mol Pharmacol 1999;56:867-74.

62. Li L, Fattah EA, Cao G, Ren C, Yang G, Goltsov AA, Chinaul ACt, Cai W-W, Timme TL, and Thompson TC. Glioma Pathogenesis-Related Protein 1 Exerts Tumor Suppressor Activities through Proapoptotic Reactive Oxygen Species c-Jun NH2 Kinase Signaling. Cancer Res 2008;68(2):434–43.

63. Kirshner JR, He S, Balasubramanyam V, Kepros J, Yang C-Y, Zhang M, Du Z, Barsoum J, and Bertin J, Elesclomol induces cancer cell apoptosis through oxidative stress. Mol Cancer Ther 2008;7(8):2319–27.

64. Baker AF, Landowski T, Dorr R, Tate WR, Gard JMC, Tavenner BE, Dragovich T, Coon A, and Powis G. The Antitumor Agent Imexon Activates Antioxidant Gene Expression: Evidence for an Oxidative Stress Response. Clin. Cancer Res., June 1, 2007; 13(11): 3388 – 3394.

65. Isham CR, Tibodeau JD, Jin W, Xu R, Timm MM, and Chaetocin KC: A promising new antimyeloma agent with in vitro and in vivo activity mediated via imposition of oxidative stress. Bible. Blood, March 15, 2007; 109(6): 2579 – 2588.

66. Bhalla S, Balasubramanian S, David K, Sirisawad M, Buggy J, Mauro L, Prachand S, Miller R, Gordon LI and Evens AM. PCI-24781 induces caspase and reactive oxygen species–dependent apoptosis through NF-κB mechanisms and is synergistic with bortezomib in lymphoma cells. Clinical Cancer Research 15, 3354, May 15, 2009.

67. Lecane PS, M. Karaman W, Sirisawad M, Naumovski L, Miller RA, Hacia JG, and Magda D. Motexafin Gadolinium and Zinc Induce Oxidative Stress Responses and Apoptosis in B-Cell Lymphoma Lines. Cancer Res., December 15, 2005; 65(24): 11676 – 11688.

68. O'Brien PJ. Molecular mechanism of quinone cytotoxicity. Chem Biol Interact 80:1–41, 1991.

69. Little JB. Cellular, molecular, and carcinogenic effects of radiation. Hematol Oncol Clin N Am **7**:337–352, 1993.

70. Borek C, Antioxidants and Radiation Therapy. J. Nutr. 134:3207S-3209S, November 2004.

71. Fang J, Sawa T, Akaike T and Maeda H, Tumor-targeted Delivery of Polyethylene Glycol-conjugated D-Amino Acid Oxidase for Antitumor Therapy via Enzymatic Generation of Hydrogen Peroxide. *Cancer Research* 62, 3138-3143, June 1, 2002.

72. Mallams JT, Balla GA and Finney JW, Regional oxygenation and irradiation in the treatment of malignant tumors. Prog Clin Cancer 1965; 1: 137.

73. Finney JW, Collier RE, Balla GA, Tomme JW, Wakley J, Race GJ, Urschel HC, D'Errico AD and Mallams JT, The preferential localization of radioisotopes in malignant tissue by regional oxygenation. Nature 1961; 202: 1172.

74. Finney JW, Balla GA, Collier RE, Wakely J, Urschel HC and Mallams JT, Differential localization of isotopes in tumors through the use of intra-arterial hydrogen peroxide: Part 1: Basic science. Amer J Roentgen 1965; 94: 783.

75. Schreiner A, Hyperbaric oxygen therapy in bactericides infections. Acta Chir Scand 1974; 140: 73-76.

76. Hampton MB and Orrenius S, Dual regulation of caspase activity by hydrogen peroxide: implications for apoptosis. FEBS Lett (1997) 414: 552-6.

77. Davies KJ, The broad spectrum of responses to oxidants in proliferating cells: a new paradigm for oxidative stress. IUBMB Life. 1999 Jul; 48(1):41-7.

78. Manakata T, Semba U, Shibuya Y, et al. Induction of interferon-gamma production by human natural killer cells stimulated by hydrogen peroxide. J Immunol 985;134(4):2449-2455.

79. Takeuchi T, Matsugo S and Morimoto K, (1997) Mutagenicity of oxidative DNA damage in Chinese hamster V79 cells. *Carcinogenesis*, 18, 2051–2055.

80. Drisko JA, Chapman J, Hunter VJ. The use of antioxidants with first-line chemotherapy in two cases of ovarian cancer. J Am Coll Nutr 2003;22:118–23.

81. Buettner GR. & Jurkiewicz BA, (1996) Catalytic metals, ascorbate and free radicals: combinations to avoid. *Radiat. Res.* 145, 532-541.

82. Halliwell B, (1990) "How to characterize a biological antioxidant", Free Radical Res. Commun. 9, 1-32.

83. Levine M, (1986) New concepts in the biology and biochemistry of ascorbic acid. New Engl. J. Med. 314,892-902.

84. Chen Q, Espey MG, Krishna MC, Mitchell JB, Corpe CP, Buettner GR, Shacter E, and Levine L, Pharmacologic ascorbic acid concentrations selectively kill cancer cells: Action as a pro-drug to deliver hydrogen peroxide to tissues. PNAS. September 20, 2005. Vol. 102. No. 38. pp. 13604-13609.

85. Chen Q, Espey MG, Sun AY, Lee J, Krishna MC, Shacter E, Choyke P, Pooput C, Kirk KL, Buettner GR, and Levine M, Ascorbate in pharmacologic concentrations selectively generates ascorbate radical and hydrogen peroxide in extracellular fluid in vivo. PNAS. May 22, 2007. Vol. 104. No. 21. pp. 8749-8754.

86. Chen Q, Espey MG, Sun AY, Pooput C, Kirk KL, Krishna MC, Khosh DB, Drisko J, Levine M, Pharmacologic doses of ascorbate act as a prooxidant and decrease growth of aggressive tumor xenografts in mice. PNAS. August 12, 2008. Vol. 105. No. 32. pp. 11105-11109.

87. Levine M, Espey MG, and Chen Q, Losing and finding a way at C: New promise for pharmacologic ascorbate in cancer treatment. Free Radical Biology & Medicine. 47 (2008) pp. 27-29.

88. Carr A and Frei B, Does vitamin C act as a pro-oxidant under physiological conditions? The FASEB Journal. 1999;13:1007-1024.

89. Zilberstein, J., Bromberg, A., Frantz, A., Rosenbach-Belkin, V., Kritzman, A. and Pfefermann R, et al. Light-dependent oxygen consumption in bacterio-chlorophyll-serine-treated melanoma tumors: On-line determination using a tissue-inserted oxygen microsensor. Photochem Photobiol 1997; 65: 1012-1019.

90. Al-Waili, NS and Butler, GJ, Phototherapy and malignancy: Possible enhancement by iron administration and hyperbaric oxygen. Med Hypotheses. 2006;67(5):1148-58.

91. Tomaselli F, et al. Photodynamic therapy enhanced by hyperbaric oxygen in acute endoluminal palliation of malignant bronchial stenosis. Eur J Cardiothorac Surg. 2001 May;19(5):549-54.

92. Agarwal ML, Clay ME, Harvey EJ, Evans HH, Antunez AR and Oleinick NL, Photodynamic therapy induces rapid cell death by apoptosis in L5178Y mouse lymphoma cells. Cancer Res 1991; 51: 5993-5996.

93. Kochevar IE, Lynch MC, Zhuang S, Lambert CR, Singlet oxygen, but not oxidizing radicals, induces apoptosis in HL-60 cells. Photochem Photobiol. 2000 Oct;72(4):548-53.

94. Luna MC, Wong S and Gomer CJ, Photodynamic therapy mediated induction of early response genes. Cancer Res 1994; 14: 315-321.

95. Korbelik M and Dougherty GJ, Photodynamic therapy-mediated immune response against subcutaneous mouse tumors. Cancer Research 1999; 59: 1441-1446.

96. Korbelik M, Induction of tumor immunity by photodynamic therapy. J Clin Laser Med Surg 1996; 14: 315-334.

97. Henderson BW and Dougherty TJ, How does photodynamic therapy work? Photochem Photobiol 1992; 55: 145-157.

98. Moan, J. and Berg, K. The photodegradation of porphyrins in cells can be used to estimate the lifetime of singlet oxygen. Photochem Photobiol 1991; 53: 549-553.

99. Wentworth P Jr, Jones LH, Wentworth AD, Zhu X, Larsen NA, Wilson IA, Xu X, Goddard WA 3rd, Janda KD, Eschenmoser A, Lerner RA, Antibody catalysis of the oxidation of water. Science. 2001 Sep 7;293(5536):1806-11.

100. Wentworth P Jr, McDunn JE, Wentworth AD, Takeuchi C, Nieva J, Jones T, Bautista C, Ruedi JM, Gutierrez A, Janda KD, Babior BM, Eschenmoser A, Lerner RA, Evidence for antibody-catalyzed ozone formation in bacterial killing and inflammation. Science. 2002 Dec 13;298(5601):2195-9.

101. Howes RM, Tumoricidal Activity of An Injectable Singlet Oxygen System Generated From Physiological Agents. (The Howes Singlet Oxygen Cancer Therapy System). In *The Medical and Scientific Significance of Oxygen Free Radical Metabolism.* © 2005. Free Radical Publishing Co. Kentwood, LA. pp. 893-912. (available at www.iwillfindthecure.org)

102. Howes RM and Farber G, Tumoricidal Activity of the Howes Singlet Oxygen Delivery System in Human Basal Cell Carcinoma. In *The Medical and Scientific Significance of Oxygen Free Radical Metabolism.* © 2005. Free Radical Publishing Co. Kentwood, LA. pp. 883-892. (available at www.iwillfindthecure.org)

103. Howes RM and Steele R H, Microsomal chemiluminescence induced by NADPH and its relation to lipid peroxidation. Res. Commun. Chem. Path. Pharmacol., July-Sept. 1971, 2; 4 & 5:619-626.

104. Howes RM and Steele RH, Microsomal chemiluminescence induced by NADPH and its relation to aryl-hydroxylations, Res Commun. Chem. Path. Pharmacol., March 1972, 3; 2:349-357,

105. Yasui, H, Deo K, Ogura Y, Yoshida H, Shiraga T, Kagayama A and Sakurai H, Evidence for singlet oxygen involvement in rat and human cytochrome P450-dependent substrate oxidations, Drug Metab. Pharmacokin. 2002, 17 (5): 416-426.

106. Howes R M, Allen RC, Su CT and Hoopes JE, Altered polymorphonuclear leukocyte bioenergetics in patients with thermal injury, the Surgical Forum, 1976, 27:558-560.

107. Howes RM, Steele RH and Hoopes JE, The role of electronic excitation states in collagen biosynthesis, Persp. In Biol. And Med., Summer 1977, 20; 4:539-544.

108. Howes RM, Steele RH and Hoopes JE, Peroxide induced chemiluminescence in an in vitro proline hydroxylation system, 1976, 8; 1:77-84.

109. Noguchi, N., Nakad, A., Itoh, Y., Watanabe, A. and Niki, E. Formation of active oxygen species and lipid peroxidation induced by hypochlorite. 2002, Arch Biochem Biophys. 397; 2:440-447.

110. Questionable methods of cancer management: hydrogen peroxide and other 'hyperoxygenation' therapies. *CA Cancer J Clin. 43 (1): 47–56. 1993.*

111. *Sweet F, Kao MS, Lee SC, Hagar WL, Sweet WE (August 1980).* "Ozone selectively inhibits growth of human cancer cells". Science (journal) *209 (4459): 931–3.*

112. *Zänker KS, Kroczek R, (1990). "In vitro synergistic activity of 5-fluorouracil with low-dose ozone against a chemoresistant tumor cell line and fresh human tumor cells". Chemotherapy. 36 (2): 147–54.*

113. *Clavo B, Pérez JL, López L, et al. (June 2004).* "Ozone Therapy for Tumor Oxygenation: a Pilot Study". *Evid Based Complement Alternat Med 1 (1): 93–98.*

114. *Kusznieruk K,* Tumor Hypoxia and Ozone Therapy".*The Stem Cell Patent Journal, October 24th, 2006.*

115. *Bocci V, Larini A, Micheli V (April 2005). "Restoration of normoxia by ozone therapy may control neoplastic growth: a review and a working hypothesis". J Altern Complement Med 11 (2): 257–65.*

116. *Clavo B, Ruiz A, Lloret M, et al. (December 2004).* "Adjuvant Ozonetherapy in Advanced Head and Neck Tumors: A Comparative Study". *Evid Based Complement Alternat Med 1 (3): 321–325.*

117. *Borrego A, Zamora ZB, González R, et al. (February 2004).* "Protection by ozone preconditioning is mediated by the antioxidant system in cisplatin-induced nephrotoxicity in rats". *Mediators Inflamm. 13 (1): 13–9).*

118. *Borrego A, Zamora ZB, González R, et al. (August 2006). "Ozone/oxygen mixture modifies the subcellular redistribution of Bax protein in renal tissue from rats treated with cisplatin". Arch. Med. Res. 37 (6): 717–22.*

119. Potanin et al., Ozonotherapy In The Early Postoperative Period In The Surgical Treatment Of The Lung Cancer. [Written in Russian] Kazanskij Medicinskij Zurnal No. 4, 263-265, 2000.

120. Gretchkanev et al., Role of Ozone Therapy in Prevention and Treatment of Complications of Drug Therapy for Ovarian Cancer. Akusherstvo Ginekologiya No 4, 57-58, 2002.

121. Kontorschikova et al., Ozonetherapy In A Complex Treatment Of Breast Cancer. In Proceedings of the 15th Ozone World Congress, 11-15th Sept 2001, Medical Therapy Conference (IOA 2001, Ed.), Speedprint Macmedia Ltd, Ealing, London, UK, 2001.

122. Tomaselli F, et al. Acute effects of combined photodynamic therapy and hyperbaric oxygenation in lung cancer. Lasers Surg Med. 2001;28(5):399-403.

123. Maier A, et al. Combined photodynamic therapy and hyperbaric oxygenation in carcinoma of the esophagus and the esophago-gastric junction. Eur J Cardiothorac Surg. 2000 Dec;18(6):649-54.

124. Chen Q, et al. Improvement of tumor response by manipulation of tumor oxygenation during photodynamic therapy. Photochem Photobiol. 2002 Aug;76(2):197-203.

125. Babior BM, Oxygen dependent microbial killing by phagocytes. N Engl J Med 1974; 298: 659-668, 721-726.

126. DeChatelet LR, Oxidative bactericidal mechanisms of polymorphonuclear leukocytes. J Infect Dis 1975; 131: 295-303.

127. Hohn DC, Oxygen and leukocyte microbial killing. Davis, J.C., Hunt, T.K. Eds. Hyperbaric Oxygen Therapy, Bethesday, Undersea Med Soc 1977; 101-110.

128. Hypoxic Prostate/Muscle pO2 (P/M pO2) Ratio Predicts for Biochemical Failure in Patients with Localized Prostate Cancer: Long-term Result." Abstract # 5136. ASCO 2009.

129. Howes M.D., PhD., R, (2009). Dangers of Antioxidants in Cancer Patients: A Review. *PHILICA.COM Article number 153*. Published 7th February, 2009.

130. Loughlin KR, Manson K, Cragnale D, Wilson L, Ball RA, Bridges KR, The use of hydrogen peroxide to enhance the efficacy of doxorubicin hydrochloride in a murine bladder tumor cell line. *J Urol.* 2001;165:1300-1304.

Randolph M Howes, PhD, MD

Randolph M Howes, PhD, MD completed residency in general surgery and plastic surgery while doing basic research in oxygen-free radicals at Johns Hopkins University. He invented the triple lumen catheter and, in 2004, published the first selective world review on oxygen metabolism in his book: UTOPIA (Unified Theory of Oxygen Participation in Aerobiosis), which was revised in 2014 and is now available at www.amazon.com.

Pro-oxidant Protection and Oxidative Self-Healing

Dr Howes believes the free radical theory is unfounded and that electronically modified oxygen derivatives (EMOD) are of low toxicity and are essential for energy production, pathogen protection, secondary messenger signaling and as tumoricidal agents. His unified theory states that EMOD deficiency levels allow for the manifestation of diseases, including neoplasia, and is integral in the aging phenomena. Dr Howes recognizes that antioxidants can commonly become pro-oxidants. He points out that antioxidants have failed to control aging and disease and that the scientific literature is increasingly showing that antioxidants can harm biological systems. Please refer to his other companion books also available at www.amazon.com.

Companion Books of Prof. R. Howes, MD, PhD:

Howes, R. M. *U.T.O.P.I.A. - Unified Theory of Oxygen Participation in Aerobiosis.* © 2004. Free Radical Publishing Co. Kentwood, LA, available at www.iwillfindthecure.org.

Howes R. M. *The Medical and Scientific Significance of Oxygen Free Radical Metabolism.* © 2005. Free Radical Publishing Co. Kentwood, LA. USA. available at www.iwillfindthecure.org.

Howes, R. M. *Hydrogen Peroxide Monograph 1: Scientific, Medical and Biochemical Overview.* © 2006; Free Radical Publishing Co. USA. 200 pages. available at www.iwillfindthecure.org.

Howes, R. M. Monograph 2: *Antioxidant vitamins A, C & E: Equivocal Scientific Studies,* © 2006; Free Radical Publishing Co. USA. 171 pages. available at www.iwillfindthecure.org.

Howes, R. M. *Cardiovascular Disease and Oxygen Free Radical Mythology,* © 2006;

Free Radical Publishing Co. USA. 308 pages. available at www.iwillfindthecure.org.

Howes, R. M. *Diabetes and Oxygen Free Radical Sophistry,* © 2006;

Free Radical Publishing Co. USA. Free Radical Publishing Co. USA. 366 pages. available at www.iwillfindthecure.org.

Howes, R. M. *Reactive Oxygen Species Insufficiency (ROSI)*

as the Basis for Disease Allowance and Coexistence:

Extraordinary Support for an Extraordinary Theory

Vol I, II & III. © 2008; 1564 pages. available at www.iwillfindthecure.org.

Howes, R. M. Volume I 501 pages #7 © 2008. Free Radical Publishing Co. USA.

Howes, R. M. Volume II 505 pages #8 © 2008. Free Radical Publishing Co. USA.

Howes, R. M. Volume III 562 pages #9 © 2008. Free Radical Publishing Co. USA.

Howes, R. M. *THE HOWES PAPERS*

© 2009; Free Radical Publishing Co. USA. 211 pages

Howes R.M. *"COFFEE TABLE MUSINGS of the*

Da Vinci in COWBOY BOOTS"

Pithy Prose and Perspicacious Aphorisms. © 2009; 103 pages

Howes, R. M. Reactive Oxygen Species vs. Antioxidants:

"The Oxypocalypse" or

"The war that never was" © 2010; Free Radical Publishing Co. USA. 550 pages. available at www.iwillfindthecure.org.

Howes R.M. *Death in Small Doses?:*

Antioxidant Vitamins A, C & E in the 21st Century

Book One: *A Health Impact Statement For The Layman*

© 2010; Trafford Publishing. Indianapolis, USA. 90 pages

Howes R.M. *Antioxidant Vitamins are Making A Killing;*

Antioxidant Vitamins A, C & E in the 21st Century

Book Two: *A Health Impact Statement For The Medical Scientist*

© 2010; 184 pages

- Death In Small Doses? Trafford Publishing, © 2010

- Antioxidant Overkill, CreateSpace and Free Radical Publishing, © 2011

- Dangers of Excessive Antioxidants in Cancer Patients, CreateSpace and Free Radical Publishing, © 2011

- Heart Disease and Antioxidant Failures, CreateSpace and Free Radical Publishing, © 2011

- Antioxidant Failures and Dangers, CreateSpace and Free Radical Publishing, © 2011

- Anti-Aging Anti-oxidant Scams, CreateSpace and Free Radical Publishing, © 2011

- Sports, Athletes, Exercise Facts and Antioxidant Myths, CreateSpace and Free Radical Publishing, © 2011

- Alzheimer's Disease: Forget Antioxidants and Supplements, CreateSpace and Free Radical Publishing, © 2012

- Sex, Performance, Reproduction, Naked Radicals And Antioxidants, CreateSpace and Free Radical Publishing, © 2012

- Antioxidants Linked To Deadly Unintended Consequences, CreateSpace and Free Radical Publishing, © 2013

- U.T.O.P.I.A.: Unified Theory of Oxygen Participation In Aerobiosis, CreateSpace and Free Radical Publishing, © 2014, revised

- Hydrogen Peroxide: A Health, Homeostatic and Protective Essentiality, CreateSpace and Free Radical Publishing, © 2014

- Reactive Oxygen Species vs. Antioxidants: The Oxypocalypse or The War That Never Was, CreateSpace and Free Radical Publishing, © 2014

- Diabetes and Oxygen Free Radical Sophistry, CreateSpace and Free Radical Publishing, © 2014, revised

All books available at www.amazon.com; www.barnesandnobles.com; www.booksamillion.com.

Companion Papers of Prof. R. Howes, MD, PhD:

Dr. Howes has authored over 350 medical publications in health related editorials.

Citation: R. Howes: Mythology of Antioxidant Vitamins?. *The Journal of Evidence-Based Alternative and Complimentary Medicine.* April, 2011. 16(2): 149-189.

Citation: R. Howes: Cancer Therapy: A Review with Scientific Validation for the Role of Electronically Modified Oxygen Derivatives in Oncologic Treatment Modalities. *The Internet Journal of Alternative Medicine.* 2010 Volume 8 Number 1.

Citation: R. Howes: Hydrogen Peroxide: A review of a scientifically verifiable omnipresent ubiquitous essentiality of obligate, aerobic, carbon-based life forms. *The Internet Journal of Plastic Surgery.* 2010 Volume 7 Number 1.

Howes M.D., PhD., R. (2009). Dangers of Antioxidants in Cancer Patients: A Review. *PHILICA.COM Article number 153*. Published 7th February, 2009. (20 pages)

Howes M.D., PhD., R. (2008). Aging and anti-aging claims: a review on antioxidant vitamins A, C & E. *PHILICA.COM Article number 116*. Published on 12th January, 2008. (16 pages)

Howes M.D., PhD., R. (2007). Sleep: An original "radical" proposal. *PHILICA.COM Observation number 42*. Published on 5th October, 2007. (1 page)

Howes M.D., PhD., R. (2007). Antioxidant Vitamins A, C & E; Death in Small Doses and Legal Liability? *PHILICA.COM Article number 89*. Published on 5th April, 2007. (23 pages)

Howes M.D., PhD., R. (2007). Cancer, Apoptosis and Reactive Oxygen Species: A New Paradigm. *PHILICA.COM Article number 86*. Published on 26th February, 2007. (11 pages)

Howes M.D., PhD., R. (2007). Antioxidant Vitamins A, C and E: Assessing Potential for Harm. *PHILICA.COM Article number 83*. Published on 15th February, 2007. (14 pages)

Howes M.D., PhD., R. (2007). The Consequent Downfall of the Free Radical Theory. *PHILICA.COM Article number 75*. Published on 22nd January, 2007. (9 pages)

Howes, R.M.: "The Free Radical Fantasy," The Annals of New York Academy of Sciences, 2006, Vol. 1067, pp. 22-26.

(Howes, 2005) (Howes, R.M. Tumoricidal Activity of An Injectable Singlet Oxygen System Generated From Physiological Agents: The Howes Singlet Oxygen Cancer Therapy System). In The Medical and Scientific Significance of Oxygen Free Radical Metabolism. © 2005. Free Radical Publishing Co. Kentwood, LA. pp. 893-912).

(Howes, Farber, 2005) (Howes, R.M. and Farber, G. Tumoricidal Activity of the Howes Singlet Oxygen Delivery System in Human Basal Cell Carcinoma. In The Medical and Scientific Significance of Oxygen Free Radical Metabolism. © 2005. Free Radical Publishing Co. Kentwood, LA. pp. 883-892).

(Howes et al, 1977) (Howes, R.M., Steele, R.H. and Hoopes, J.E., The role of Electronic excitation states in collagen biosynthesis, Persp. In Biol. And Med., Summer 1977, 20; 4:539-544).

(Howes, Steele, 1976) (Howes, R.M., Steele, R.H. and Hoopes, J.E., Peroxide induced Chemiluminescence in an in vitro proline hydroxylation system, 1976, 8; 1:77-84).

(Howes et al, 1976) (Howes, R. M., Allen, R.C., Su, C.T. and Hoopes, J.E., Altered polymorphonuclear leukocyte bioenergetics in patients with thermal injury, the Surgical Forum, 1976, 27:558-560).

(Howes, Steele, 1972) (Howes, R.M. and Steele, R.H., Microsomal chemiluminescence induced by NADPH and its relation to aryl-hydroxylations, Res Commun. Chem. Path. Pharmacol., March 1972, 3; 2:349-357).

(Howes, Steele, 1971) (Howes, R. M. and Steele, R. H., Microsomal chemiluminescence induced by NADPH and its relation to lipid peroxidation, Res. Commun. Chem. Path. Pharmacol., July-Sept. 1971, 2; 4 & 5:619-626).

**I despise precious time wasted,
for it alone, is the unfinished canvas
displaying the portrait of my life.
R. M. Howes, M.D., Ph.D.
9/7/09**

"We are what we repeatedly do. Excellence then, is not an act, but a habit." ~Aristotle

OTHER BOOKS

PUBLISHED: Partial list. The Fire Eaters, Molding your own destiny more easily, Carnivore Press, © 1982
Uplift, The Answer Book to your plastic and cosmetic surgery questions, Carnivore Press, © 1986
The Pundit Speaks, vol. I. An Anthology of Neoclassical Poetic Philosophy, Carnivore Press, © 1990
The Pundit Speaks, Volume II, An Anthology of Neoclassical Poetic Philosophy, Free Radical Press, © 1994
The Pundit Speaks, Volume III, An Anthology of Neoclassical Poetic Philosophy, Free Radical Press, © 1996
The Pundit Speaks, Volume IV, An Anthology of Neoclassical Poetic Philosophy, Free Radical Press, © 2000
The Fable of the Chocolate Covered Strawberry Coloring Book, Free Radical Press, © 2001
The Pundit Speaks, Volume IV, An Anthology of Neoclassical Poetic Philosophy, Free Radical Press, © 2003
The Pundit Speaks, Volume V, An Anthology of Neoclassical

Poetic Philosophy, Trafford Publishing, © 2009
Coffee Table Musings of The DaVinci In Cowboy Boots, Trafford Publishing, © 2010

Available at: www.philica.com
www.medi.philica.com
www.iwillfindthecure.org
www.amazon.com

If you believe the implausible,
you will accept the indefensible and
not recognize the inexcusable.
R. M. Howes, M.D., Ph.D.
6/5/11
DOC
R_x ANDOLPH
HOWES

RAD!CAL

www.ingramcontent.com/pod-product-compliance
Lightning Source LLC
Chambersburg PA
CBHW051623170526
45167CB00001B/38

* 9 7 8 1 4 9 9 5 6 7 9 2 2 *